OXFORD MEDICAL PUBLICATIONS

Global Anaesthesia

Oxford Specialist Handbooks published and forthcoming

General Oxford Specialist Handbooks
Addiction Medicine
Applied Medicine and Surgery in Dentistry
Day Case Surgery
Infection in the Immunocompromised Host
Perioperative Medicine, 2e
Pharmaceutical Medicine
Postoperative Complications, 2e
Renal Transplantation
Retrieval Medicine

Oxford Specialist Handbooks in Anaesthesia
Anaesthesia for Emergency Care
Global Anaesthesia
Neuroanaesthesia
Obstetric Anaesthesia, 2e
Paediatric Anaesthesia, 2e
Regional Anaesthesia, Stimulation and Ultrasound Techniques
Thoracic Anaesthesia
Vascular Anaesthesia

Oxford Specialist Handbooks in Cardiology
Adult Congenital Heart Disease, 2e
Cardiac Catheterization and Coronary Intervention
Cardiovascular Computed Tomography, 2e
Cardiovascular Imaging
Cardiovascular Magnetic Resonance
Echocardiography, 2e
Fetal Cardiology, 2e
Heart Disease in Pregnancy
Heart Failure, 2e
Hypertension
Inherited Cardiac Disease
Nuclear Cardiology
Pacemakers and ICDs, 2e
Pulmonary Hypertension
Valvular Heart Disease

Oxford Specialist Handbooks in Critical Care
Advanced Respiratory Critical Care
Cardiothoracic Critical Care

Oxford Specialist Handbooks in End of Life Care
Dementia
Heart Failure
Kidney Disease
Respiratory Disease

Oxford Specialist Handbooks in Infectious Disease
Infectious Disease Epidemiology

Oxford Specialist Handbooks in Neurology
Parkinson's Disease and Other Movement Disorders, 2e
Stroke Medicine, 2e

Oxford Specialist Handbooks in Oncology
Practical Management of Complex Cancer Pain

Oxford Specialist Handbooks in Paediatrics
Community Paediatrics
Manual of Childhood Infections, 4e
Paediatric Dermatology 2e
Paediatric Endocrinology and Diabetes
Paediatric Gastroenterology, Hepatology, and Nutrition, 2e
Paediatric Intensive Care
Paediatric Nephrology, 3e
Paediatric Neurology, 3e
Paediatric Palliative Medicine, 2e
Paediatric Radiology
Paediatric Respiratory Medicine
Paediatric Rheumatology

Oxford Specialist Handbooks in Pain Medicine
Spinal Interventions in Pain Management

Oxford Specialist Handbooks in Psychiatry
Addiction Medicine, 2e
Forensic Psychiatry
Medical Psychotherapy

Oxford Specialist Handbooks in Radiology
Head and Neck Imaging
Interventional Radiology
Musculoskeletal Imaging
Thoracic Imaging

Oxford Specialist Handbooks in Surgery
Burns
Cardiothoracic Surgery, 2e
Colorectal Surgery
Current Surgical Guidelines
Gastric and Oesophageal Surgery
Hand Surgery, 2e
Oral and Maxillofacial Surgery, 2e
Otolaryngology and Head and Neck Surgery
Plastic and Reconstructive Surgery
Surgical Oncology
Urological Surgery
Vascular Surgery, 2e

Oxford Specialist Handbooks in Anaesthesia

Global Anaesthesia

EDITED BY

Dr Rachael Craven

Consultant Anaesthetist, University Hospitals Bristol, United Kingdom; Volunteer Anaesthetist Médecins sans Frontières

Dr Hilary Edgcombe

Consultant Anaesthetist, Oxford University Hospitals NHS Trust, UK

Dr Ben Gupta

Consultant Anaesthetist, University Hospitals Bristol, United Kingdom; Volunteer Anaesthetist Médecins sans Frontières

OXFORD
UNIVERSITY PRESS

OXFORD
UNIVERSITY PRESS

Great Clarendon Street, Oxford, OX2 6DP,
United Kingdom

Oxford University Press is a department of the University of Oxford. It furthers the University's objective of excellence in research, scholarship, and education by publishing worldwide. Oxford is a registered trade mark of Oxford University Press in the UK and in certain other countries

First Edition Published in 2020

Impression: 1

Published in the United States of America by Oxford University Press
198 Madison Avenue, New York, NY 10016, United States of America

British Library Cataloguing in Publication Data
Data available

Library of Congress Control Number: 2019950133

ISBN 978–0–19–880982–1

Printed and bound in China by
C&C Offset Printing Co., Ltd.

It has been our privilege while visiting many low- and middle-income countries to meet and work with anaesthesia providers of all cadres in providing care, training, and teaching. These professionals have taught us how to work in their setting with patience, kindness, and expertise. This book is gratefully dedicated to them all.

Foreword

The World Federation of Societies of Anaesthesiologists unites hundreds of thousands of anaesthesiologists in 150 countries to improve patient care and access to safe anaesthesia and perioperative medicine. My experience from being involved in the international anaesthesia community is that we all have much to share, much to learn from each other. That certainly is the case when we are travelling to work in an unfamiliar setting.

Five out of seven billion people in this world do not have access to safe, accessible and affordable anaesthesia, and worst is the situation in South East Asia and Sub-Saharan Africa. Many anaesthesiologists practising in privileged circumstances want to help by travelling to work in low- and middle-income countries, far from their own safe home work environment. That is positive for many reasons, but good intentions are not always paired with competence and skills.

As health workers, we are all familiar with the term "First, do not harm". There are only too many examples of well-intending colleagues working abroad who do more harm than good, not understanding the context nor properly respecting their local colleagues. This is often due to lack of understanding of local culture and habits, difficulties to work with unfamiliar resources and conditions and too low self-insight. Some are so used to having all sorts of monitoring and fancy tools available that their clinical skills are suffering, and they are helpless without the fancy support.

Not all of this can be mitigated by a written text, but a one-place-to-go-to comprehensive resource is a good start. The *Oxford Specialist Handbook of Global Anaesthesia* is the book I was looking for thirty years ago when I first worked in an environment that was less resourced than I was used to.

Dr Rachael Craven, Dr Hilary Edgcombe and Dr Ben Gupta are all based in the United Kingdom, but have recruited an impressive group of authors from high, middle and low income countries. These authors are all experienced in working in different environment from their home base, or they have experience in welcoming foreign colleagues to their home base.

With this book, newcomers will not have to reinvent the wheel, and by that creating unstable and sometimes unsafe conditions for our patients. The book covers all fields from cultural awareness to detailed practical instructions in how to provide safe anaesthesia in different situations. I will not be surprised if providers living permanently in low resource setting will also find it useful as a supplement to ordinary textbooks in anaesthesia.

Jannicke Mellin-Olsen, MD, DPH,
Consultant anaesthesiologist,
Department of Anaesthesiology and Intensive Care Medicine,
Baerum Hospital, Sandvika,
Norway and President World Federation of Societies of
Anaesthesiologists

Foreword

Preface

The *Oxford Specialist Handbook of Global Anaesthesia* is written for trained anaesthetists who are planning to work in low-resource settings. As anaesthetists, our practice is inextricably linked to the drugs, equipment, colleagues, and culture with(in) which we work. When these things change, our approach must change. This book aims to bridge that potential knowledge gap for anaesthetists accustomed to working in high-resource settings.

The book is designed for anaesthetists who are trained and competent to anaesthetize a wide range of patients without direct supervision. As such, much basic knowledge is assumed: the focus is rather on key differences between settings, and how to adapt your practice accordingly.

We hope that this book will be useful to anaesthetists moving from high-income countries to work in low- and middle-income countries. We also hope it will prove useful to those who have trained in urban centres and then moved to work in remote or rural areas, where working conditions can be radically different. Lastly, we hope that it may be of use to anaesthetists working in conflict and catastrophe settings where circumstances inevitably lead to severely constrained resources.

The book has been written and reviewed by anaesthetists with a wealth of experience in practising and teaching in low-resource settings. However, the nature of the 'make do and adapt' approach to working in these settings means that many of the anaesthetic techniques and drug doses described are necessarily based on expert opinion and experience. Furthermore, anaesthetic techniques may be recommended that would fall below the expected standard in a high-resource setting. We urge the reader, therefore, to exercise their own professional judgement when using the book in their own context. The best source of expertise in most low-resource settings is those who already work there.

Wherever in the world you find yourself practising, providing consistently safe anaesthesia and analgesia when resources are scarce can be difficult, stressful, and tiring, but ultimately extremely rewarding. We hope that the addition of this book to your 'back pocket' will make the situation a little less stressful and a lot more rewarding.

R Craven
H Edgcombe
B Gupta

Preface

Acknowledgements

A book like this would not be possible without the goodwill and hard work of very many people from around the world. We are first tremendously grateful to all our contributors, chapter editors, and to those who have offered feedback and support to them and us throughout the writing and editing process. We are also very grateful to OUP, especially to Geraldine Jeffers and Fiona Sutherland, who have supported this project from its inception and provided us with much-needed advice and guidance.

We would like to name in particular Iain Wilson, for his insight and encouragement, and Eric Vreede, who heroically read and commented on the entire manuscript once drafted, to its, and our, vast advantage.

Finally, we hugely appreciate the support of our colleagues and families, who put up with all the travel and stories on our return and display the flexibility required of those who work and live with people like us. Without them too, this book would not exist.

Thanks

The production of this book has been financially supported in part by Diamedica (www.diamedica.co.uk), who design, provide, and service anaesthesia and critical care equipment suitable for use in low-resource settings. Their tireless work to promote safer anaesthesia worldwide is recognized and reflected in the assistance they have given to bring this book to publication.

Thank you also, in advance, to the readers of this book. We would be glad to hear of any suggestions, omissions, errors, or areas for improvement. Please do e-mail us at OSHGA@outlook.com.

All royalties received by the editors as a result of sales of the *Oxford Specialist Handbook of Global Anaesthesia* will be donated to Médecins Sans Frontières.

Contents

Contributors

Dr Christine Bartulec (Organizing Your Environment)
Senior Anaesthesiologist
International Committee of the Red Cross
Geneva
Switzerland

Dr Tom Bashford (Context, Perioperative Care)
President, World Anaesthesia Society
Research Fellow, NIHR Global Health Research Group on Neurotrauma, University of Cambridge
Cambridge
UK

Dr Phil Blum (Drugs and Transfusion)
Senior Staff Anaesthetist
Royal Darwin Hospital
Darwin
Australia

Dr Adrian Bosenberg (Regional Anaesthesia)
Professor of Anesthesiology and Consultant Pediatric Anesthesiologist
Seattle Children's Hospital, University of Washington
Seattle, WA
USA

Dr Chris Bowden (Drugs and Transfusion)
Clinical Director, Department of Anaesthesia and Pain Management
Frankston Hospital
Melbourne
Australia

Dr Nick Boyd (Paediatrics)
Consultant Paediatric Anaesthetist
Bristol Royal Hospital for Children
Bristol
UK

Dr Rachel Collis (Obstetrics and Gynaecology)
Consultant Anaesthetist
University Hospital of Wales
Cardiff
UK

Dr Tom Coonan (Drugs and Transfusion)
Professor, Departments of Anesthesia and Surgery
Dalhousie University
Halifax, NS
Canada

Dr Ibironke Desalu (Paediatrics)
Professor of Anaesthesia, College of Medicine, University of Lagos
Consultant Anaesthetist, Lagos University Teaching Hospital
Lagos
Nigeria

Dr Michael Dobson (Anaesthesia Equipment and Utilities)
Consultant Anaesthetist
University of Oxford
Oxford
UK

Dr Faye Evans (chapter lead Paediatrics)
Senior Associate in Perioperative Anesthesia, Boston Children's Hospital
Assistant Professor of Anesthesia, Harvard Medical School
Boston, MA
USA

Dr Paul Firth (Paediatrics)
Pediatric Anesthesiologist
Head of the Division of Community and Global Health
Massachusetts General Hospital
Boston, MA
USA

Dr Rachel Freedman (Organizing Your Environment)
Senior Registrar in Anaesthesia
Imperial School of Anaesthesia
London
UK

Julian Gore-Booth (Context)
Chief Executive Officer
World Federation of Societies of Anaesthetists
London
UK

Dr Lara Herbert (General and Urological Surgery)
Consultant Anaesthetist
Royal Cornwall Hospitals NHS Trust
Treliske
Cornwall
UK

Dr Sarah Hodges (Paediatrics, Trauma)
Head of Department of Anaesthesia
CoRSU Rehabilitation Hospital
Kampala
Uganda

Dr Victoria Howell (Tropical Medicine for Anaesthetists)
Consultant Anaesthetist
The Queen Elizabeth Hospital NHS Foundation Trust
King's Lynn
UK

Dr Amy Hughes (Organizing Your Environment)
Lecturer in Emergency and Humanitarian Response
Humanitarian and Conflict Response Unit
University of Manchester
Manchester
UK

Dr Jo James (Context)
Bernard Johnson Advisor—Global Partnerships
Royal College of Anaesthetists
London
UK

Dr Sanja Janjanin (Organizing Your Environment, Trauma)
Lead Anaesthetist
International Committee of the Red Cross
Geneva
Switzerland

Dr Jey Jeyanathen (chapter lead Regional Anaesthesia)
Consultant in Anaesthesia and Intensive Care
Humanitarian Lead for Defence Anaesthesia
Defence Lecturer, Academic Department of Military Anaesthesia and Critical Care
Queen Victoria Hospital NHS Foundation Trust
London
UK

Dr Rebecca Jones (Obstetrics and Gynaecology)
Locum Consultant Anaesthetist
University Hospitals Bristol NHS Foundation Trust
Bristol
UK

Dr Judith Kendell (Trauma)
Anaesthesia Referent
Médecins Sans Frontières (Operational Centre Brussels)
Brussels
Belgium

Dr Nur Lubis (chapter lead Trauma)
Consultant Anaesthetist, Whipps Cross Hospital
Volunteer Anaesthetist Médecins Sans Frontières
London
UK

Dr Polly Marshall-Brown (Critical Care)
Senior Registrar in Anaesthesia
Peninsular School of Anaesthesia
Southwest England
UK

Dr Francesca Mazzola (Critical Care)
Senior Registrar in Anaesthesia
Royal Marsden Hospital NHS Trust
London
UK

Dr Bruce McCormick (chapter lead Critical Care, Organizing Your Environment)
Consultant Anaesthetist
Royal Devon and Exeter NHS Foundation Trust
Exeter
UK

Dr Rachel McKendry (The Difficult Airway)
Consultant Anaesthetist
University Hospitals Bristol NHS Foundation Trust
Bristol
UK

Dr Wayne Morriss (Organizing Your Environment, Perioperative Care)
Director of Programmes—World Federation of Societies of Anaesthesiologists
Consultant Anaesthetist
Christchurch Hospital
Christchurch New Zealand

Dr Mary Nabukenya (Paediatric Anaesthesia)
Lecturer and Registrar in Paediatric Anaesthesia
Makerere University
Mulago Hospital
Kampala
Uganda

Dr Susane Nabulindo (Paediatric Anaesthesia)
Consultant Paediatric Anaesthesiologist
University of Nairobi
Nairobi
Kenya

Robert Neighbour (Anaesthesia Equipment and Utilities)
Managing Director
Diamedica (UK) Ltd
Barnstaple
UK

Mr David Nott (Trauma)
Consultant Surgeon, Imperial College London
Volunteer Surgeon: International Committee of the Red Cross, Médecins Sans Frontières, and Syria Relief
London
UK

Dr Sarah O'Neill (Obstetrics and Gynaecology)
Consultant Anaesthetist
Salford Royal NHS Foundation Trust
Volunteer Anaesthetist, Médecins Sans Frontières
Manchester
UK

Dr Nelson Olim (Trauma)
Regional Advisor for Emergency Medical Teams Initiative
WHO Eastern Mediterranean Regional Office
World Health Organization
Geneva
Switzerland

Dr Becky Paris (Context)
Consultant Anaesthetist
Hereford County Hospital
Hereford
UK

Dr Stephen Pickering (Context)
Consultant Anaesthetist
United Mission Hospital
Tansen
Nepal

Dr Andrea Reis (Organizing Your Environment)
Senior Anaesthesiologist
International Committee of the Red Cross
Geneva
Switzerland

Dr Clare Roques (Perioperative Care)
Consultant Anaesthetist and Inpatient Pain Lead
Heatherwood and Wexham Park Hospitals
SloughUK

Dr Oliver Ross (Context)
Consultant Anaesthetist
University Hospital Southampton
Southampton
UK

Dr Naomi Shamambo (Context, Perioperative Care)
Senior Registrar in Anaesthesia and Lead for Primary Trauma
University Teaching Hospital
Lusaka
Zambia

Dr Kate Stephens (chapter lead, Critical Care)
Consultant in Critical Care and Anaesthesia
Nevill Hall Hospital
Abergavenny
UK

Dr Ruth Tighe (General and Urological Surgery)
Consultant Intensivist and Anaesthetist
East Kent Hospitals Universities Hospitals Trust
Ashford
Kent
UK

Dr Isabeau Walker (chapter lead, Paediatric Anaesthesia)
Consultant Anaesthetist
Great Ormond Street Hospital
London
UK

Dr Matt Wilkes (Anaesthesia Equipment and Utilities, Perioperative Care)
Research Fellow
Centre for Altitude, Space and Extreme Environment Medicine
University College London
London
UK

Symbols and Abbreviations

➲	go to page
AAGBI	Association of Anaesthetists of Great Britain and Ireland
ABCD	airway, breathing, circulation, disability
ABG	arterial blood gas
AC	alternating current
ACE	angiotensin-converting enzyme
ACS	acute coronary syndrome
ACT	artemisinin-based combination therapy
AF	atrial fibrillation
AIN	acute interstitial nephritis
AKI	acute kidney injury
ALS	advanced life support
APH	antepartum haemorrhage
APL	adjustable pressure limiting
APLS	advanced paediatric life support
APTT	activated partial thromboplastin time
ARDS	acute respiratory distress syndrome
ARM	anorectal malformation
ART	antiretroviral therapy
ASA	American Society of Anesthesiologists
ASD	atrioseptal defect
ASM	anterior scalene muscle
Atrac.	atracurium
AVPU	alert, verbal, pain, unresponsive
BBB	bundle branch block
BiPAP	bilevel positive airway pressure
BMI	body mass index
BMV	bag mask ventilation
BP	blood pressure
BSA	body surface area
CBF	cerebral blood flow
CDC	Centers for Disease Control and Prevention
CG	compressed gas
CLP	cleft lip/palate
$CMRO_2$	cerebral metabolic requirement oxygen
CMV	cytomegalovirus
CNS	central nervous system
CO	cardiac output
CO_2	carbon dioxide
CPAP	continuous positive airway pressure
CPD	citrate, phosphate, dextrose
CPD	continuing professional development
CPD-A1	citrate, phosphate, dextrose with added adenine
CPP	cerebral perfusion pressure
CPR	cardiopulmonary resuscitation

CPSP	chronic post-surgical pain
CS	Caesarean section
CSF	cerebrospinal fluid
CT	computerized tomography
CVS	cardiovascular system
CXR	chest x-ray
DC	direct current
DDI	decision to delivery interval
DDV	Diamedica drawover vaporizer
DIC	disseminated intravascular coagulation
DKA	diabetic ketoacidosis
DOT	direct observation of therapy
DPA	Diamedica portable anaesthesia system
DVT	deep vein thrombosis
EBV	estimated blood volume
ECG	electrocardiogram
ED	emergency department
EMO	Epstein Macintosh Oxford vaporizer
EMT	emergency medical team
ENT	ear, nose, and throat
EPM	essential pain management
ERPC	evacuation of retained products of conception
ETAT	emergency triage assessment and treatment
$ETCO_2$	end-tidal carbon dioxide
ETT	endotracheal tube
FA	femoral artery
FAST	Focused Assessment with Sonography for Trauma
FB	foreign body
FBC	full blood count
FFP3	filtering face piece
FGM	female genital mutilation
FiO_2	fractional inspired oxygen concentration
FLACC	Face Leg Activity Cry Consolability
FMJ	full metal jacket
FN	femoral nerve
FRC	functional residual capacity
FV	femoral vein
GA	general anaesthesia
G&S	group and save
GBS	Guillain–Barré syndrome
GCS	Glasgow coma score
GMC	General Medical Council
GTN	glyceryl trinitrate
HACE	high-altitude cerebral oedema
HAPE	high-altitude pulmonary oedema
Hb	haemoglobin
HbF	foetal haemoglobin
HbS	sickle haemoglobin
Hct	haematocrit
HDU	high dependency unit
HIC	high-income countries
HIV	human immunodeficiency virus

HME	heat moisture exchanger
HTIG	human tetanus immune globulin
HUS	haemolytic uraemic syndrome
Hz	Hertz
IASP	International Association for the Study of Pain
ICP	intracranial pressure
ICU	intensive care unit
IL1	interleukin-1
IM	intramuscular
IO	intraosseous
IPPV	intermittent positive pressure ventilation
IV	intravenous
IVC	inferior vena cava
IVI	intravenous infusion
KCl	potassium chloride
LA	local anaesthetic
LBW	low birth weight
LD	latissimus dorsi
LFT	liver function tests
LMA	laryngeal mask airway
LMIC	low- and middle-income countries
MABL	maximum allowable blood loss
MAC	minimum alveolar concentration
MAP	mean arterial pressure
MDR	multi-drug resistant
MEWS	medical early warning score
MI	myocardial infarction
MILS	manual in line stabilization (of c spine)
MN	median nerve
MRI	magnetic resonance imaging
MSF	Médecins Sans Frontières
MSM	middle scalene muscle
NAAT	nucleic acid amplification test
NG	nasogastric
NGO	non-governmental organization
NIV	non-invasive ventilation
NNRTI	non-nucleoside analogue reverse transcriptase inhibitor
NPA	nasopharyngeal airway
NRTI	nucleoside analogue reverse transcriptase inhibitor
NSAID	non-steroidal anti-inflammatory drug
NSTEMI	non-ST elevation myocardial infarction
ODP	operating department practitioner
OIB	Oxford inflating bellows
OLV	one lung ventilation
OMV	Oxford miniature vaporizer
ORS	oral rehydration solution
OSA	obstructive sleep apnoea
PA	popliteal artery
PAC	Portable Anaesthesia Complete vaporizer
Panc.	pancuronium

PaO_2	partial pressure of arterial oxygen
PAP	physician anaesthesia provider
PCA	patient controlled analgesia
PCI	percutaneous coronary intervention
PDA	patent ductus arteriosus
PEP	post-exposure prophylaxis
PEEP	positive end expiratory pressure
PET	pre-eclamptic toxaemia
PI	protease inhibitor
PO	per oram (oral)
PP	placenta praevia
PPH	postpartum haemorrhage
PR	per rectum
PSARP	posterior anorectoplasty
PTSD	post-traumatic stress disorder
PV	popliteal vein
RAE	
RAT	Recognize, Assess, and Treat
RCD	residual current device
RDT	rapid diagnostic test
ReSoMal	Rehydration Solution for Malnutrition
Rh	Rhesus
RN	radial nerve
RR	respiratory rate
RRT	renal replacement therapy
RSI	rapid sequence induction
RTA	road traffic accident
RTI	respiratory tract infection
RUQ	right upper quadrant
SA	subclavian artery
SC	subcutaneous
SCD	sickle cell disease
SJ	semi-jacketed
SIADH	syndrome of inappropriate ADH secretion
SIRS	systemic inflammatory response syndrome
SN	sciatic nerve
SpO_2	oxygen saturation
SSFFC	substandard, spurious, falsely labelled, falsified, and counterfeit
STEMI	ST elevation myocardial infarction
Sux.	suxamethonium
SV	spontaneous ventilation
SV	subclavian vein
SVP	saturated vapour pressure
SVR	systemic vascular resistance
SVT	supraventricular tachycardia
TAP	transversus abdominis plane
TAT	transanastomotic tube
TB	tuberculosis
t.d.s.	ter die sumendum
TFT	thyroid function test
TIVA	total intravenous anaesthesia
TNF	tumour necrosis factor

TO4	train of four
TOF	tracheo-oesophageal fistula
TRALI	transfusion-related lung injury
U&E	urea and electrolytes
UA	unstable angina
UAM	universal anaesthesia machine
UHC	Universal Health Coverage
UK	United Kingdom
UN	ulnar nerve
UN	United Nations
UPS	uninterruptable power supply
URTI	upper respiratory tract infection
V	volts
VACTERL	vertebral, anal, cardiac, tracheal, oesophagus, renal, and limbs
Vec.	vecuronium
VP	ventriculoperitoneal
VRII	variable rate insulin infusion
VSD	ventriculoseptal defect
WCC	white cell count
WFSA	World Federation of Societies of Anaesthesiologists
WHO	World Health Organization
XDR	extensively drug resistant

Chapter 1

Context

Tom Bashford, Julian Gore-Booth, Jo James, Stephen Pickering, Becky Paris, Oliver Ross, and Naomi Shamambo

Anaesthesia in the global context

In high-income countries (HICs) anaesthesia mortality has steadily decreased over the past 70 years, but in many low- and middle-income countries (LMICs) this improvement is not evident. In some countries anaesthesia mortality has been found to be as high as 1:133, one to two *thousand* times higher than it is in a hospital in a HIC. It is no exaggeration to state that—in the global context—anaesthesia is in crisis.

There are many contributory factors to such high mortality rates, but the question remains: if we know how to deliver safe surgery and anaesthesia, why is this same care not available to over 70% of the world's population?

2015—a breakthrough year

In 1980 the Director General of the World Health Organization (WHO) described surgical care as an essential component of 'Universal Health Coverage' (UHC). Since that time there has been limited progress in advancing universal access to safe surgery and anaesthesia; however, 2015 gave rise to some key drivers for change with the publication of:

- *Disease Control Priorities 3—volume 1, Essential Surgery*
- *Global Surgery 2030: The Lancet Commission on Global Surgery.*

And at the 68th World Health Assembly meeting, the unanimous approval, by Member States, of a Resolution:

- 'Strengthening emergency and essential surgical care and anaesthesia as a component of universal health coverage.'

These set out the extent of the crisis, and the case for investment in surgery and anaesthesia, with potential solutions and recommendations for countries, institutions, and individuals. Key messages include:

- Five out of seven billion people lack access to safe, affordable surgical and anaesthesia care when needed.
- An estimated 16.9 million lives were lost in 2010 from conditions requiring surgical care (four times the combined number of lives lost from HIV/AIDS, tuberculosis, and malaria).
- Provision of 44 essential surgical procedures at first level (often called 'district') hospitals would avert 1.5 million deaths per year.
- Scaling up surgical and anaesthesia services to reach a surgical volume target of 5,000 procedures per 100,000 population would cost US$420 billion by 2030, but realize a saving, in LMICs, of US$12.3 trillion.

Safe anaesthesia—the ingredients

The WHO-World Federation of Societies of Anaesthesiologists' (WFSA) International Standards for a Safe Practice of Anaesthesia define safe anaesthesia as a product of:

- workforce
- medicines
- equipment and infrastructure.

Workforce

A recent WFSA workforce survey estimated that there are around 450,000 physician anaesthesia providers (PAPs) in the world. In HICs PAP density is almost 18 per 100,000, whilst in LMICs this drops to just 0.19 per 100,000. A significant and urgent scale-up of both physician and non-physician anaesthesia providers is needed across LMICs.

Medicines (and safety)

Cost, legislation, logistics, safety—there is little data available, but we do know that in many LMICs often the only anaesthetic drug consistently available and administered in local hospitals is ketamine. Even in larger hospitals only one volatile agent might be available (usually halothane), and nitrous oxide is a rarity. A study of 555 LMIC health facilities found that ketamine anaesthesia was available in 72.9%, whilst volatile general anaesthesia was only available in 56.2%.

Over 80% of the world's population lives in countries with very limited access to analgesics.

Infrastructure and equipment

A study of hospitals in 22 LMICs revealed that only 60% had reliable access to running water and electricity, only 45% had reliable access to oxygen, and just 50% had reliable access to anaesthesia machines and pulse oximetry. Other literature indicates that in some sub-Saharan African countries, as many as 90% of anaesthesia departments do not have the facilities to give a safe anaesthetic to a child; one study in Papua New Guinea showed that only 57% of hospitals always have resuscitation bags and masks available.

Conclusion

The global crisis in anaesthesia is real. Addressing it requires urgent scaling up of the anaesthesia workforce (with various levels of trained provider), an aligned response in terms of equipment and infrastructure, and adequate availability of medicines. Safe anaesthesia is essential for safe surgery and should be an integral part of all health systems.

Humanitarian and developmental principles

Definitions

- In healthcare, humanitarian action and international development represent efforts by the international community to respond to failures of native healthcare systems either as a result of an acute event, or due to chronic deficiencies, or both.
- Humanitarian action has been defined as aid that seeks to save lives, alleviate the suffering, and maintain the dignity of a crisis-affected population.
- Development, by contrast, may be defined as the work done in resource-poor settings to improve the long-term wellbeing of their populations and to contribute to their capacity to look after themselves.

Humanitarian action

- In healthcare, this entails the immediate short-term provision of medical services to those whose health systems have failed due to man-made or natural disasters.
- United Nations (UN) General Assembly Resolution 46/182:
  - lays out four fundamental humanitarian principles: humanity, impartiality, independence, and neutrality
  - advocates to provide humanitarian assistance with full respect for the sovereignty of the recipient State.
- Following an acute event, agencies engaged in humanitarian relief should be coordinated via the UN cluster system.
- The WHO leads the Health Cluster in addition to coordinating emergency medical teams (EMTs).
- EMTs have three levels: levels 2 and 3 require anaesthetic input.
- Humanitarian work is governed by humanitarian principles and protected by humanitarian law, a branch of international law pertaining to armed conflict.

Development

- In healthcare, development work often focuses on training, health system strengthening, and population health, with an emphasis on the sustainability and scalability of the interventions delivered.
- Equally important are advocacy, partnership, and academic collaboration.
- Unlike humanitarian work, the legal framework for development work is less clear-cut.

The humanitarian–development nexus

- This term has been used to describe the interface between humanitarian action and development.
- The two approaches often have different funding sources, immediate priorities, ways of working, and rhetoric, but they are increasingly interrelated.

- Humanitarian emergencies are more likely and more severe, when existing systems are already weak, requiring development.
- If a humanitarian response cannot hand over to a functional national health system, then the problem is also one of development.
- In practice, significant overlap often occurs: humanitarian action and development projects are required to co-exist, and their harmonization should be pursued.
- For anaesthetists, the line between providing immediate humanitarian assistance through clinical care, and involvement in development through health systems strengthening will often be blurred.

Ethical considerations

- Both forms of aid have faced criticism for:
  - undermining native healthcare systems
  - wastage or misappropriation of funds
  - failure to deliver their objectives
  - failing to work with each other.
- A failure to appreciate the humanitarian–development context in which you are working can undermine efforts to improve care from an ethical, legal, and practical standpoint.
- Standards have been proposed for international partnerships, quality improvement, humanitarian assistance, and EMTs.
- For anaesthetists, there are defined international clinical standards in addition to best practice guidelines for emergency surgical responses.
- Visiting anaesthetists should consider their standards of practice both in relation to their own licensing body, but also international guidelines and those of their host country.
- Legal and ethical accountability in both arenas is complex and, in practice, often very dilute.
- It is impractical for all anaesthetists to be experts on the extensive theory and rhetoric around development and humanitarian work; however, an appreciation of the complexity of the field is vital to inform the funding, design, delivery, and evaluation of efforts in global health.

Understanding your context

- The following 20 questions can be posed when considering the context of any global health work to be undertaken.
- They may be very difficult to answer but attempting to do so is a useful exercise in itself.
  - 1. Is my primary role to provide direct care or improve services?
  - 2. To whom is my duty of care?
  - 3. Who are my colleagues?
  - 4. Who wants me here and why?
  - 5. What does my organization and/or their donor want to achieve?
  - 6. What do I want to achieve?
  - 7. What other visitors are here and what do they want?
  - 8. What do my local partners want and need?
  - 9. What is the local capacity—am I supporting or undermining it?
  - 10. Why has the local system failed?
  - 11. What does the local system need to be functional?

- 12. How long do I have here?
- 13. What can I do that is meaningful in that time?
- 14. What happens when I leave?
- 15. Who continues this work?
- 16. Who am I accountable to?
- 17. What does best practice here look like?
- 18. Am I competent to deliver best practice?
- 19. Can the current system support my interventions?
- 20. What are the risks to me, my partners, and my patients?

Adapting your practice

Case 1—Caesarean section, consent, and cross-match

It's the cold season in a remote mountainous district. A young woman in labour has travelled a full day to reach the hospital. Even on arriving at the hospital, labour analgesia is not offered to her, because none is available. The local doctor says an urgent Caesarean section (CS) is necessary. Her husband, terrified of allowing anyone to cut his wife, refuses to sign consent. Whilst the local staff counsel the husband, your thoughts go to the logistical challenge of anaesthetizing in this kind of environment.

- It's very cold—there is a tiny heater in theatre that barely takes the chill off. You are concerned about intraoperative heat loss, neonatal resuscitation, and maternal haemorrhage.
- Referral is not an option—the nearest hospital is a 5-h drive away and has little more than you can offer here.
- The usual choice of preoperative tests is unavailable.
- You check her haemoglobin and try to cross-match blood, but there is no blood bank—the availability of blood depends on a 'walking donor'—usually a family member.
- The staff have obtained consent for the surgery. They remind you that every test and intervention is also a financial burden to the husband (he must pay for everything); however, he agrees to have his blood checked for compatibility and donates 1 unit.
- The process of anaesthesia resembles that back home: cannulation, intravenous (IV) fluids, preparation of drugs, and insertion of the spinal.
- In this cold, dusty environment you try to maintain a strict sterile field. The needle is contained within an autoclaved 'spinal pack', each item cleaned and sterilized, but re-used from another patient—nothing is thrown away here unless absolutely necessary.
- As surgery begins you monitor the maternal vital signs closely. The baby is delivered and handed to a nurse. There is silence.
- You take a few steps over to see the baby, lying limp on a trolley. Helping the nurse deliver rescue breaths, dry, wrap, and stimulate the baby—his colour and tone improve and he lets out a cry.
- Immediately your attention returns to the mother. The surgeon tells you the uterus is boggy, she is haemorrhaging.
- You add oxytocin to the IV fluids and start the blood transfusion. It is fresh, warm, whole blood and in combination with oxytocin the patient improves.

This time the lives of both mother and baby have been saved.

Success! This word, its definition and concept, will be challenged often by other cases where one life may be lost and one saved, or worse. Allow yourself time to process these difficult cases.

Leaning points 1: Know your environment

- Local culture impacts greatly on medical practice in all settings. Endeavour to understand it deeply where you are.
- For example, in some cultures, consent for surgery comes from the husband, father, or another relative. Patients themselves may be

unwilling or disempowered to make these decisions themselves. Lack of understanding and suspicion of medical interventions puts additional pressure on emergency situations.

- Prepare for your new environment:
  - Read, talk to colleagues, use online resources, courses, and conferences.
  - Learn ketamine anaesthesia and blocks with landmark/nerve stimulator techniques.
  - Gain some experience with draw-over anaesthesia machines.
- In your new environment:
  - Understand what is already there, what is already done, and what is already known.
  - Acknowledge local expertise and think carefully before attempting to change practice. Local workers are often very experienced, knowledgeable, and have adapted techniques to the environment.

Case 2—'Thank goodness you're here'

'Thank goodness you're here,' said the visiting orthopaedic surgeon, 'a woman has fallen down the cliff, shattering her skull, please anaesthetize her so we can do a thorough debridement.'

- You have just arrived as sole anaesthetist in a small, remote hospital.
- You go to the operating theatre and find a functioning self-inflating bag and mask, a laryngoscope, some endotracheal tubes, and a scanty selection of anaesthesia drugs.
- Reminding yourself of the basics you plan the case: ketamine, pancuronium, and pethidine. Not exactly a familiar combination.
- Monitoring consists of a pulse oximeter, manual sphygmomanometer, and clinical signs. There is an oxygen concentrator and cylinder for back-up in case of electricity failure. The suction machine must be shared with the surgeons but relies on electricity.
- Your limited language skills make preoperative assessment tricky. You rely on local staff and careful examination. Her Glasgow coma score (GCS) is 12, chest is clear, heart sounds normal. She is in her 30s but weighs barely 45 kg.
- You feel out of your comfort zone. You wish for a skilled assistant, a(nother) consultant, or an intensivist, but there are none so you brief a co-volunteer on how to assist you.
- Carefully pre-oxygenating the patient you consider how all your usual anaesthesia techniques must be adapted.
- You give the best anaesthetic you can, carefully titrating ketamine throughout, ventilating the patient by hand, and monitoring closely.
- As surgery finishes you have no idea of neuromuscular activity or end-tidal CO_2.
- After some time, the patient begins to breathe spontaneously, is extubated, and after an hour is returned to the ward.

Early the following morning you discover the patient awake, sitting in bed, and asking for water. With no adverse surgical or anaesthesia effects she is keen to go home.

Learning points 2: Working in isolation

- Isolation may be physical, cultural, medical, educational, or emotional. It is important to prepare for each of these.
- Even in isolated settings modern communication technology is helping to bypass traditional senses of isolation, making the world smaller—remember there is almost always someone who can help or support, whether local or international.
- Make plans to decrease all forms of isolation: find others who have worked or are working near you, who are happy to be consulted.
- Learn some of the local language and the basic non-verbal communication of the culture in which you are working.
- You may not have skilled assistance or back-up options so work out emergency plans early.
- Have all your additional equipment (bougie, oro-pharyngeal airways, etc.) and emergency drugs laid out and within reaching distance when anaesthetizing—there may be no-one to pass you things in an emergency.
- With the correct instruction, anyone can be co-opted to assist you, medical or not.

Case 3—Joining an established team

You are to work in a larger hospital, 10 h from the main city. It has seasonally hindered access from flooding, landslides, and political rallies. You are responsible for the smooth running of three major operating theatres. Your team has six experienced nurse anaesthetists and three student nurse anaesthetists, but no skilled assistants. You have already observed the skills of the senior nurse anaesthetist (20+ years' experience) in calmly and proficiently anaesthetizing every patient, neonate to geriatric, ASA1 to ASA4. Despite your own experience you realize that you are going to learn more than you will teach.

- There is an established anaesthesia service that seems to work.
- You mitigate your temptation to point out every deviation from your norms, by asking questions to understand the rationale for how and why things function here as they do.
- You make notes on areas for quality improvement, safety issues, and successful techniques and routines already in place.
- Local staff are keen to learn and advance their skills.
- The organization is good; patients come in the night before and are prepared for theatre.
- You review the high-risk patients and those attending for major surgery early each morning.
- Most patients are poor, and their attendance to hospital for anything other than life-threatening illness is dictated by the farming calendar.
- Stoical patients present late, with sepsis or inoperable tumours that may have been amenable to curative resection if treated earlier. Chronic diseases are often only diagnosed at the time of preoperative assessment, and may be uncontrolled.
- Risk–benefit assessments require consideration of a much wider range of variables than you are used to.

- Discussions with patients and families are crucial and they may opt for non-operative treatment despite advice for surgery.
- Back-up options are restricted here; referral pathways less established, and transportation and referral of patients often result in huge financial and social burdens to the family.
- Support for higher level care is challenging, and protracted periods in theatre or recovery may be a substitute for those requiring it.

Learning points 3: Practical adaptations

- Globally, anaesthesia is provided by a range of practitioners: physician anaesthetists, nurses, and medical officers.
- Understanding your role is essential—find the balance between your own knowledge and experience and that of local healthcare providers. Take time to watch and learn before jumping in. There is usually a reason why things are done the way they are. Staff have found that it works that way in their situation. Change without understanding the reasons may be dangerous and lead to deaths.
- Do the standards you are aiming for differ from local expectations?
- Work is always a compromise between what you consider safe in your hospital and what is necessary under the circumstances. Cleanliness, pre-op preparation, and drug and equipment availability may all fall below what you would normally accept.
- Be sensitive in instigating change and gain support from local colleagues, or else it will last, at best, for the time you are there.
- Maintain basic safety; embrace the WHO Surgical Safety Checklist principles to enhance communication and planning.
- Perioperative care is difficult: consider carefully which tests will give essential information. Patients may have undiagnosed or uncontrolled disease; recovery care and ward skill varies greatly.
- The decision to operate, or not, should be made with the surgeon, patient, family, and theatre team. Often, especially when the service is in the hands of non-physician providers, surgeons will be in charge and push for surgery when perhaps it shouldn't take place. Failed surgery or death on the table may have significant repercussions, not only for the patient and their family, but also for the community and work of the hospital. On the other hand, death on the table may well be an accepted occurrence.
- Referral pathways are often unestablished, and there may be no functional relationship between referring and receiving hospitals.
- The communication and handover of patient care or acceptance of patient care is often non-existent. Where will you refer to, and what is the capacity of the receiving hospital? How will the patient be transferred? Can they be optimized beforehand?

Preparation and self-care

Working in a low-resource setting can be a rewarding experience for any anaesthetist. It is important, however, to adequately prepare yourself before, during, and after a visit, to reduce risks to your physical and psychological health—not only for your own sake but also for the sake of your colleagues and patients.

Where to go?

- There is a variety of options, including short surgical 'camps', educational projects, and longer clinical placements.
- If you have no experience working in low-resource settings it is sensible to try a short placement first, e.g. 1–2 weeks, preferably where you can work alongside someone more experienced.
- Even if experienced you may not have practised in some specialties for some time. Confirm what's expected and update before travelling.
- E-learning resources are freely available on the internet (see Further Reading). Face-to-face training courses are also available.
- The longer you stay, the more productive your trip will tend to be.
- Give yourself plenty of time to apply for a post—up to a year is often required to gain permissions, medical registrations, and visas, etc.
- Only ever undertake work in a conflict zone or 'fragile state' with an established organization, e.g. Médecins Sans Frontières (MSF).
- Know as much as possible about the place where you are going to work: the clinical environment, staff, patient mix, local culture.
- Have realistic aims and objectives and be aware of your limitations.

What is a 'good-quality' placement?
Although no guarantee, the following may be indicators that a placement is likely to have good governance processes in place.

- Well reviewed by previous attendees and/or running for some time.
- It is with a well-established organization, for instance, a substantial non-governmental organization (NGO) with a good reputation.
- The post is affiliated to reputable bodies such as the Association of Anaesthetists in your home or the host country.
- There is evidence of proper induction, mentorship and clinical support, adequate accommodation, and a requirement for mandatory personal travel insurance and in-country medical registration.

Physical health

The main causes of damage to your physical health are infectious diseases and trauma. Minor conditions such as sunburn rarely have long-term effects but can ruin a short trip.

General

- Ensure you have all required vaccinations—allow time to complete these before travel.
- If you have a pre-existing medical condition consider whether this can be treated safely should there be a worsening of the condition.
- Avoid the temptation to regularly work excessive hours—fatigue may predispose you to physical and psychological illness.
- Use caution in self-treating with drugs acquired in the country visited as there may be no guarantee of their safety and efficacy.

- Make sure there is someone you can contact in the unit you are working in should your personal safety be in danger, e.g. due to acute illness or threat of assault.

Infectious diseases

Advice changes all the time and it is important to obtain the latest recommendations from travel health advisers, infectious disease departments of your hospital, or trusted websites (see Further Reading).

Traveller's diarrhoea

- Can be debilitating and completely ruin the entirety of a short trip.
- Avoid high-risk foods and water. Be meticulous with hand hygiene.
- Make sure you have access to treatment, including antidiarrhoeal medication, rehydration salts, and antibiotics.

Malaria

- Ensure you have appropriate prophylaxis, and always complete this on returning home.
- The best way to avoid malaria is to avoid being bitten—follow recommendations, e.g. cover up, use bed nets, etc.

Human immunodeficiency virus (HIV)

Ideally you should:

- Wear robust footwear in theatre (take your own if in doubt).
- Use high-quality surgical sterile gloves.
- Be familiar with management of needle-stick injury.
- Know the whereabouts of post-exposure prophylaxis (PEP) packs (find out if available in-country—you may wish to take your own).

Other diseases

- Be aware of other infectious and tropical diseases in the country you are visiting (see 'fitfortravel' in Further Reading); know what to look out for so symptoms are not overlooked and treatment delayed.
- There appears to be an increase in sexual activity in aid workers. Make sure you are aware of the symptoms and signs of sexually transmitted diseases. Take appropriate precautions if engaging.

Carry a bag with you every day containing: water, snacks, antidiarrhoeal medication, simple analgesics, insect repellent, sunscreen, a hat, alcohol hand gel, toilet tissue, bacterial wipes, sanitary products, a torch, good-quality theatre shoes, gloves, and face masks.

Trauma

This can vary from slips and trips, to road traffic accidents (RTAs) and assault, both physical and sexual. Risks are high in many LMICs. The following points will help to reduce risks:

- If using a driver, make sure they are sober, safe, recommended, and have appropriate insurance.
- Do not drive yourself unless you have experience and confidence in that country. If you do, make sure the vehicle is in good condition and insured, and travel with someone else, preferably during the day.
- Carry a functioning phone.

- When travelling, in most circumstances, you will be safer if accompanied by a friend. Inform someone of your whereabouts, your phone number, and estimated time of arrival.
- Behave and dress in a manner that is appropriate to the culture of the country.
- The incidence of RTAs, other trauma, and all types of assault is significantly increased during the hours of darkness.

Psychological health

Working in a low-resource environment you may be exposed to considerable psychological stress that may lead to trauma/post-traumatic stress disorder (PTSD). The impact will be lessened if you are prepared and aware.

Home and family

- Sort out any financial matters before leaving. Long-term trips may cause considerable financial strain, which is unwanted added stress.
- Pre-arrange ways to communicate with loved ones whilst away.

When you are away

- Look after yourself. Burn-out will be unpleasant for you and you will be of no further use to the people you are working with.
- Loneliness and homesickness are very common. Some placements are very isolated. Try to form a social support network in country as well as maintaining communication links with home.
- Difficulties with communication, poor living standards, and intolerance to the climate can all contribute to anxiety and stress.
- Disappointment may replace your initial enthusiasm and expectations when you are exposed to a very different culture. We go out with dreams of glory and improving the world, but the reality is different. Talk to someone who has been in a similar environment.
- Avoid recreational drugs and excess alcohol.
- Find something to occupy yourself when not working: exercise, reading. Write a diary or blog.
- Make sure you have some down time, relaxing and enjoying the country.

When you are working

- You may find the conditions very challenging and may have to make very difficult clinical decisions without the support you are used to.
- You may experience animosity from staff. Try to understand the hierarchy and adapt.
- Increasing stress may lead to insomnia, irritability, loss of concentration, and agitation. Make sure there is someone in country or at home you can discuss this with, such as a mentor or supervisor.
- You have a duty of care to patients—if too tired to work, don't.
- Overwork, a stressful and challenging environment, and fatigue may lead to a form of PTSD. Know the signs and symptoms and discuss with your mentor.
- The organization you are working for may have a support network to help you.

Coming home

- 'Re-entry syndrome' is common and more likely after a long trip.
- You may be filled with enthusiasm but no-one seems interested in talking to you about your experience—you may feel very isolated.
- You may feel shocked at the culture changes when returning to a more materialist society, including the apathy to LMIC problems.
- Discuss any anxieties with those who have been on similar placements. You will find it is very common; it will go in time.

Insurance and registration

Personal travel insurance

- Ensure that your cover includes repatriation costs should you need to be returned to your home country for continuing treatment.
- Fully disclose your working conditions with your insurance company and get this confirmed in writing.
- If working for an organization ask for advice on insurance. They may have a recommended provider.

Registration

- It is essential you are registered with the medical regulatory body of the country you are visiting.
- Failure to register may, in the worst-case scenario, lead to imprisonment, if you have been involved with a serious clinical incident.

Teaching anaesthesia

General considerations

- The mantra 'If you visit a LMIC, you must teach' is repeated often, but needs some softening before it is considered a hard-and-fast rule.
- Can you qualify to be a teacher where the diseases, drugs, equipment, presentations, and protocols are completely different to your normal working life?
- Initial exposure to working in a LMIC is a steep learning curve, but despite this, the request is often to teach.
- The learners may be new to anaesthesia (pre-service) or in need of continuing professional development (CPD is especially important for educationally isolated rural workers).
- How can this be done best when we are in an unfamiliar environment ourselves, feeling like a novice?
- Like all the other aspects of resource-poor working, it will require preparation, flexibility, realistic goals, and a good dose of humility.

Preparation

- Do a 'train the trainer' course before you leave home—become a better teacher.
- Contact someone who is familiar with your destination—how anaesthesia works and how teaching is conducted.
- Prepare material thoroughly, simplifying as you go.
- Find out what the people would like to learn, relying particularly on those with authority and experience, to direct you on subject matter.
- If teaching is to be ad hoc, try to define agreed targets. Recognize that this will evolve over time.
- Learn local terminology, drugs, and anaesthetic techniques.
- Take resources digitally, e.g. USB sticks, but have a plan for failed/no computer/projector scenarios.
- Learning even a few words in the local language builds rapport.
- Create the learning environment carefully, maximizing potential for discussion and interaction and minimizing distractions.

The target audience and skill sharing

- Low-resource setting hospitals have often developed a series of simple anaesthetic recipes. Don't judge what you consider to be an inappropriate or unsafe routine practice on the spot. Take the time to uncover its history. Earn your right to speak about it.
- Teaching from visitors is often welcomed but be careful not to attempt to fix that which is not broken, or blur the simple recipes with irrelevant subtleties.
- In many places anaesthesia providers have a non-medical background and assumptions about level of understanding of anatomy, physiology, or pharmacology cannot be made.
- This context means that starting with the basic sciences may not work. It's often better to begin with skills and 'what to do'.

- Occasionally experienced providers may make seemingly odd requests: 'Teach us about GA for MRI'. Respect the request. Technology and opportunities change quickly.
- Your talk on spinal anaesthesia may be good but the recipients may have done more spinals already than you'll do in your whole career.

Teaching or learning in a second language

- Speak slowly and clearly, pause often, use short simple sentences.
- If there is written material, say the exact words written.
- Learn the local terminology for medical English. Refer to drugs and equipment using the exact words the local providers use.
- Use a dictionary or the most fluent bilingual person to clarify confusing words.
- Take frequent breaks.

What to teach

- Rigid rules and guidelines used in well-equipped anaesthesia services, although evidence-based, may not be directly applicable in resource-poor settings.
- 'Single use', 'refer to higher-care centre', 'invasive monitoring', or 'send to ICU' are privileges not available worldwide.
- Teaching content must reflect local realities. Case-based teaching forces the teacher to stick to local diseases, drugs, and available techniques.

Teaching in theatre

- Ensure your presence is approved by the hospital authorities.
- Choose moments and cases appropriately.
- Students will watch you carefully and, whilst they may not understand all you say, they will see all you do—do not cut corners, skip steps, or contradict what you teach.
- Demonstrate practical skills without commentary initially. A second or simulated situation is better for verbal instruction, discussion, and explanation.
- Be clear about who is ultimately responsible for the anaesthetic, and be ready to immediately hand over the case to a local senior provider if necessary.
- Cameras are distracting and intrusive—beware of cultural and personal sensitivities. Informed consent is required for all photographs.

Setting up a teaching programme

Syllabus creation

- The syllabus must balance the need to focus on the kind of knowledge and skills required for the graduate in their work life and the need to cover areas that are aspirational, anticipating improvements and modernization.
- The first is the most important and syllabus writers must have a very clear idea of the work environment and responsibilities that a graduate will face.

- Syllabus writers should visit peripheral hospitals to understand precisely what is needed in the most difficult environments, before creating the syllabus.
- Syllabuses from similar countries may be adapted for use.

Government approval/recognition

- A programme that has the potential to be used nationally should be established through official government channels, allowing recognition of training.
- This may be a slow process but helps to create a career path, standardizes teaching across a whole system, and will give a better chance of longevity of the educational programme.

Models of learning

- Education models differ throughout the world. Rules that determine how a classroom, textbook, or computer-based presentation should be structured may not apply in other settings, or may even be counter-productive, especially where there is a language barrier.
- The much maligned 'rote-learning' educational model may actually be a local strength, to be exploited and used as a platform for more analytical thinking and teaching.
- Case studies based on common local scenarios are superior to traditional subject-based teaching, and make a good connection between the 'book theory' and the real work.
- Use of manikins, simulation, computer-based e-learning, and videos (locally made or from internet resources) have all been used effectively throughout the world.
- Low-fidelity simulation (simple and low-cost) can bring teaching to life.
- Mentors do not have to be confined to the local trainers. Mentoring by phone and internet has been used successfully.

Practical and theoretical

- The syllabus should balance the practical skills of anaesthesia and the theoretical knowledge that underpins it. The challenge in syllabus development is to have these two elements interact as much as possible, and dismantle the 'theory and practice' division.
- The list of skills included should reflect the environment of the workplace plus realistic aspirations.

Being a good visitor

We have all had visitors. Some of the visitors we have had, we have liked their company, and we would not have minded them staying longer or coming back. But then there are those of our relatives or friends we would rather shorten their visits or not come at all. The same is true for those of us receiving visitors to our hospitals. The question is: what makes one a good visitor and another a bad visitor? What pitfalls may we fall into as visitors?

Saviour mentality

- Here visitors think they already have the solution to a problem and can come in and quickly save the world. In fact, they have no idea of what the real problem is, much less the solution.
- The visitor is going to 'show them how it should be done' … truthfully, you can't. As you will often find out, there are reasons why it's not being done like that. A lot of times it ends up being the local staff showing you how it's done.
- The God complex is exhausting, you burn out and waste resources, and ultimately offend the very people you are trying to help.

The know it all!

- Sometimes visitors think they know it all. Some may be justified in their thinking, but I am yet to meet them.
- You will learn more and also share your ideas better if you acknowledge that the people you are visiting may know a few tricks.
- The know-it-all attitude does not cultivate relationships that are needed to effect change.
- It is really important to ask the people you are visiting what the norm is for them and the reasons behind the norms.
- It is good to learn from those who have gone before us; however, it is also worth having an open mind. If you base all your actions on previous reports, you are likely to miss out on new opportunities.

Spreading yourself thin

- Here visitors become very ambitious—they think they can sort out all the problems, or indeed teach everyone.
- Learn to realize you are but one person and can't do all the things that need doing; hence the importance of partnership with local residents.
- Be selective about what you want to achieve. You only have one set of hands: find one or two things to do and do them well.
- Make it clear to the people you are visiting what your visit intends to achieve. If you are good at what you do, you will be needed and called from all directions, leading to burn-out and mistakes.
- You must, however, be flexible: expect anything! Don't be rigid to the point of being useless to those you are visiting because of earlier set goals.

One size fits all

- The developing world is not one country! The problems are as diverse as the climate and terrain.
- Each place will demand a different approach with different norms.
- There are certainly some similarities but never assume that what worked for one place will work for another.

Give them money/equipment

- You may feel overwhelmed: the natural inclination is to give money without understanding the extent of the problem.
- This is not sustainable, we lose our independence and become dependent on handouts.
- Your effort may countermand the efforts of the local authority in the development of their people.

Reinventing the wheel

- Sometimes as visitors, we may have a plan or intervention we thought of implementing before getting to know what is in existence.
- This has led to reinventing the wheel, which can be frustrating for those visiting and those being visited.
- Thus, one has to know what exists locally and what knowledge gaps or deficiencies are there for effective change to take place.

My way is the best!

- There is an African saying that 'One who does not travel will always say, their mum is the best cook.' Sometimes we may be set in our ways and think our way is the best!
- Unfortunately, that's not usually the case, as we all know there are definitely several ways of skinning a cat!
- Your way or opinion may not be the best for the environment you are in, thus instead of helping, one actually destroys.

When in Rome do what they do!

- As a visitor, we may alienate ourselves from those we are visiting, because we are different and our culture is different.
- However, when in Rome, do what the Romans do! This applies to developing world countries as well. Get in the dirt with us and learn from us too! This creates or helps build team spirit, which is needed for any change to be effected.

The developing world has many different terrains, climates and cultures. When you visit you may be overwhelmed. It's important to remember that the approaches required are as different as the colours of the rainbow. The developing world is rich in its people. You will find warmhearted and happy people despite the problems with which they may co-exist.

Further reading

Anaesthesia in the global context

Debas HT et al. (2015) *Essential Surgery. Disease Control Priorities*, 3rd ed., vol. 1, Washington, DC: World Bank.

Meara JG et al. (2015) Global surgery 2030: evidence and solutions for achieving health, welfare and economic development. *Lancet* 386 (9993): 569–624.

Kempthorne P et al. (2017) The WFSA Global Anesthesia Workforce Survey. *Anesth Analg* 125 (3): 981–990. https://www.wfsahq.org/workforce-map

Humanitarian and development principles

WHO (2008) Glossary of humanitarian terms. http://www.who.int/hac/about/reliefweb-aug2008.pdf

Barnett M (2011) *Empire of Humanity: A History of Humanitarianism.* Ithaca, NY: Cornell University Press. ISBN-10 0-8014-7879-0

Ooms G (2006) Health development versus medical relief: the illusion versus the irrelevance of sustainability. *PLoS Med* 3 (8): e345.

Editorial (2011) Natural disasters—taking a longer term view. *Lancet* 377 (9764): 439.

Adapting your practice

THET principles of partnership: http://www.thet.org.uk

Preparation and self-care

http://www.fitfortravel.scot.nhs.uk/destinations.aspx
http://www.aagbi.org/international
http://www.rcoa.ac.uk/global-partnerships
http://www.aagbi.org/international/thet
http://www.rcoa.ac.uk/e-la/anaesthesia-humanitarian-austere-environments

Teaching anaesthesia

Dobson S, Dobson M, Bromiley L (2011) *How to Teach: A Handbook for Clinicians*. Oxford: Oxford University Press.

Bullock I et al. (2015) *Pocket Guide to Teaching For Clinical Instructors*, 3rd ed. Oxford: Wiley-Blackwell.

Chapter 2

Organizing Your Environment

Christine Bartulec, Rachel Freedman, Amy Hughes, Sanja Janjanin, Bruce McCormick, Wayne Morriss, and Andrea Reis

Minimum standards for equipment and monitoring

International standards

- Minimum standards for equipment and monitoring are described in the World Health Organization-World Federation of Societies of Anaesthesiologists International Standards for a Safe Practice of Anaesthesia 2018 (see 'Further Reading' in this chapter). This section is based on these standards.
- The standards are relevant to any healthcare facility anywhere in the world in which general anaesthesia (GA), sedation, and/or regional anaesthesia (spinal, epidural, major limb blocks) are performed.
- The minimum standards are appropriate for a range of simple surgical procedures and management of most anaesthetic emergencies.
- Higher standards are required for more advanced facilities where complex surgery is performed.

General considerations

- In low- and middle-income countries (LMICs), equipment for the provision and monitoring of anaesthesia may be unavailable or scarce.
- In some settings, minimum standards may not be met. In these settings, only emergency, life- or limb-saving anaesthesia and surgery should be performed, and urgent efforts should be made to correct the equipment and monitoring deficiencies.
- When resources are scarce, it is vital to consider the cost versus benefit of using consumables, e.g. electrocardiogram (ECG) electrodes, or single-use equipment. In many facilities, repeated use of single-use equipment (e.g. endotracheal tubes) is common.

Minimum standards for non-monitoring equipment

- All anaesthetizing locations should be equipped with the following:
  - an oxygen supply (oxygen concentrator, cylinders, or pipeline)
  - facemasks and oropharyngeal airways (adult and paediatric)
  - laryngoscope with a range of blades
  - endotracheal tubes (adult and paediatric)
  - intubation aids (e.g. bougie or stylet)
  - suction device and suction catheters
  - self-inflating bags (adult and paediatric)
  - equipment for intravenous infusions and injection of medications
  - equipment for spinal anaesthesia and/or regional blocks
  - sterile gloves.
- All locations should have access to a defibrillator.
- If inhalational anaesthesia is performed, a safe delivery system (draw-over or plenum) is required. A plenum system should be equipped with safety features to prevent misconnection or the delivery of a hypoxic mixture.
- If resources allow, additional available equipment should include:
  - laryngeal mask airways
  - automated ventilator
  - pressure infusor device

- blood warmer
- patient warming device.

Minimum standards for monitoring

- The most important monitor is a trained and vigilant anaesthesia provider who is continuously present during the anaesthetic.
- There is no substitute for clinical observation of:
  - pulse rate and quality
  - peripheral perfusion
  - respiratory rate and pattern (chest, breathing system bag)
  - breath sounds
  - heart sounds.
- The following monitoring equipment should be used during every anaesthetic:
  - pulse oximeter
  - intermittent non-invasive blood pressure monitor.
- Many anaesthetists working in low-resource settings advocate the continuous use of a mono-aural praecordial (taped to chest) or oesophageal stethoscope, especially when anaesthetizing children. The stethoscope allows monitoring of heart rate and rhythm and ventilation as well and gives an indication of cardiac output.
- Carbon dioxide monitoring is currently problematic because of the lack of appropriately robust and suitably priced devices.
  - Carbon dioxide detection (e.g. colorimetry or non-waveform capnography if waveform capnography is not available) should be used to confirm correct placement of an endotracheal tube.
  - If resources allow, continuous capnography should be available and used in all patients undergoing a general anaesthetic.
- Urine output monitoring should be used in appropriate cases.
- If resources allow, additional available monitoring equipment should include:
  - inspired oxygen concentration monitor
  - ECG
  - temperature monitor.

Paediatric equipment and monitoring

- See 'Equipment for Paediatric Anaesthesia', Chapter 7 (pp. 117–18).

Triage

Establishing priorities for treatment amongst many casualties is difficult and presents ethical and medical dilemmas. The importance of triage is even greater when resources are limited.

Example triage system

Category 1/Red

- Requires immediate surgery or other life-saving intervention and has a good chance of recovery. Should be first priority.

Examples

- Airway burns or injuries causing airway obstruction.
- Tension pneumothorax.
- Compressible major haemorrhage.
- Traumatic amputation.

Category 2/Yellow

- Patients require an intervention but not immediately.

Examples

- Head injury without airway compromise.
- Penetrating wounds without major haemorrhage.
- Compound fractures.
- Major soft tissue wounds.

Category 3/Green

- Patients do not require immediate intervention—'walking wounded'.

Examples

- Minor and superficial wounds.
- Minor, closed fractures with no neurovascular compromise.

Category 4/Black

- Patients with likely unsurvivable injuries or likely to have very poor quality of survival (within context).

Examples

- Penetrating head injuries with low Glasgow coma score (GCS), e.g. <8.
- Quadriplegia.
- Burns >50% body surface area.
- Major blood loss with no blood available.

Setting up a triage area

Consideration should be given to the following.

The space around and inside the triage facility

- Topography, water and power supply, shelter from the elements.
- Best access and egress routes, patient drop-off points.
- 'Pop-up' space outside facility to treat excess casualties, e.g. tents.
- Security and crowd control—how will this be achieved?
- Culture—are separate male and female treatment areas required?

Equipment

- Mobile trolleys/boxes with basic emergency equipment, e.g. gloves, dressings, splints, bandages, tourniquets, tetanus prophylaxis, analgesia, intravenous (IV) access, fluids, blankets.
- Materials to be used as lightweight stretchers for patient transport.

Communication and flow

- Erect a board (local language) informing people about the situation.
- A small battery-powered loud speaker may be useful.
- Clearly marked routes for internal and external flow of patients.
- A single point of entry to the health facility can help control flow.
- Have a system in place for resupply of materials and staff.
- Documentation for triage, patient labelling methods, record keeping.
- Think about communication between different areas (theatres, triage area, ward). Two-way radios can be useful.

Organization of the triage area

- Know who your team will be and when possible, train your team in triage. Local healthcare workers may not have triage experience or may have more experience than you, depending on the area.
- Consider running a mass casualty simulation to test your systems.
- Allocate team roles and, if necessary, create diagrammatic and written action cards for your team.
- Aim to designate Red (Category 1), Yellow (Category 2), Green (Category 3), and Black (Category 4) areas for triaged patients. These can be created using string and tape.
- Allocate individuals to care for patients in these specific areas.
- Provide a central patient reception area (desk and shelter) where every patient treated is documented and tagged. Location is important as many patients may be treated outside and not enter the health facility. A mobile reception system could be considered.
- Know your equipment and personnel limitations. Pre-plan as much as possible and understand your equipment resupply options.
- Keep patients and family members informed as much as possible.
- Consider the consequences of a mass casualty event occurring within the health facility itself.

Practical points

- Initial triage should be done by an experienced clinician familiar with triage, or by two experienced clinicians working together, which can help share the burden of difficult decision making.
- Permanent markers are a simple way to designate triage categories.
- Clinical conditions can change—patients should be routinely reassessed and triage categories changed if necessary.
- Category 4 patients present an ethical dilemma. Whilst you may not want to use precious resources for them such as oxygen, they must, nonetheless, be treated with dignity.

Emergency room

- Across different global health contexts, human and material resource availability within emergency rooms (ERs) varies considerably.
- Many healthcare facilities may not have a designated ER, nor any individuals trained to deliver emergency medical care.
- Power, lighting, water, sanitation, and fuel may not be available.
- Equipment and pharmacy should be adaptable to this context and consideration given to improvisation, providing it can be performed safely, ethically, and is clinically indicated.
- If you are the clinician responsible for the emergency care of patients, your remit may include:
  - designation of a space to be used as the ER
  - identifying the minimum equipment and pharmaceutical resources required to deliver basic emergency care
  - establishing an inventory of ER equipment and pharmaceuticals
  - establishing a standardized ER layout and equipment plan (see Figure 2.1)
  - local healthcare worker training.

Examples of improvisation

- Pelvic/limb splints can be made using sheets and/or wooden poles.
- Bed traction for femur fracture using hanging sock/small sandbag filled with sand/pebbles to approx. 10% of patient's weight. Fluid bags can also be used. Wide sticky tape can be used to attach to leg.
- Cotton wool soaked in saline can be used as ECG 'dots', alternatively gel can be applied to old (dried) ECG stickers or crocodile clips can be attached to coins taped onto the chest.
- Fabric hanging from ceiling for patient privacy screens.
- String attached to ceiling for hanging fluids.
- Empty clean plastic bottle adapted as a 'spacer' for salbutamol.

Equipment to consider if resources and experience permit

- Ultrasound machine and probe.
- Battery-powered combined patient monitor +/− defibrillator.
- Nebulizer and mask.
- Doppler probe.
- ECG recording machine.

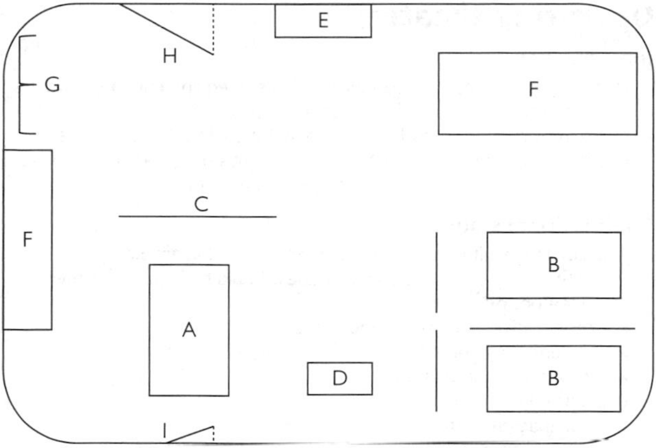

Fig. 2.1 Example of a basic emergency room set-up. (A) Trolley allocated for resuscitation patient. If possible use a trolley with an optional 45° back rest. (B) Trolley for patients needing emergency care. (C) Patient screens. (D) Emergency cart or table. This cart should contain all the kit required for the immediate treatment of acutely unwell patients. A summarized list of suggested equipment is as follows: airway equipment, including foot pump-driven suction. This can be as advanced (laryngoscope, tracheal tubes, bougies, etc.) or as basic (oropharyngeal airway and self-inflating bag) as resources and expertise allow. Oxygen source: concentrator, cylinder or both and oxygen masks. Intravenous (IV) and intra-osseous access equipment and sharps bin. IV fluid and giving sets, syringes and needles. Emergency drugs. Splinting devices for pelvic and limb trauma. Tourniquets, bandages, pressure dressings, and occlusive dressings for chest wounds. Chest drain, equipment to site drain and collection bags. Sutures and suture set. Nasogastric tube, urinary catheter. Monitoring equipment, including manual blood pressure monitor and battery powered oxygen saturation (SpO_2) probe. Blood sugar monitor, finger-prick haemoglobin tester, and thermometer, if available. Head-torch and spare batteries. Gloves, visor, stethoscope, and trauma shears or scissors. (E) Healthcare worker desk. Blackboard or similar. Patient injuries and treatment documentation sheets. (F) Storage area—dark and cool for pharmacy items: Pharmacy stock which does not require cold chain. Stock equipment in expiry date order. Towels, bedpans, toilet rolls, bowls, cleaning products. Sheets/blankets, patient gowns, patient ID bands. Additional items not on emergency cart, e.g. sanitary towels, tongue depressors, otoscope and ophthalmoscope, weighing scales, vaginal speculum, urine dipsticks, pregnancy test, plaster (fractures) and bandages, dental set, crutches. (G) Seating for patients waiting to be seen. (H) Doorway to emergency room. This may be a single door to the outside or to another part of the health centre. Often doors are single breadth. This can cause problems if a patient arrives on a stretcher. (I) Window. If there is no power or fuel available the generator may not work and lighting will not be available. Having head torches, batteries, and natural light from the window is very beneficial.

Operating theatre

Introduction

- In low-resource settings, certain standards of equipment and drugs are required for the safe conduct of anaesthesia.
- More importantly, anaesthesia personnel should be present in the room throughout anaesthesia and the patient's oxygenation, ventilation, circulation and temperature continually monitored.

International standards

- In accordance with the Helsinki Declaration on Patient Safety in Anaesthesiology, protocols and facilities should be in place for the management of:
  - preoperative assessment and preparation
  - checking equipment and drugs and syringe labelling
  - difficult/failed intubation
  - anaphylaxis
  - local anaesthetic toxicity
  - massive haemorrhage
  - infection control
  - postoperative care and pain relief
  - malignant hyperpyrexia (even in the absence of dantrolene).
- The international standards applicable depend on the size of the hospital and the range of surgery carried out.
- Below is outlined the minimum standards for general surgery in an environment with limited resources, i.e. the most basic facility. Even this however will be highly aspirational for many.

Operating theatre equipment

The anaesthesia cart

- Beware of reorganizing the cart to suit your personal preference. If it has already been set up by a local provider, ask and discuss first.
- The anaesthesia cart serves as storage for consumable equipment and drugs for anaesthesia and resuscitation in the theatre. Everything must be easily accessible in an emergency.
- You may choose to have a separate 'emergency/resuscitation cart' or to have an 'emergency/resuscitation section' on your main cart.
- One drawer can be used for IV fluids and giving sets, or an additional box can serve this purpose.
- Depending on case load you may choose to have a separate paediatric cart, including a box for newborn resuscitation.
- It is sensible to organize all carts the same way to ensure quick and easy access to kit in case of an emergency.
- The cart(s) should be simple, easy to clean, and mobile as it will be in daily use. Do not clutter with unnecessary kit.

Checklists for suggested essential drugs and equipment for the anaesthesia cart can be found in the Appendix.

Other equipment in the operating theatre

Operating theatre furniture

- General equipment includes IV stands, tables for monitor/s and table for sterile preparation (spinal/regional anaesthesia), and voltage stabilizers to protect equipment from unstable electricity supply.
- Operating table (preferably tilting), plastic board (pat-slide) or plastic sheeting for transferring patients.
- Torches and spare batteries for emergency lighting.
- Foam/wooden 'wedge' to position patients head up and/or tilt pelvis.

Anaesthesia, resuscitation, and monitoring

- See 'Minimum Standards for Equipment and Monitoring', in this chapter (pp. 22–3). Additional equipment under ideal circumstances includes:
  - peripheral nerve stimulator
  - ultrasound machine (regional anaesthesia, IV access)
  - all in one monitor: automated blood pressure (BP), ECG, end tidal carbon dioxide, and anaesthetic gas monitoring.

Patient warming

- Warm drapes/blankets (or foil blankets) to cover patients.
- Warmed fluids for irrigation (all open surgical cavities).
- Adjustable room temperature (air-con off to keep patients warm).
- Warmed IV fluids.
- External heat packs, e.g. warm bags of saline warmed in buckets of warm water or a microwave can be wrapped in drapes and placed around the neck, axillae, and groin. Be careful not to place hot fluid bags in direct contact with skin—risk of burns.

Neonatal resuscitation (may be kept in dedicated box/cart)

- Insulating blanket.
- Manual suction pump.
- Suction tubes, different sizes.
- Self-inflating bag + mask (sizes 0 and 1)
- Oxygen tubing.
- Feeding tubes (for umbilical IV access and nasogastric (NG) tube).
- Vicryl suture.
- Laryngoscope handle + blade: Miller 0/Macintosh 0.
- Endotracheal tubes, different sizes.
- Oro-pharyngeal airways, different sizes.
- IV cannulae (butterfly).
- Syringes, needles.
- Adrenaline, glucose 50%.
- Adhesive tape.
- Sterile gloves, sterile gauze.

Recovery area

- The immediate postoperative recovery period is of paramount importance in the safe conduct of anaesthesia.
- In many parts of the world, the recovery area is no more than a corridor near the operating theatre and staff are untrained.
- The challenge is to use what you have available to you in terms of human and material resources to create the safest possible recovery area under the circumstances.
- Anaesthetic techniques may need to be modified to accommodate poor recovery area staffing or equipment. For example, regional techniques to facilitate awake surgery may be safer than GA.

Admission criteria

- GA including ketamine anaesthesia.
- Spinal anaesthesia.
- Moderate to deep sedation.
- Note: patients with regional limb block with light or no sedation and minor surgery may be able go straight back to the ward, bypassing recovery, as long as they do not need observation from a surgical point of view, i.e. for post-op bleeding.

Layout

- The recovery area should be centrally located inside the theatre complex with easy access from the operating theatre and separate access for transfer of patients to the ward.
- A communication system with the operating theatre and wards is helpful, e.g. two-way radios/internal telephone, and an emergency alert system (may be simple, e.g. shouting, air horn).
- Doorways minimum 1.2 m wide.
- Minimum two recovery beds (for one to two operating theatre tables).
- If more than two operating tables are in use, increase recovery beds by one for each additional operating table.
- Adjustable beds/trolleys, positioned to allow access to patient's head from behind the bed/trolley.
- Separations (screens) between beds for patient privacy.

Human resources

- An anaesthetist always has overall responsibility, even if not present.
- Recovery room minimum staff:patient ratio of 1:3.
- It is rare in low-resource settings to have a trained, dedicated anaesthetic recovery nurse. It is more likely that there will be healthcare workers who can be trained in anaesthetic recovery.
- As a result, protocols for routine post-anaesthetic observations and thresholds for calling for help should be simple and clear.
- It is also sensible, if recovery staff have only basic training, to ensure that all patients have a secure, patent airway and pain is well controlled before transferring from the operating theatre.

- Staff with only basic training may not be able to administer strong analgesics and/or maintain an airway in an emergency.
- If there is no-one competent to staff the recovery room you will need to recover your own patients (can slow down a list).

Equipment

- A trolley or box with equipment for emergency airway management should be present, e.g. bag valve mask, oropharyngeal airways.
- The emergency equipment from the operating theatre should be mobile and immediately available to the recovery area.
- Glucose meter, haemoglobin meter, thermometer as available.

Drugs

- Recovery staff may not have the training to independently assess patients and give IV medication. Aim for recognition of problems in the first instance—you can attend and treat from theatre as able.
- Useful drugs to have available in recovery room include:
  - antiemetics, e.g. ondansetron, cyclizine
  - midazolam/diazepam for treating ketamine hallucinations
  - morphine and tramadol
  - flumazenil, naloxone, and neostigmine/atropine.

Observation in recovery

- A time-based sheet to record patient observations should be in place.
- Vital signs, level of consciousness, and pain scores should be clearly recorded and acted upon if necessary.
- Output from any drains, catheters, and wound sites should be recorded and fluid balance recorded as necessary.

Discharge criteria

- Discharge criteria should be explicit and agreed with the anaesthetist beforehand but should ideally be nurse-led.
- No mandatory minimum length of stay.
- Ensure the patient has a responsible caretaker to accompany them.
- Nurse-led discharge criteria could include:
  - awake, able to communicate normally
  - vital signs stable (set limits for oxygen saturation (SpO_2), respiration rate (RR), BP, heart rate (HR))
  - urine output adequate
  - normal temperature
  - surgical drain checked
  - wound unremarkable
  - pain adequately controlled
  - no nausea and vomiting
  - IV cannula working and flushed
  - records completed including proposed further treatment.

Critical care

Introduction

- **High dependency units** (HDUs) are for patients who require closer observation than those on a normal ward. They may have one failing organ system. Complex interventions such as non-invasive ventilation or invasive monitoring may occasionally be provided.
- **Intensive care units** (ICUs) are for patients who require mechanical ventilation or have two or more failing organ systems.
- In many low-resource settings the above definitions are completely meaningless. The HDU/ICU is best described as any area that can provide a higher level of care than the regular ward.
- Often the HDU/ICU is only differentiated from the normal ward by a slightly better nursing ratio and/or possible access to oxygen.
- In this section the term HDU refers to any form of higher care area.

Location

- HDU may be a separate ward or one or more specific beds in a general ward. There may be several HDUs, e.g. adult and paediatric.
- It is generally more efficient to have all unwell patients in one place.
- There should be easy access to HDU in an emergency: if possible HDU should be close to the emergency department and theatres.

Set-up

- Large enough to allow free movement of staff around each bed, with space to carry out procedures and screens or curtains for privacy.
- Well lit (windows), with bedside lights, and torches for power cuts.
- Oxygen should be available: piped, concentrator, or cylinders.
- Side rooms are helpful for barrier nursing immunosuppressed or infectious patients, or for privacy, but more nurses may be required in order to observe patients adequately.
- Aim for a separate equipment storage area and sluice. A dedicated treatment room may also be helpful for more mobile patients.

Water, sanitation and hygiene

- Ensure a safe water supply including drinking water, using a water filter system if necessary.
- Sinks or plastic bowels and soap should be easily accessible for handwashing. Everyone (staff and visitors) should wash their hands on entering the unit, before and after every patient contact.
- White coats should be removed (source of cross-infection). Aprons and gloves should be worn for contact with patients if available.
- Hand towels should be disposable or laundered regularly.
- Facilities for aseptic technique should be present if possible including surgical scrub, sterile gloves and gowns, hats, and masks.
- Leak-proof, puncture-resistant sharps containers should be available.

Equipment

Suggested equipment for an HDU is detailed below. It may be aspirational for many low-resource settings. Strive to source and retain equipment that is robust, simple to use, easy to maintain, and has a ready supply of spare parts/consumables. Ensure back-up options are available, e.g. oxygen cylinders, torches, and battery-powered pulse oximeters for use during power cuts.

Suggested HDU equipment

- Resuscitation trolley equipment:
  - oxygen cylinder
  - IV cannulae and fluids
  - resuscitation drugs
  - bag valve mask and basic airway equipment
  - supraglottic airways
  - intubation equipment
  - torch, tape, scissors, gloves, sharps box.
- General equipment:
  - defibrillator
  - monitors
  - infusion pumps
  - fluid warmer
  - procedure trolleys.
- Equipment by each bed:
  - oxygen concentrator or cylinder, tubing and masks
  - bag valve mask and oropharyngeal airways
  - suction equipment (single-use)
  - gloves, aprons, and hand disinfectant
  - patient observation charts
  - table and seat for nurse
  - drip stand.
- Beds:
  - Should be mobile, able to tilt head up/down, and have removable sides. Pressure-relieving mattresses are ideal if available.
- Monitoring:
  - The most important monitor is a trained and attentive nurse.
  - A pulse oximeter, sphygmomanometer, and stethoscope should always be available.
  - Thermometers, urimeters, glucometer, and capnography should also be available if possible.
  - ECG monitoring and automatic blood pressure (with correct sized cuffs) are helpful.
  - Portable monitors, which can also be used for transfers, are ideal.

Drugs

- Depending on training and equipment there may be the capacity to administer drugs that cannot be given on a general ward, including:
  - inotrope infusions: see 'Cardiovascular Support' in Chapter 12 (pp. 271–2)
  - intravenous opioid boluses
  - oxytocin infusions postpartum
  - intravenous magnesium (pre-eclampsia)
  - sedatives, e.g. diazepam for seizure control post head injury.

Staffing

- Attention to staff training and nurse–patient ratios is key to delivering high-quality critical care.
- There should be clear leadership in the HDU and staff should be supported to look after critically ill patients with education and an appropriate level of supervision from clinicians.
- Ideally, there should be one trained nurse for every two patients, plus a nurse in charge and nursing assistants. This is rarely achievable, but with supervision and simple guidelines even non-clinical hospital workers can be trained to work in HDU.
- HDU doctors should review patients twice daily at a minimum.
- Responsible surgeons or physicians should work closely and communicate with HDU staff.
- Input from physiotherapists, microbiologists, pharmacists, and dieticians should be encouraged if available.

Observations

- Increased frequency of observations, and appropriately acting on them, is central to HDU care.
- Ideally, HDU patients should have continuous monitoring with observations recorded every 2 h.
- Establish context-appropriate guidelines according to the available monitoring and staffing levels.
- Set clear parameters for when a clinician should be called.
- Pulse, blood pressure, respiratory rate, oxygen saturation, conscious level, urine output, and pain score should be recorded.
- Consider using or adapting a context-appropriate medical early warning score (MEWS) to help detect deteriorating patients.

Ventilation

- It is rare that an HDU will have the equipment and staffing to allow safe prolonged ventilation of patients.
- Even if a ventilator is available it may be safer to extubate a patient postoperatively rather than rely on poorly trained/distracted staff.
- For more on the pros and cons of ventilating patients postoperatively in low-resource settings see 'Respiratory Support' in Chapter 12 (pp. 268–70).
- There are a number of ways of providing continuous positive airway pressure (CPAP) to patients postoperatively on HDU. See 'Respiratory Support' in Chapter 12 (pp. 268–70).

The surgical safety checklist

- Surgical care is a vital and cost-effective intervention but comes with associated morbidity and mortality. Estimates suggests that at least half of all surgical complications are avoidable.
- In 2008, the World Health Organization's (WHO) Safe Surgery Saves Lives Study Group published a checklist aiming to reduce the rate of major surgical complications.
- The checklist aims to reduce the rate of major surgical complications. The checklist can be modified to suit any location and is used successfully in LMICs.
- An example checklist for adaptation can be seen in the Appendix.

Concept

- The WHO Surgical Safety Checklist is a three-part process, used to standardize delivery of care in the operating theatre. It advocates essential safety checks intended to improve communication between operating theatre team members.
- Additionally, it can be helpful to have a team brief and debrief at the start and finish of every operating list.
- The checklist comprises three parts:

Sign in

- Before induction of anaesthesia.

Time out

- Before skin incision.

Sign out

- Before the patient leaves the operating room.

Implementation in LMICs

- The checklist was designed to be modified for the local environment. Context-specific alterations should be made.
- It can be delivered as a paper checklist to be placed in the patient's notes, or using a blackboard/whiteboard or poster on the wall.
- A single 'checklist coordinator' should lead the checklist process. This may be hard to achieve in understaffed operating theatres.
- Use of the checklist requires support from government, hospital management, and local staff for it to fully embed into the ethos of an operating theatre department. This is difficult.
- Listen to local comments or objections, they may be well founded: try to engage local team members in designing their own solutions.

Possible barriers to the use of a surgical safety checklist

Team brief

- Insufficient/changing staff members present at brief.
- Emergency work often makes up the majority of theatre caseload, so the plan for the day may be rapidly changeable.

Sign in

- Language barriers between staff and patients hinder communication.
- Lack of identity wristbands (can use sticky tape and a marker pen).
- Full names, dates of birth, and hospital numbers may not be available, or even known to the patient (dates of birth especially).
- Written consent forms may not be used, and/or communication difficulty may hinder informed consent in emergency settings.

Time out

- Established hierarchies and/or urgency of surgery may make it difficult to complete checks prior to surgery starting.

Sign out

- Non-standardized instrument sets make counts laborious.

Team debrief

- Reflective practice may not be embedded into the culture of the department. This can take decades to change.
- Without available solutions to problems the process may feel futile.

General

- Lack of 'buy in' from senior team members will make implementation difficult in cultures with steep hierarchical structures.

Further reading

Minimum standards for equipment and monitoring

Gelb AW, Morriss WW, Johnson W, et al. (2018) World Health Organization—World Federation of Societies of Anaesthesiologists (WHO-WFSA) international standards for a safe practice of anesthesia. *Anesth Analg* 126: 2047–2055.

Triage

International Committee of the Red Cross (2010) *War Surgery Part 1*: http://www.icrc.org/eng/assets/files/other/icrc-002-0973.pdf

Emergency room

WHO emergency care resources: http://www.who.int/emergencycare/en

Operating theatre

ICRC Geneva (2017) *Anaesthesia Handbook*. Geneva: ICRC.

Mellin-Olsen J et al. (2010) The Helsinki declaration on patient safety in anaesthesiology. *Eur J Anaesthesiol* 27 (7): 592–597.

Recovery area

Australian and New Zealand College of Anaesthetists (2006) *Recommendations for the Post Anaesthesia Recovery Room*, Review PS4: http://fpm.anzca.edu.au/documents/ps4.pdf

Whitaker DK et al. (2013) Immediate post anaesthesia recovery: AAGBI guideline. *Anaesthesia* 68: 288–297.

Critical care

Faculty of Intensive Care Medicine: Guidelines for the provision of intensive care services (2016): https://www.ficm.ac.uk/sites/default/files/gpics_ed.1.1_2016_ _final.pdf

The surgical safety checklist

Gawande AA et al. (1999) The incidence and nature of surgical adverse events in Colorado and Utah in 1992. *Surgery* 126: 66–75.

World Alliance for Patient Safety (2008) *WHO Guidelines for Safe Surgery*. Geneva: World Health Organization.

Further reading

Minimum standards for equipment and monitoring

[illegible]

Trauma

[illegible]

Emergency room

[illegible]

Operating theatre

[illegible]

Recovery area

[illegible]

Critical care

[illegible]

[illegible] checked

[illegible]

Chapter 3

Anaesthesia Equipment and Utilities

Michael Dobson, Robert Neighbour, and Matt Wilkes

Draw-over anaesthesia

Draw-over techniques deliver inhalational anaesthesia using room air as the carrier gas and provide the following advantages, which are particularly pertinent in low-resource settings:

- Draw-over systems never deliver a hypoxic gas mixture.
- No need for compressed gases.
- No need for electricity.
- Supplementary oxygen used ultra-economically—1 l/min yields fractional inspired oxygen concentration (FiO_2) >30%.
- No need for oxygen or agent monitoring.
- Can be maintained and serviced locally.
- Economical (capital and running costs < compressed gas machines).

Components of a draw-over system

See Figure 3.1 for a diagrammatic representation of the key components and basic function of a draw-over system.

Notes

- All components must have a low resistance to breathing.
- The same draw-over system can be used for either spontaneous ventilation (SV) or intermittent positive pressure ventilation (IPPV) without any alterations. During SV the patient can breathe 'through' the bag/bellows. To convert to IPPV simply start squeezing the bag/bellows.
- Bags/bellows commonly used for draw-over incorporate a unidirectional valve to prevent reverse flow into the vaporizer during IPPV.
- A suitable ventilator can be used in place of the bag/bellows but is for convenience rather than a requirement.

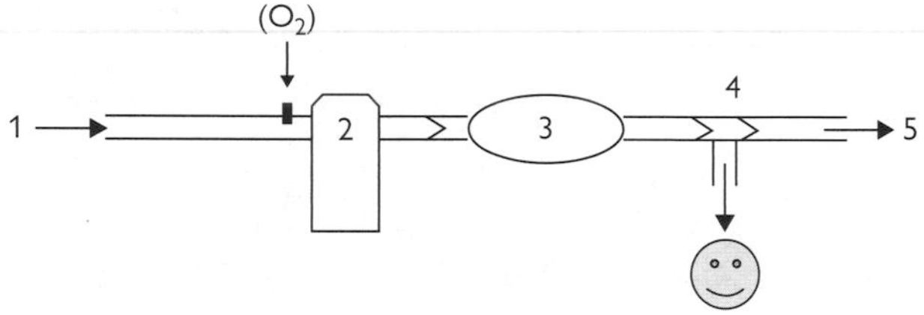

Figure 3.1 Components of a basic draw-over system. Gas moves through the system from left to right. It is drawn through either during inspiration, or by the recoil of the self-inflating bag or bellows (3). Air enters through an open-ended tube or port (1). Note that inspired oxygen concentration cannot fall below atmospheric (less 1–2% to account for the addition of the volatile agent). Supplementary oxygen may be added to the system from an oxygen concentrator or cylinder upstream of the vaporizer. As gas is drawn though the vaporizer (2) volatile anaesthetic is added to the gas mixture. A unidirectional valve (4) must be incorporated to ensure that gas only flows one way through the system. See the Appendix for pictures of suitable valves. When the patient exhales, gas is vented from the system (5).

- The system may be portable/self-assembly (the Triservice anaesthetic apparatus, Diamedica portable anaesthesia system—DPA) or incorporated into a full-capability unitary machine with built-in oxygen concentrator and possibly ventilator (Glostavent, Glostavent Helix, and Universal Anaesthesia Machine (UAM)).
- Used with any agent other than ether (ether increases ventilation), oxygen supplementation to >25% and/or controlled ventilation will be required.

Oxygen enrichment

- An open-ended reservoir stores the oxygen delivered during expiration (when there is no forward flow in the system). It must be upstream of the vaporizer.
- This can simply be a length of open-ended tubing with standard oxygen tubing inserted into the end and taped in place to stop it falling out.
- For convenience, most systems have a small 't-piece' nipple attachment for oxygen on the upstream reservoir tubing, close to the vaporizer, as indicated in Figure 3.1.
- Alternatively, a bag-type oxygen reservoir system is supplied with Diamedica and UAM systems. The bags will move during breathing and allow free entrainment of air, if required, during inspiration. They cannot be used to ventilate the lungs.

Table 3.1 shows the achievable delivered oxygen concentrations at a minute volume of 5 l/min. Some sort of open oxygen reservoir, e.g. tubing/bag, is required for this. Higher concentrations (up to 80%) are achievable with higher flow rates. Higher minute ventilation lowers the FiO_2 whereas lower increases it.

Draw-over vaporizers

- Have a low resistance to flow.
- Characteristics of common vaporizers are summarized in Table 3.2.
- Typically, vaporizers are fitted with 22 mm connectors, as they form part of the breathing system.
- Mostly do not have keyed fillers. This can be useful (see isoflurane/halothane on (pp. 61–63) but is also a potential hazard.
- Isoflurane and halothane have similar vapour pressures, so the scale on the vaporizer is accurate for either agent, but note that they are not equipotent! You must know what is in your vaporizer and its contents must be correctly labelled.

Table 3.1 Achievable oxygen concentration in draw-over systems.

Supplementary oxygen flow	Fractional inspired oxygen concentration (FiO_2) (if miniature vaporizer = 5 l/min) (%)
500 ml/min	28
1 l/min	37
2 l/min	52

Table 3.2 Commonly found draw-over vaporizers.

Vaporizer*	Agent†	Agent volume (ml)	Thermal buffering	Thermo-compensation
OMV	Hal./Iso.	20–50	Y	Y
EMO	Ether only	800	Y	Y
DDV	Hal./Iso./Sevo.‡	150	Y	Y
UAM/OES	Hal./Iso.	200	Y	N
PAC	Hal./Iso.	150	Y	Y

*OMV, Oxford miniature vaporizer; EMO, Epstein Macintosh Oxford vaporizer; DDV, Diamedica drawover vaporizer; UAM/OES, Universal Anaesthetic Machine vaporizer manufactured by OAS Medical; PAC, Portable Anaesthesia Complete vaporizer.

†Hal., halothane; Iso., isoflurane; Sevo., sevoflurane.

‡The DDV sevoflurane vaporizer is a different version to the standard halothane/isoflurane DDV.

When using sevoflurane in the OMV, maximal output is just over 3% and not sufficient for an inhalational induction. To circumvent this problem, two OMVs with Sevoflurane can be used in series, the outputs are additional.

- Performance is comparable with plenum vaporizers. Different vaporizers achieve this by a mix of thermal buffering and thermocompensation. In very warm environments the vaporizer may over-deliver with respect to dialled concentration and in very cold environments it may under-deliver.
- Always turn off or disconnect the vaporizer when filling, to prevent a sudden rise in delivered concentration if air is drawn directly into the open vaporizing chamber.
- In the absence of an agent monitor make regular, documented checks on the filling level of your vaporizer to reduce any risk of awareness during IPPV.
- Most manufacturers mark the direction of gas flow by an arrow inscribed on the top or front of the vaporizer.
- If you are unfamiliar with a vaporizer, go to the manufacturer's website and read the instructions.
- See the Appendix for pictures of common draw-over vaporizers.

Breathing systems

- You do not *attach* a breathing system. Draw-over *is* a breathing system. Different draw-over set-ups vary only in valve position.
- Functionally, two valves are needed in the system:
  - A unidirectional valve to prevent retrograde flow when delivering controlled ventilation (usually incorporated in either the vaporizer outlet or the bag/bellows inlet).
  - A breathing valve to direct gas into the patient during inspiration, and out during expiration.
- Note the Oxford inflating bellows (OIB) has an extra unidirectional valve on the outlet (patient) side. It was designed for use with an expiratory spill (Heidbrink) valve, which is rarely used nowadays. To

prevent airlocks in the system, disable the bellows outlet valve with the magnet supplied or by removing its metal disc. If the valve is not disabled and an airlock occurs the patient will not be able to exhale—briefly disconnect the patient from the system to allow exhalation, then correct the fault.
- Draw-over is a one-way system, so the output concentration of the vaporizer is always the patient's inspired concentration.
- In a draw-over system anaesthesia is deepened either by increasing the vaporizer setting or (in IPPV) by increasing minute ventilation.
- If you hyperventilate, the patient will be deeper than expected, and hypocapnic, so will be slow to resume breathing postoperatively.
- Compared with circle systems, when altering the vaporizer setting, the inspired concentration alters to match it very quickly—within a few breaths.

Breathing valves
- In the most basic system, the breathing valve comprises a single unit, placed next to the mask or airway device/tube, and to which a scavenging tube can be attached directly. Suitable valves include:
  - Ambu E1 valve (the Ambu E2 is not suitable because it is a resus valve with only one leaflet that allows entrainment of ambient air). E1 has two leaflets and E2 has only one. Be aware!
  - Laerdal valve
  - Ruben valve.

See the Appendix for pictures of the above valves.
- There are many other valves, most unsatisfactory and some (copies of the above valves) that are downright dangerous. If in doubt check by breathing through the valve before using (clean first).
- To reduce drag from the weight of such valves, Diamedica and Gradian produce two-limb (or coaxial) systems, in which all the valve components are situated at the machine end, away from the patient's face. The principle is the same though—it is not a circle system!

Checking a draw-over circuit
- See the Appendix for a draw-over equipment checklist.

Children and draw-over systems
- Unmodified adult draw-over systems can be safely used for children above 20 kg and down to 15 kg if IPPV is used.
- Below these thresholds, flow rates (not volumes) through the vaporizer may be too low to allow the vaporizers to generate an adequate concentration of anaesthetic. This may occur in two circumstances:
  - The low flow rates generated by a spontaneously breathing child.
  - Use of adult bags/bellows, especially in smaller children and babies, which generate lower flow rates at small volumes when compared with paediatric bag/bellows delivering the same volume.
- Note that this is a guide. The exact weight limits at which clinically relevant under-delivery of volatile agent occurs are not set in stone and may be slightly lower than stated here.

Solutions

- Use IPPV, preferably with a paediatric bag/bellows and paediatric breathing valve.
- Use ketamine. See 'Ketamine' in Chapter 4 (pp. 56–60).

Using draw-over in plenum ('push-over') mode in children

Draw-over vaporizers can be used in plenum mode to allow use of a T-piece with SV or IPPV, using one of the two following options:

Option one

- See Figure 3.2.
- Connect oxygen to the inlet of an Oxford miniature vaporizer (OMV) with an airtight connector.
- Run oxygen at 4 l/min minimum (higher flow rates can be used without a problem).
- Directly attach an Ayres T-piece to the vaporizer outlet. Back pressure (via the vaporizer) on the oxygen concentrator is not a problem as long as there is no circuit leak upstream of the vaporizer.

Option two

- Attach an Ayres T-piece, or similar, downstream of the bellows. Use the OIB at a frequency of about six to eight times/min to generate a 'background' flow, allowing the T-piece to be used for ventilation. The distal valve of the OIB will need to be operational. A similar effect can be achieved with a self-inflating bag. May be easiest with two people.

Notes

- Most vaporizers will under-deliver—approx. 80% of indicated concentration—in plenum mode. Be vigilant for adequate anaesthesia and increase dialled volatile concentration as necessary.
- Plenum mode is useful when performing a gas induction on small children as a continuous flow of volatile is delivered to the patient.
- The DPA, which is in common use and uses the Diamedica drawover vaporizer (DDV), does not require altering in any way to convert from draw-over to plenum mode at small tidal volumes, it will do so automatically.
- Epstein Macintosh Oxford vaporizer (EMO) requires at least 10 l/min inflow of oxygen to work in plenum mode.
- The Portable Anaesthesia Complete vaporizer (PAC) does not work in plenum mode.

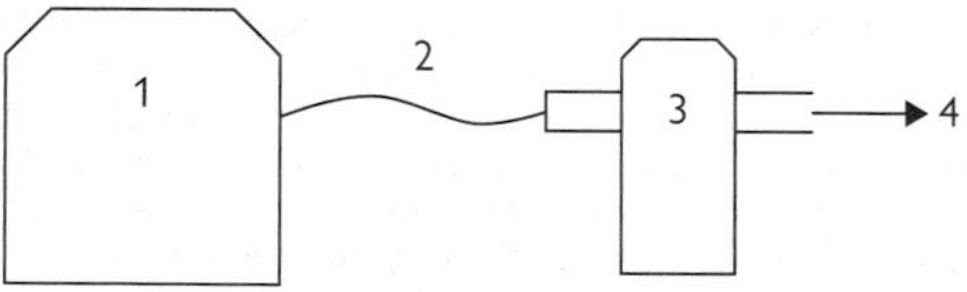

Figure 3.2 Example of draw-over vaporizer in plenum mode. (1) Oxygen source (4 l/min minimum). (2) Double walled. (3) Vaporizer. (4) Vaporizer output attached directly to T-piece as per option 1 above.

Gas induction with draw-over anaesthesia

- A close fit with the facemask is essential, or the child will draw in room air round the mask and dilute your anaesthetic.
- For the reason above, using halothane to induce a child with draw-over can be difficult as it is slow and requires a cooperative child to maintain a good seal. A useful compromise is to give ketamine 5 mg/kg IM first, after which a facemask can be more tightly held.

Unitary draw-over machines

- Diamedica Glostavent and UAM machines are suitable for use with controlled ventilation for any size of child, but their performance with spontaneous breathing in small children has not been assessed.

Care and maintenance

General principles

Cleanliness

- Regular external cleaning is vital.
- Don't leave anything open-ended (e.g. a vaporizer, tubing) as insects can easily get in. Store equipment in a clean cupboard or sealed plastic bag and/or put clean gauze in the end of tubing.
- Check any air filters weekly, daily in the dry season.

Cleaning and sterilizing the breathing system

- Draw-over systems are not designed to be disposable/single-use.
- Use a heat moisture exchanger (HME) filter/humidifier if you can.
- The patient's exhalations only pass downstream, so even an infected patient is unlikely to contaminate the bag/bellows or vaporizer.
- If a valve such as an Ambu/Laerdal is contaminated, you must disassemble and clean all the components separately (the yellow neoprene leaflets are surprisingly tough and withstand autoclaving well) then reassemble and test the valve yourself. Most Ruben valves cannot be disassembled, and are not able to be effectively sterilized.
- Contaminated rubber tubing can be autoclaved. Polythene tubing will probably melt in an autoclave—sterilize it chemically.

Vaporizer care

- Your vaporizer is the heart of your draw-over system. Simple regular care will give you many years of trouble-free use.
- Regular draining of the vaporizer is vital, especially for halothane vaporizers and especially if not being used for a period of time. Halothane contains additives that do not evaporate, and leave a sticky residue that will eventually make your vaporizer inoperable.
- Liquid drained must be discarded and not put back in the bottle.
- A stuck halothane vaporizer can be filled with an organic solvent (ether, alcohol, or halothane itself) and inverted several times. This will temporarily soften the deposits. It must be fully emptied and dried before re-use and will require full cleaning according to the manufacturer's instructions to prevent further recurrence.

Compressed gas machines

If you find a compressed gas (CG) (Boyles) machine in a low- and middle-income country (LMIC), it could be hazardous, regardless of age, for the following reasons:

'New' machines (frequently donated)

- Any machine designed to run on 60 Hz (e.g. those originating in the USA) will fail in a matter of months if run on 50 Hz mains.
- Most CG machines will be probably be unusable in the event of a power outage, which is liable to disrupt patient, oxygen, and CO_2 monitoring, and cause the ventilator to stop. If the machine has battery back-up, this seldom exceeds 30 min.
- Most will be fitted with a circle/absorber system, but soda lime may be unobtainable.
- Oxygen monitors depend on fuel cell sensors, which last <6 months if exposed to high oxygen concentrations.
- Many ventilators on this type of machine use large volumes (10–20 l/min) of oxygen as a power source for the ventilator.
- Nitrous oxide and cylinders of medical air are hard to obtain.
- The final destiny of such machines is usually giving halothane in 100% oxygen with no capacity for mechanical ventilation.

Old machines (sometimes more than 50 years old)

- Require no electricity.
- Often lack mechanical gas interlocks and oxygen sensors, so risk giving hypoxic gas mixtures.
- Leak—leading to inadequate gas flows and oxygen wastage.

Checking your machine

The World Federation of Societies of Anaesthesiologists (WFSA) publishes approved checklists but in addition you need to think about the following in resource-poor settings.

'What if' check

- Before every case, think '*what if*':
  - The mains electricity supply fails and is not restored?
  - The oxygen cylinder or pipeline fails?
- You must have a back-up plan for both these common situations—involving at least having a self-inflating bag to keep the patient alive; you also need to know how you will continue the anaesthetic.

Checking your machine for leaks

- Unexpectedly short cylinder life is pathognomonic of a leak.
- Check by getting a paintbrush and jar of soapy water. With the machine connected, and a set gas flow of 5 l/min, paint the entire gas pathway—cylinder, regulator, hoses, connections to the CG machine, all the pipework of the machine, flowmeters, backbar, vaporizer connections, and breathing system (look for bubbles). Double check by fitting a 2-l reservoir bag at the patient outlet—it should fill completely in 24 s.

Oxygen

Reliable oxygen supplies are a problem for many, if not most hospitals in the world. Traditionally oxygen is manufactured by fractional distillation of air, an energy-consuming process with high associated costs. In LMICs, oxygen may cost ten times more per litre than in high-income countries (HICs).

Common problems with cylinder supplies

- Hospital unable to afford them.
- Leaks from poorly maintained cylinders and regulators.
- Incorrect and faulty regulators.
- Large cylinders used unrestrained/free standing.
- Non-standard marking of cylinders/incorrectly labelled contents.

Oxygen concentrators

- Oxygen concentrators produce good quality (95%) oxygen (the remainder is inert argon) from room air via zeolite adsorption.
- This is a low-energy, therefore economical, process.
- The zeolite does not become exhausted—it regenerates during each adsorption cycle.
- A typical small concentrator uses about 350 watts (W) of power, and can produce 8 l/min of oxygen. The typical capital cost is US$600–1,000.
- Small concentrators are vulnerable to power cuts: risks can be reduced by having a protected electrical supply such as an uninterruptible power supply (UPS) (see 'Electricity' in this chapter (pp. 48–9) and/or a low pressure (up to 5 bar) oxygen storage system.
- Large concentrators are available that can be used to run a hospital pipeline system and to fill cylinders.
- The current generation of small concentrators produce oxygen at an outlet pressure of only 1.3 bar, so can only be used for draw-over.

Reliability

- Nominal service interval is 5,000 h of use, but this requires no more than a filter change.
- If well cared for, these machines can be expected to run trouble-free for up to 20,000 h (8 years of use, at 8 h/day, 6 days/week!)

Troubleshooting

- If left unused, the zeolite will nonetheless slowly adsorb moisture from the air; once a column has become fully saturated with water it will not recover. Using the concentrator regularly will keep the zeolite in good condition. If a machine is not in regular use, running it for 30 min/week is enough.
- Even operating theatres are dusty places, and if the inlet filter becomes clogged the concentrator will fail—indeed this is the commonest cause of failure. The inlet filter is normally a piece of plastic foam, requiring no more than a good rinse under the tap to clean it.
- Where ambient humidity is high, more of the zeolite column is required for water adsorption, leaving less for nitrogen, and a decrease in oxygen output concentration. This can usually be corrected by modestly reducing the flow of oxygen.

Electricity

Introduction

- Mains or 'grid' electrical supply systems around the world fall into two main alternating current (AC) ranges: 100–127 volts (V) and 220–240 V, at frequencies of either 50 or 60 Hertz (Hz).
- The two most common systems are those that are nominally 110 V at 60 Hz and 230 V at 50 Hz.
- The majority of electrical equipment is power supply-specific, requiring the correct voltage and frequency to function correctly.
- In low-resource settings there are three principal issues that contribute to a reduction in life and eventual failure of medical equipment: unstable electrical supply, poor maintenance of electrical infrastructure, and variation in the supply requirements of donated equipment.

Unstable electrical supplies

- If voltage or frequency is too high, equipment is likely to run hot. If voltage or frequency is too low then any cooling fans will run slow, also resulting in equipment running hot.
- The consequence of both situations is a reduction in the useful life of the equipment. Additionally, sudden failure and reestablishment of supply can also adversely affect electrical equipment.

Poor maintenance of electrical infrastructure

- Common problems include lack of earthed supplies, incompatible plugs and sockets, and the reversal of live and neutral connections.

Donated equipment

- When equipment is donated from a location outside the recipient's standard supply, e.g. 110 V equipment donated to a 230 V supply area, a step transformer is often used. Whilst this resolves the voltage issue, it does not change the frequency and the result is also a reduction in the life of the equipment or its failure. Frequency conversion is much more difficult and expensive to achieve.

Personal safety

- Electrical shock is at best unpleasant and at worst fatal but there are a number of simple ways to reduce or eliminate this risk.
- For someone to receive an electrical shock they must be part of a circuit; for an injury to result, they must be part of a circuit with sufficient current for a long enough period to cause harm.
- In low-resource settings the three major risk factors for inadvertently becoming part of a circuit are:
  - Poor or modified wiring.
  - Inappropriate (or no) protection devices, such as circuit breakers and fuses.
  - Liberal application of water (or other conducting fluids), particularly prevalent in an operating theatre environment.

Reducing risk

- Look for, and avoid, exposed wiring and inappropriate or overloaded sockets and plugs. Avoid multiple extension leads, particularly those on the floor where they are exposed to water and other liquids.
- Fuses and circuit breakers are more difficult to check but residual current devices (RCDs) are cheap to purchase and worth considering as a travel accessory.
- Before leaving for a low-resource setting, research the voltage requirements and plug/socket configuration of the destination and always use fused adaptors where possible.
- Consider the purchase of a socket testing device to identify the correct wiring and earth connection of sockets at your destination.

Equipment protection devices

A range of voltage correction and stabilization devices are available for equipment protection. Some provide simple line conditioning ('voltage smoothing') and others provide wide-ranging protection against power surges, spikes (very large surges, e.g. due to lightning strike) as well as providing limited power back up for the equipment. Selection of the most appropriate solution should be referred to a competent person in that field.

- Automatic voltage switchers: prevent damage to electrical and electronic equipment from power fluctuations. Some provide for high-voltage protection, some for low-voltage protection, and some for both as well as protection for power-back surges, which can happen when voltage is restored following a period of loss.
- Surge and spike suppressors: protect electronics by diverting unwanted energy away from the device during a voltage surge.
- UPS: provides back-up power (usually from a battery) to a device when the mains power fails or dips. Also generally provides surge protection. A number of differing types exist ranging from 'off line', 'on line', 'line interactive', to 'on line/double conversion'. The last of these is the most comprehensive, converting AC power to direct current (DC) and then reconverting to AC to provide very stable power.

Alternative electrical supply systems

Many low-resource settings with unreliable or intermittent electrical power will have an alternative or back-up supply solution. The most common at present is a petrol or diesel generator supply, but limited solar power systems are increasingly being introduced.

- Electrical output from a generator may be variable depending on its level of maintenance and the available technical support; it may also take some time to take over when the grid power supply fails.
- Some locations may have back-up solutions for short-term power interruptions, usually involving a bank of 12–24 V batteries, charged when mains power is available (or via solar) and discharged through an inverter to convert the low-voltage DC to suitable voltage AC power when required.

Hygiene and sterilization

Whilst most of this should be second nature to you, some aspects may be carried out by an assistant at home and may be less familiar. Common chemical solutions are detailed in Table 3.3. Approaches to sterilizing anaesthetic equipment are summarized in Table 3.4.

General hygiene and waste disposal measures

- Adopt universal precautions if there is any possibility of contact with bodily fluids, non-intact skin, or mucous membranes.
- Dispose of sharps in designated bins.
- Smash all ampoules prior to disposal to avoid them being recovered and resold as counterfeit medicines.

It is your responsibility to make sure your equipment is safe for re-use through cleaning, disinfection, and/or sterilization (Table 3.4). Cleaning, the physical removal of contamination without necessarily destroying infectious agents, is the most important part of the process.

Table 3.3 Common chemical solutions for disinfection/sterilization.

Chemical	Immersion time at 20C		Notes
	Disinfection	Sterilization	
Ethanol 70% (alcohol)	20 min	Not indicated	Stable, damages rubber
Formaldehyde (formalin)	10 min	> 24 h	Mutagenic, carcinogenic
Formaldehyde vapour	Not indicated	8 h	Place instruments in sealed bag with tablets
Gluteraldehyde >2% (CIDEX)	20 min	10 h	Coagulates blood and fixes tissue to surfaces
Hydrogen peroxide 7.5% (SPOROX)	30 min	6 h	Caution with brass, copper, zinc, nickel/silver plating
Hydrogen peroxide 7.35% with peracetic acid 0.23% (METREX)	15 min	3 h	Caution with lead, brass, copper, zinc
Ortho-phthalaldehyde 0.55% (CIDEX OPA)	12 min	Not indicated	Stains proteins grey
Povidine iodine 10%	20 min	Not indicated	Degrades silicone
Sodium hypochlorite 0.5% (bleach)	10 min	Not indicated	Corrosive

Table 3.4 Sterilization of common anaesthetic equipment.

Item	Association of Anaesthetists of Great Britain and Ireland (AAGBI) standard	Alternative suggestions
Airway adjuncts	Single-use	Reject if grossly contaminated. Clean, then autoclave, chemical sterilization or boiling
Ambuvalves	Single-use	Clean, then autoclave if no heat moisture exchanger (HME) filter used
Anaesthetic machine surfaces	Low-level disinfection of all surfaces daily or immediately if visible contamination	Wipe down with 0.05% sodium hypochlorite*
Bougies	High-level disinfect or sterilize up to five times or single-use	Clean, then high-level disinfection or boiling
Breathing circuits	Change circuits weekly if a new HME filter used for every patient. Change immediately if visible contamination or an infectious case	If no HME filter, then clean and autoclave/high-level disinfected between cases. Change circuit if contamination or infectious case, particularly tuberculosis
Catheter mounts	Single-use	Clean followed by high-level disinfection or boiling
Endotracheal tubes	Single-use	Most red rubber and silicone tubes autoclavable. If not—clean, high-level disinfection or boiling
Facemasks	Single-use or sterilization	If reusable then autoclave or chemical sterilization. If single-use then clean, high-level disinfection or boiling
Laryngoscope blades	Autoclave or single-use	Clean, then autoclave or chemical sterilization or boiling
Laryngeal mask airways	Single-use	Reusable: clean, then autoclave. Can re-use up to 40 times. Single-use: clean then high-level disinfection or boiling
Monitoring equipment	Clean with neutral-pH wipe between cases	Wipe with 0.05% sodium hypochlorite*
Ventilator	HME filter on the ventilator expiratory port and change with the breathing circuit	Use an HME filter if possible. If not, try to clean according to manufacturer's instructions

*0.05% sodium hypochlorite is a 1 in 10 dilution of bleach.

- **Non-critical equipment** contacts healthy skin only (e.g. finger pulse oximeter) and cleaning at the point of use is sufficient.
- **Semi-critical equipment** contacts mucous membranes or non-intact skin (e.g. laryngoscope blades) and requires cleaning followed by disinfection or sterilization.
- **Critical equipment** enters sterile tissue or the vascular system (e.g. intravenous cannulae) and requires cleaning followed by sterilization.

Cleaning

Cleaning by hand

Wash at 50–60C in a neutral (pH 7) detergent with stiff brushes, ideally nylon rather than steel wool. Open and close hinged instruments when both washing and rinsing. Rinse in sterile water at 40–50C. Air dry in a closed cabinet at 65–75C to retard microbial growth.

Ultrasonic washer

Uses bursting bubbles (cavitation) to clean instruments. Do not place dissimilar metals in the same cleaning cycle. Fully submerge the instruments under the cleaning fluid but do not place items directly on the bottom of the tank. Wash off the cleaning fluid at the end of the cycle with sterile water and change the fluid frequently.

Chemical disinfection and sterilization

Immerse the instruments for the required time (see Table 3.3) then rinse with sterile or boiled water. Do not let the rinsing water stand. Many of these chemicals are pungent: be sure to take appropriate precautions.

If no chemicals are available then boil items in water for 30 min. A home microwave oven (600 W) will disinfect compatible materials in 5 min and may sterilize after > 45 min.

Making sterile water for rinsing

- Strain the water through a muslin filter/tights.
- Run it through a ceramic or carbon 0.2 μm filter (most water purifiers).
- Bring to a boil in a clean lidded pan for 5 min.
- Use immediately or store in a sterilized container.

Alternatively, strain and filter then leave in bright sunlight for > 4 h in a polyethylene terephtalate container.

Further reading

Dobson M (2000) *Anaesthesia at the District Hospital*, 2nd ed. Geneva: WHO.
Dobson M (2017) *The Right Stuff. Anaesthetic Equipment and Techniques That Work Best in Low-Resource Countries*. London: World Anaesthesia Society.
Association of Anaesthetists of Great Britain and Ireland (2008) Infection control in anaesthesia. *Anaesthesia* 63 (9): 1027–1036.
Rutala WA, Weber DJ (2008) *Healthcare Infection Control Practices Advisory Committee Guideline for Disinfection and Sterilization in Healthcare Facilities*. http://cdc.gov/infectioncontrol/pdf/guidelines/disinfection-guidelines.pdf

Further reading

Chapter 4

Drugs and transfusion

Phil Blum, Chris Bowden, and Tom Coonan

Ketamine

In many low-resource settings ketamine is the mainstay of anaesthetic practice because it is inexpensive and versatile. It can be used relatively safely in the absence of complex monitoring, reliable electricity, and oxygen supplies. In addition, its sympathomimetic properties make it particularly useful for shocked patients.

Presentation

- Presented as 10, 50, or 100 mg/ml (includes preservative benzalkonium chloride) solutions.
- The most commonly available commercial ketamine solution is a racemic mixture of R (−) and S (+) isomers.
- All doses in this chapter refer to the racemic mixture.
- S (+) ketamine (rarely available, more expensive) is a single optical isomer solution. S-ketamine, compared with the racemic mixture, is:
  - presented in 5 and 25 mg/ml solutions
  - approximately twice as potent—halve doses for S(+) ketamine
  - associated with fewer central nervous system (CNS) side effects and shorter recovery time.

Pharmacodynamics

Primarily an *N*-methyl-D-aspartate (NMDA) glutamate receptor antagonist, ketamine has analgesic, amnesic, psychomimetic, and neuroprotective effects. Classic ketamine anaesthesia is described as a dose-dependent CNS depression leading to a dissociative state, characterized by profound analgesia and amnesia, but not necessarily loss of consciousness.

Although not asleep, the patient seems completely unaware of their environment and is uncommunicative. Varying degrees of facial grimacing, vocalization, hypertonus, and purposeful skeletal muscle movements often occur independently of surgical stimulation.

CNS effects

- Anaesthesia/analgesia/amnesia.
- Traditionally thought to increase cerebral blood flow (CBF) and therefore intracranial pressure (ICP). However recent literature suggests there is no increase in ICP with controlled ventilation.
- Anticonvulsant.
- Hallucinations and delirium (not universal).

Cardiovascular effects

- Via its sympathomimetic action: increases in systemic and pulmonary blood pressure and heart rate and consequently in cardiac output.
- Also causes direct myocardial depression. Although generally outweighed by sympathomimetic effects, this may be unmasked in the maximally compensated shocked patient, causing hypotension.

Respiratory

- Minimal respiratory depression.
- Transient apnoea is possible if large/rapid intravenous (IV) injection and/or concurrent opioid/benzodiazepine is administered.
- Upper airway skeletal muscle tone maintained.

- Increased salivary secretions.
- Potent bronchodilator secondary to increased catecholamines.

Uterus and placenta
- Uterine tone preserved.
- Ketamine readily crosses the placenta in pregnancy.

Contraindications
- Few, if any, absolute contraindications in austere environments. Caution with:
  - ischaemic heart disease
  - severe/poorly controlled hypertension
  - pulmonary hypertension
  - concurrent use of thyroxine (exaggerated hypertensive response).

Disadvantages in clinical use
- Hallucinations/emergence delirium.
- Hypersalivation.
- Instrumentation of the airway is possible but may be complicated by mastication/biting/increased jaw muscle tone and requires adequate opiate (laryngospasm is still possible with ketamine).
- Increased or maintained skeletal muscle tone; patient may move (requires experienced surgeon).
- Assessment of depth of anaesthesia can be challenging.

Practical use

Indications and dosing

Ketamine is extremely versatile and can be used in the following ways:

Procedural sedation, e.g. burns dressing changes
- 0.1–0.5 mg/kg IV, 2–4 mg/kg IM.
- PO: Adult 500 mg, child 15 mg/kg.

Pre-medication, e.g. prior to gas induction in children
- Give 30 min to 1 h prior to induction of anaesthesia if giving PO.
- 8 mg/kg PO (can use IV preparation but tastes bitter, dilute in a small volume of suitable clear fluid).
- 5 mg/kg IM a few minutes prior to induction, wait for effect (may be painful, adding lidocaine can help).

Induction of anaesthesia
- 1–2 mg/kg IV over 30 s. Onset 60 s. Duration 15–20 min.
- Less in shocked patients, 0.5–1 mg/kg and not more than 1 mg/kg in neonates and infants; risk of apnoea.
- 8–10 mg/kg IM. Onset 5 min. Duration 20–30 min.

Maintenance of anaesthesia
- Can be used in spontaneously breathing patients or paralyse and intubate for longer procedures.
- Repeat bolus doses of 0.5 mg/kg PRN, e.g. every 15–20 min.
- IV infusion: 50 μg/kg/min initially, titrated to effect. If no infusion pump is available (common), an infusion can be given using a standard IV fluid set-up:

- Add 500 mg ketamine to 500 ml IV fluid (1 mg/ml solution).
- Identify the type of giving set (usually 20 or 15 drops/ml).
- Start the rate initially at 1 drop/kg/min.
- This works fine as a starting rate for both 20 drops/ml giving sets and 15 drops/ml (less common) giving sets.
- Titrate drop rate down or up as required. Note that for any given drop rate a 15 drops/ml giving set will deliver proportionally more ketamine to the patient. This may or may not be clinically relevant.
- For example, for a 50 kg person and a 20 drops/ml giving set: 50 drops/min = 2.5 mg/min = 50 μg/kg/min. If using a 15 dropsl/ml giving set the rate works out to be 67 μg/kg/min.
- For induction with this infusion: run at 2 drops/kg/min until anaesthetized then reduce to 1 drop/kg/min. Again, this works fine for both 20 drops/ml and 15 drops/ml giving sets.

Post-op analgesia

- IM for acute pain in doses of 2–4 mg/kg.
- IV for acute pain: bolus of 50–100 μg/kg bolus until pain controlled then infusion of 1.5–5 μg/kg/min if pump available. Or, (for adults) put 100 mg ketamine in 1,000 ml crystalloid and run over 12 h. For safety consider putting 50 mg in 500 ml and running over 6 h. If the whole bag runs in quickly in error, the patient will receive 50 mg max. rather than 100 mg.
- PO: 50–100 mg t.d.s. (adults). Useful for post-amputation pain.

Treatment of severe asthma

- Well reported but usually only used when conventional therapy has failed. Suggested regimen: 0.1 –0.5 mg/kg IV bolus, 10 μg/kg/min infusion for 3 h, to be continued as required.

Attenuating side effects

Hypersalivation

- Less of a problem in adults and in short procedures (<30 min).
- Pre-medicate with antisialagogue, e.g. atropine 5–20 μg/kg IV pre-induction. Gentle suction of secretions throughout procedure. Note: rarely necessary for short procedures, can have unpleasant side effects, and may be dangerous in fever. More commonly used for longer cases where hypersalivation is more of a problem.

Hallucinations/emergence delirium

- Can be very distressing for patient and relatives. Is less of a problem with short procedures requiring a single bolus of ketamine.
- Chance of developing emergence phenomena is reduced by co-induction with benzodiazepines, e.g. midazolam 0.07 mg/kg or diazepam 0.1 mg/kg. Note that diazepam is painful when injected IV—add small amount of 1% lidocaine to reduce discomfort and inject slowly or give after the ketamine.
- Concurrent use of opioids (both at induction and intra-operatively) also seems to reduce emergence problems and is recommended, perhaps as it reduces amount of ketamine required intra-operatively. Note there

may be a risk of post-op respiratory depression—check your recovery facilities.

- Allowing patients to recover in a calm, quiet environment is reported to reduce incidence of emergence phenomenon.
- Treat distressing symptoms in recovery with further small boluses of benzodiazepine or opioids if obviously pain related.

Patient movement intra-operatively

- If patient appears light, deepen anaesthesia with further ketamine bolus or increasing infusion rate.
- If movement is in response to painful stimulus, try small opioid boluses.
- Benzodiazepines may help if patient appears to be hallucinating.
- Restraints may be required, ensure pressure areas are protected.

Special circumstances

Single syringe field anaesthesia technique

- Requires syringe driver, useful for transfers.
- Suggested recipe below can be adapted according to drugs available, e.g. substitute diazepam for midazolam, opioid may be added.
  - Ketamine 200 mg, midazolam 10 mg, vecuronium 10 mg, made up to 50 ml with 0.9% saline.
  - Appropriate separate induction dose of IV ketamine/vecuronium (or any induction agent and muscle relaxant).
  - Infuse mixture at 0.5 ml/kg/h (= 2 mg/kg/h ketamine).
  - Cease 20 min prior to waking patient.

'Ketofol'

- For procedural sedation:
  - Mix 50 mg propofol with 50 mg ketamine and add water for injection to a total volume of 10 ml; this gives 5 mg propofol and 5 mg ketamine per ml.
  - IV bolus dose technique is as for procedural sedation according to the ketamine component, e.g. 0.1–0.5 mg/kg titrated to effect.
  - Ketamine and propofol seem to act synergistically.
  - Side effects of each drug (hypotension, respiratory depression for propofol, emesis and agitation for ketamine) are attenuated as doses are lower for both.
  - For the elderly, make up with 25 mg propofol instead and bolus as above—reduces propofol dose administered (less hypotension).

Hemodynamically unstable patients

- Be aware that in severely shocked patients, hypotension can still occur following induction of anaesthesia with ketamine.
- Reduce induction dose to a maximum of 0.5 mg/kg.
- Strongly consider continuing anaesthesia with ketamine—switching to a volatile anaesthetic post induction can lead to precipitous drops in blood pressure.

Apnoea and ketamine

- When giving ketamine, transient apnoea is not uncommon, especially with larger, rapidly delivered IV boluses, shocked patients, neonates, and/or if opioids and/or benzodiazepines have been given.
- In most instances support the airway, administer oxygen (if not already doing so), wait, and the patient will commence spontaneous ventilation. If the patient shows signs of desaturation, gently ventilate until they start breathing again.
- Although it is reasonable to use ketamine in an emergency without supplemental oxygen, you must always have a means to ventilate the patient immediately to hand, e.g. self-inflating bag and mask.

Ketamine and drug control

- Ketamine can be a drug of abuse but is not currently scheduled under international drug control conventions—this may change.
- International laws to restrict illicit drug use (e.g. morphine, ketamine) potentially result in lack of essential medicines in low- and middle-income countries (LMICs).

Volatile agents

See Table 4.1.

Halothane

- A very safe agent as long as the anaesthetist is aware of its cardiac effects compared with newer agents.
- Pleasant smelling, thus a useful agent for inhalational induction.
- Respiratory effects similar to newer agents (depressant).
- Most halothane vaporizers can deliver up to 5% (approx. 7 minimum alveolar concentration (MAC)).

Specific issues

Arrhythmias

- Ventricular ectopic beats and bigeminy are very common and are usually caused by high concentrations of halothane.
- Higher concentrations of halothane can produce ventricular tachycardia and fibrillation.
- Halothane sensitizes the myocardium to the effects of adrenaline particularly in the presence of acidosis and hypercapnoea. The concomitant use of adrenaline containing solutions of local anaesthetic is not absolutely contraindicated but care must be taken:
    - Avoid infiltrating more than 100 µg of adrenaline in under 10 min in an adult (1:200,000 solution = 5 µg/ml).
    - Maintain normo- or hypocapnoea.
    - Avoid deep halothane anaesthesia during infiltration: you may consider IV supplementation of anaesthesia at this point.
    - Adrenaline and noradrenaline infusions at rates >0.15 µg/kg/min will provoke arrhythmias.
- Light anaesthesia or inadequate analgesia can cause sympathetic activation, precipitating abnormal rhythms. Increase ventilation if the patient is hypercapnoeic; administer IV opioid and/or deepen anaesthesia as required.
- Halothane can also cause bradycardias: consider correcting hypercapnoea and reducing depth of anaesthesia. Atropine may help but can provoke a worse tachycardia: if the patient is otherwise stable, avoid treating the number.

Table 4.1 Properties of volatile agents.

	MAC (%)	SVP at 20°C (mmHg)	Boiling point (°C)	Blood gas partition coefficient
Halothane	0.75	243	50	2.4
Ether	1.9	425	35	12.0
Isoflurane	1.15	238	49	1.4
Sevoflurane	2.0	162	59	0.6

MAC, minimum alveolar concentration; SVP, saturated vapour pressure.

Hepatitis

- Type 1: reversible, subclinical increase in serum transaminases levels. Occurs in up to 25% of patients.
- Type 2: fulminant hepatic necrosis ('halothane hepatitis'). Very rare, incidence 1:35,000 in largest study to date, mortality 50%.
- Diagnosis of exclusion—exclude viral hepatitis, malaria and other tropical diseases, other hepatotoxic drugs, transfusion reactions, and surgical hepatic pathology.
- Risk factors include multiple exposures, female sex, middle age, obesity, and liver enzyme-inducing drugs, e.g. alcohol. Less common in children.
- Avoid repeated halothane anaesthesia within 3 months if possible. In reality, this is unrealistic in many parts of the world where halothane is the only volatile anaesthetic agent available.

Thymol

- Halothane is decomposed by light so is presented in a brown bottle and contains thymol 0.01% to prevent oxidative decomposition.
- Thymol can accumulate and cause the vaporizer dial to stick. See 'Draw-over Anaesthesia' in Chapter 3 (pp. 40–5) for solutions.

Practical tips

- Paediatric inhalational induction: although slower in onset than sevoflurane, halothane is particularly useful for the paediatric difficult airway as it allows the anaesthetist more time to secure the airway before the patient lightens.
  - Approach: increase by 0.5% every three breaths until you reach 3–4%, maintain till pupils are midpoint and central (about 3 min), then decrease to 2% for spontaneous ventilation.
  - Inhalational halothane induction can be very slow via draw-over systems. Consider adding IM ketamine (see 'Ketamine' in this chapter (pp. 56–60)
  - Noticeably slower wake-up compared with sevoflurane especially if used without nitrous oxide: consider turning the halothane off sooner than with new agents—e.g. as peritoneum is being closed during a laparotomy.
- In LMICs, volatile agent analysis will commonly not be available. The vaporizers may not have been calibrated for many years. When using an unfamiliar vaporizer for the first time, watching the local practitioners and observing clinical signs will guide you as to what percentage of agent needs to be dialled up to achieve safe anaesthesia.
- With no agent analysis and often no keyed index filling systems, be aware that what is in the vaporizer (or what's in the volatile agent bottle itself) may not correspond to the label.
- The saturated vapour pressures (SVPs) of halothane and isoflurane are similar (Table 4.1)—they can be used interchangeably in the same vaporizer (but never mixed). Many anaesthetists insist that they are able to smell the difference between agents but in practice this is not reliable.

Diethyl ether

Although rare in most anaesthetists' experience, ether is still used for anaesthesia in some remote areas of Africa and Asia.

Ether:

- Is flammable in air and explosive in higher concentrations of oxygen, thus contraindicated if diathermy is used.
- Boils at 35°C at sea level. This makes its use clinically impractical when the shaded ambient temperature is above 32°C. At 2,500 m above sea level you may start to find your ether boiling away.

Practical use

- The Epstein Macintosh Oxford (EMO) vaporizer is designed specifically for ether draw-over anaesthesia.
- Inhalational ether induction is slow and nauseating for the patient, solutions include:
    - Intravenous induction followed by ether maintenance.
    - Inhalational halothane induction using the Oxford miniature vaporizer (OMV) connected to the outlet (*not* inlet) port of the EMO, followed by ether maintenance.

Properties

- Ether's pharmacodynamic properties make it a particularly safe sole anaesthetic agent. This is especially true for anaesthetic practitioners with limited training looking after sick patients in remote locations.
- It can be thought of as the 'volatile equivalent' of ketamine.

Cardiovascular

- Weak sympathomimetic properties—reduction in blood pressure is less, particularly in hypovolaemic patients, compared with modern volatile agents. Dysrhythmias are uncommon.

Respiratory

- Less respiratory depression and better preserved minute ventilation compared with other volatiles. Spontaneous ventilation at a surgical plane of anaesthesia can be conducted without supplemental oxygen.

CNS

- Analgesic, which is useful where opioid supply may be limited.

Musculoskeletal

- Produces some muscle relaxation that allows a surgeon to perform a laparotomy or Caesarean section without the need for neuromuscular blocking agents and positive pressure ventilation.

Gastrointestinal

- Causes salivation, nausea, and vomiting, particularly if ether inhalational induction is used. No toxic hepatic or renal metabolites.

Obstetric

- There is anecdotal evidence that ether is less tocolytic than modern agents.

Muscle relaxants

Suxamethonium, vecuronium, and atracurium are on the World Health Organization (WHO) Essential Drugs list, but may or may not be present. Pancuronium is often available. Rocuronium is relatively rare. See Table 4.2.

When to paralyse

- Note that most ventilators are gas driven and require high flow oxygen, which may be in short supply.
- Hence, when using muscle relaxants, the patient will usually need to be hand ventilated, unless you are lucky and have an electrically driven or oxygen-frugal ventilator.
- Surgeons with experience in low-resource settings may be used to operating on spontaneously breathing patients and patients under ketamine, who are not quite still. Paralysis may not be required.

General considerations

- Neuromuscular monitors are expensive as well as fragile. It is unlikely one will be available.
- Consider factors that may prolong the action of muscle relaxants:
  - Acute/chronic kidney injury—laboratory testing may not be available.
  - Hypothermia—can be a problem even in warm environments.
  - Hypercapnoea—often no end-tidal carbon dioxide ($EtCO_2$) monitoring.
  - Medications that can prolong the duration of muscle relaxants, e.g. magnesium, gentamicin, and steroids.
- Lack of suxamethonium or rocuronium may make a conventional rapid sequence induction (RSI) difficult. See 'Absent Drugs and Workarounds' in this chapter (pp. 65–6) for solutions.

Table 4.2 Properties of muscle relaxants commonly found in LMICs.

	Sux.	Atrac.	Vec.	Panc.*
Intubating dose (mg/kg)	1–2	0.5	0.1	0.1
Onset (min)	1	3	3	3
Minimum time prior to attempting reversal (min)	n/a	35	30–40	70–120
Time until TO4 > 0.9 (min)	n/a	55–80	50–80	130–220
Max. time can remain unrefrigerated (days)	14	14	n/a	180

Sux., suxamethonium; Atrac., atracurium; Vec., vecuronium; Panc., pancuronium; TO4, train of four (using nerve stimulator).

*Pancuronium causes a 10–15% increase in heart rate. The pancuronium supplemental dose is 0.01–0.02 mg/kg and lasts 30–60 min.

Absent drugs and workarounds

Anaesthetic drugs are in short supply in many LMICs. The steady, reliable supply of many routine anaesthetic drugs found in high-resource environments often does not happen for the following reasons:

- Inconsistent funding at national, district, and hospital levels.
- Storage, stock-keeping, and ordering systems are less than optimal.
- Expense (patients may have to fund their own drugs).
- In-country restrictions on certain drugs, e.g. strong opioids.

General principles

- Local anaesthesia providers will have often adapted their techniques to work without certain drugs—observe and learn from them.
- Use of regional anaesthesia, either spinal, peripheral limb block, or use of local infiltration, will often circumvent the lack of drugs required for safe general anaesthesia.
- Sharing ampoules between patients is not ideal but is commonplace out of necessity in many low-resource settings. It should be avoided for neuraxial anaesthesia—risk of meningitis from cross-infection.

Vasopressors

- Ephedrine may be available; metaraminol and phenylephrine often unavailable.

Solution

- Adrenaline is usually available—dilute to 10 μg/ml: bolus 1 ml as required.

Suxamethonium

- Lack of suxamethonium and/or rocuronium is common and limits your ability to perform a 'traditional' RSI.

Solutions

- The solution chosen will depend on the individual patient circumstances, your experience, and perception of risk. None is perfect.

Use regional technique

- For example, spinal or nerve block.

Use normal 'non-RSI' technique

- Accept the increased risk of regurgitation and induce anaesthesia, paralyse, and intubate as normal.
- Take non-pharmacological precautions against regurgitation:
  - Place nasogastric tube pre-op.
  - Position patient head up until intubated.
  - Apply cricoid pressure post induction of anaesthesia.
  - Bag mask ventilate gently, using the oro-pharyngeal airway.

Timing method

- In this technique a (non-rocuronium) non-depolarizing muscle relaxant is given prior to the induction agent, in order to shorten the time from loss of consciousness to intubation.

   - Pre-oxygenate as normal and consider giving a small dose of IV benzodiazepine and/or fentanyl as a pre-med.
   - If possible, site two IV lines in case one is lost during induction.
   - Fully brief the patient that they may experience a mild sensation of weakness prior to going to sleep.
   - Give atracurium 0.75 mg/kg or vecuronium 0.15 mg/kg.
   - At the onset of clinical weakness (ptosis, lack of grip strength) give an induction dose of thiopental, wait 60 s, intubate.
   - Note that with a large dose of muscle relaxant, paralysis will be prolonged.

Pancuronium

- Pancuronium is sometimes the only muscle relaxant available. It has a slow onset and long duration of action so a priming dose is required to facilitate rapid tracheal intubation. Paralysis will last up to 1 h; longer if magnesium has been given (obstetrics).
   - Give 0.01 mg/kg pancuronium during pre-oxygenation.
   - After 3 min pre-oxygenation, give induction agent followed by 0.15 mg/kg pancuronium, wait 60 s, intubate.

Long-acting local anaesthetics

- Bupivacaine is quite widely available but sometimes lidocaine is the only available local anaesthetic.

Solutions

- Add adrenaline to 1% lidocaine (1:200,000) to prolong duration of peripheral limb blocks. Can produce surgical anaesthesia lasting over an hour and often longer.
- 1% and 2% lidocaine can be used for spinal anaesthesia but must be preservative free. A total of 3–4 ml 2% lidocaine or 8 ml 1% lidocaine will produce a block acceptable for Caesarean section and should last up to 45 min. See 'Spinal Anaesthesia' in Chapter 8 (pp. 167–71) for further details.

Propofol

- Propofol is frequently unavailable, making the use of laryngeal mask airways (LMAs) more difficult as other IV induction agents do not depress airway reflexes in the same manner. Total intravenous anaesthesia (TIVA) as practised in high-income countries (HICs) is also more challenging without propofol.

Solutions

- Ketamine can be used by infusion to provide TIVA (see 'Ketamine' in this chapter, (pp. 56–60).
- Options if keen to use an LMA:
   - Gas induction, bolus opioid, then place LMA.
   - Pre-medicate with opioid (may need larger than normal dose), induce with thiopental or ketamine and place LMA. If difficult, deepening anaesthesia with volatile or spraying LA onto the oropharynx may help.

Glycopyrronium/neostigmine

- Pre-mixed reversal is usually unavailable. Add atropine to neostigmine, e.g. add 1 mg atropine to 2.5 mg neostigmine.

Procurement, transport, and storage

- If you are part of a short surgical mission you should provide the vast majority of the drugs you are planning to use during your visit. Depleting the resources of your host in a matter of days is not helpful.
- If you are embedded in a country's healthcare system for an extended period of time you will be dependent on in-country drug procurement, transport, and storage systems. Let your practice be guided by how the locals overcome constraints inherent in their system.

Drug procurement

- Obtain supplies officially. Do not obtain drugs 'under the counter'.
- Involve a qualified pharmacist who can source, package, and prepare an invoice.
- Avoid donated medication that is out of date. If the quality of a drug is not suitable for use in your own country, it is not suitable for use in the recipient country. The donation of out-of-date medicines is prohibited by the WHO.
- Consider how the medication is packaged in relation to transportation. Plastic ampoules are much more robust than glass vials.
- Powdered medications, such as vecuronium, generally have much longer shelf lives, are more tolerant of temperature variation, and are lighter to transport than their counterparts presented in solution.

International transportation of medication

- Documentation is vital. A list of what you are carrying and in what quantities will facilitate prompt clearance through customs.
- Often official documentation of approval of importation of medicines needs to be obtained from the host country embassy prior to travel. Supplies can be confiscated by customs officials if the paperwork isn't correct.
- There may also be export regulations that you must adhere to when departing from home.
- Avoid transporting narcotics, ketamine, or ephedrine across international borders. No matter how much documentation you have it will often still be problematic.
- Anaesthetic volatile agents are classified as Dangerous Goods/ Hazardous Materials when shipped by air. Transportation without meeting specific requirements is illegal.
- Out-of-date medications will often be confiscated by customs at the host country border.
- Be aware of extremes of temperature during transport. The temperature inside a locked car in the tropical sun can easy reach over 70°C.
- Re-importation of drugs to the home country may also be a problem.

Storage

- It is common sense to store medications out of direct sunlight, avoiding freezing temperatures and excessive heat (defined as >40°C).
- Narcotics will require added security and documentation of usage.
- Some medications require refrigeration, which can be problematic; for example, based on spectroscopy, suxamethonium degrades:
  - 0.3% per month at 4°C
  - 2% per month at 21–25°C
  - 8% per month at 37°C.
- Current guidelines recommend that suxamethonium can remain out of the fridge for 14 days.
- Based on the above figures, suxamethonium will only lose 10% of its activity after about 5 months at room temperature.

Minimum standards

- The International Standards for a Safe Practice of Anaesthesia 2010 (see 'Further Reading') includes the availability of key anaesthetic drugs that are sourced from the WHO Essential Medicines List. For LMICs this is often aspirational and, as a result, not all commonly used anaesthetic drugs may be available.
- Essential Medicines, as defined by the WHO, are intended to be available in healthcare facilities at all times, in the appropriate dosage forms, with assured quality, and at a price that the individual and community can afford.
- Essential anaesthesia and pain management drugs listed by the WHO are detailed in the Appendix.
- The WHO list is a guide for the development of national and institutional essential medicine lists—thus exactly which medicines are regarded as essential remains a national responsibility.
- If you are part of a non-governmental organization (NGO) surgical team, then a list of available anaesthesia drugs should be available for review pre-deployment.

Poor-quality drugs

- Counterfeit medicines are now reclassified as substandard, spurious, falsely labelled, falsified, and counterfeit (SSFFC) medical products.
- Falsified medical products may contain no active ingredient, the wrong active ingredient, or the wrong amount of the correct active ingredient.

Practical points for anaesthetists

- Beware of the possibility of exposure to SSFFC medical products.
- Consider whether it is necessary to ensure safe access to personal medicines prior to departure, especially if you have a chronic health condition.
- Lack of adequate drug storage may lead to altered drug activity.
- Use of expired medications is common in LMICs out of necessity.
- Private purchase of drugs by patients is common in LMICs—there is a higher risk of SSFFC drugs than when sourced through official routes.

Blood transfusion

Introduction

- Anaesthesia providers working in low-resource settings will need to prepare themselves for creative solutions to the desperate situation of acute blood loss without the easy availability of blood components that is commonplace in HICs.
- Fresh whole blood is often the only option. This is not a bad thing! It is warm and full of clotting factors, which is particularly useful in bleeding with clotting abnormalities.
- When blood transfusion is needed acutely, consider the timing. Transfusing blood when there is still active bleeding may mean wasting precious blood (may only be 1 or 2 units available in the hospital).
- Otherwise healthy individuals will tolerate an Hb of 50 g/l.

Blood collection, typing, and cross-matching

General guidance

- In general, it is not appropriate for visitors to a country to undertake blood collection and cross-matching. Always work within the existing national blood collection/distribution systems and regulations.
- It is illegal to take blood collection equipment into some countries.
- Even in an emergency situation, you should not embark on blood collection and cross-matching unless you have undergone specialist training recognized in the country in which you are working.
- The information here on blood collection and cross-matching is for background information only. It is not intended as a how-to guide.

Collection

- If appropriate, ensure that a means of collecting and anticoagulating donated blood is available in your hospital, e.g. packs of 450 ml blood collection bags containing CPD (citrate, phosphate, dextrose, preserves blood for 21 days) or CPD-A1 (added adenine, preserves blood for 35 days).
- Heparin can be used for anticoagulation in doses of 2–4 units for each cc of donated blood. Note that this will entail a heparin load for the recipient.

Typing

- If there are reagents and equipment for blood typing available, there will often be local technical expertise in their use. Seek it out.
- Consider sourcing, and gaining familiarity with, bedside blood typing cards. In some countries, these are used as a bedside 'last check' before administering bank blood to a patient.

ABO antibodies

- While a full cross-match is desirable, it is not always feasible.
- Whenever possible, transfusion should be with type-specific blood.
- The administration of type O whole blood entails loading with Anti-A and Anti-B IgM, which is potentially dangerous for a non-type O recipient. This risk is relative however, and dependent on an unusually high titre of antibody in the plasma of the donor.
- It is considered justifiable to transfuse type O blood in the presence of exsanguination.

Non-ABO antibodies

- In general, IgG antibodies (such as anti D (Rh) and other non-ABO antibodies) are unlikely to bind complement and cause acute haemolytic reactions. A total of 97% of the non-Caucasian populations are D antigen positive (85% positivity in Caucasian populations).
- It is important that the Rh status of a recipient of a blood transfusion is determined, even if only after the fact. If the transfusion of Rh pos. blood to a Rh neg. recipient is unavoidable, Rh (D) immunoglobulin should be administered within 72 h if possible.

Transfusion-transmitted infections and toxins

- Donors should be screened using readily available, highly sensitive rapid screening tests for:
  - HIV1 and 2
  - HbS (sickle haemoglobin)
  - hepatitis C virus
  - syphilis.
- Directed questionnaires to the donor should include any medications that may become active, or allergenic, in recipients.
- Positive results in these instances will still lead to difficult risk/benefit decisions in the context of catastrophic blood loss.
- Testing donated blood for malaria is difficult for a number of technical reasons, although a rapid test can be done on the donor.
- Expectant treatment for post transfusion fevers in high malaria prevalence areas is recommended.

Donors

- Donations, if possible, should be from men, or from women who have never been pregnant—to greatly decrease the likelihood of antibody transfer, and to mitigate the probability of transfusion-related acute lung injury (TRALI).
- This may not be practical in a context where donors and donations are in short supply. It must also be noted that potential female donors are often chronically anaemic.

Graft vs host disease

- If possible, genetically related donors should be avoided as there is a higher risk of graft vs host disease (fever, rash, abdominal pain, diarrhoea, and vomiting).
- This is particularly true for premature neonates and other immunocompromised recipients.
- In low-resource settings this is commonly not practical as family members might be the only readily available donors and the risk/benefit ratio favours transfusion.

Special paediatric considerations

- Antibodies in children under 6 months old are of maternal origin, and potential donations should be compatible with both neonatal and maternal blood.
- Theoretically, cardiac contractility in neonates is relatively unresponsive to circulatory overload, putting them at risk of over-transfusion.

However, a more common clinical problem in low-resource settings is that children succumb from a lack of blood.

- In austere settings, cytomegalovirus (CMV) negative blood for neonates may not be available. The primary consideration is the avoidance of exsanguination.

Additional caveats in emergency blood transfusion

- Tranexamic acid should be administered, 1 g over 10 min, then 1 g over 4 h (adult dose).
- The desperate nature of emergency transfusions in austere environments requires judicious communication of risks and benefits. The alternative to a risky transfusion is often the death of a patient.
- If more than 2–4 units of incompatible type O blood have been given, it is commonly recommended that the patient should not be switched back to compatible blood.

Emergency autotransfusion

- Although there are many concerns with rudimentary cell saver set-ups, in certain circumstances they can be life-saving. See Figure 4.1.

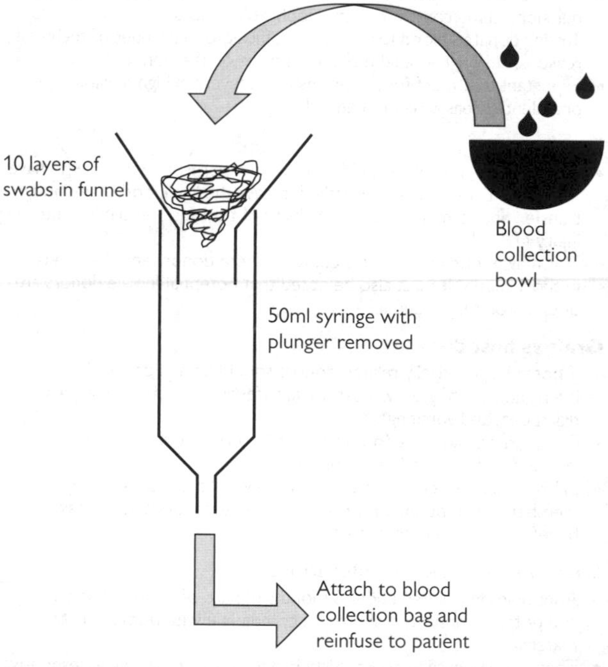

Figure 4.1 'Field' cell saver. Note: all components should be sterile.

- Blood is collected into a bowl either by gentle aspiration (<100 mmHg), scooped with a gallipot, OR by abdominocentesis with a 14 gauge needle (especially for ectopic pregnancy).
- Blood can be collected directly from a chest drain in a sterile fashion. See Figure 4.2.
- It is best to anticoagulate with CPD in the collection bag or add 2–4 units of heparin/ml blood scavenged in the bowl (1,000 units heparin/450 cc blood).
- Anticoagulation may not always be necessary, especially if blood is to be reinfused immediately.
- The collected blood is passed through a filter of four or more layers of sterile gauze placed in a funnel, into a 50 ml syringe, which is in turn connected to a blood collection bag.

Contraindications to autotransfusion

- Contamination, e.g. with amniotic fluid, bacteria, bile, gastric fluid, urine/faeces, cancer cells, or foreign matter. All are relative and a matter of degree—weigh up risk of contaminant vs risk of death by exsanguination.

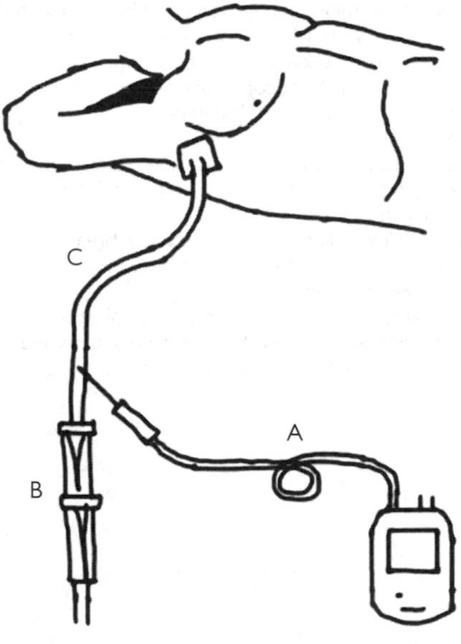

Figure 4.2 Cell salvage from a chest drain. (A) blood collection bag, needle inserted directly into (C) chest drain, (B) Heimlich valve or underwater seal. Clamp the chest drain below the collection needle only if no risk of tension pneumothorax.

- Haemostatic agents in operative field.
- Antiseptics (iodine, chlorhexidine) or large amounts of water in collected blood.
- Blood that is not fresh (over 6 h since bled).

Keep it simple!

Blood warming

- If stored bank blood is available, the means to warm it during infusion are unlikely to be available and may rely on electricity.
- Blood bags can be warmed in bowls of hot water prior to infusion but take care not to overheat them (<40°C).

Transfusion reaction

- The term encompasses a wide spectrum of reactions.
- Less severe reactions lead to fever, rash, urticaria, and mild shortness of breath/wheeze.
- Severe reactions can cause rapid, complete cardiovascular collapse, disseminated intravascular coagulation (DIC), multi-organ failure, and death. They tend to occur soon after starting a transfusion, e.g. due to ABO incompatibility or anaphylaxis.
- Patients should have their vital signs checked before and during a blood transfusion (first set within 15 min of transfusion starting).
- If only the feature of a reaction is a temperature rise of <1.5°C or rash:
  - Stop transfusion and check compatibility of blood.
  - Give paracetamol and/or anti-histamine.
  - Re-check vital signs.
  - Continue transfusion at a slower rate and observe the patient closely.
- If there are any other or additional signs of transfusion reaction:
  - Stop transfusion.
  - Assess patient immediately using the airway, breathing, circulation, disability (ABCD) approach.
  - Treat according to findings.
- Don't forget acute sepsis from bacterial contamination (may present during transfusion) as a cause of transfusion reactions and TRALI, which tends to present some hours after the transfusion.

Further reading

Ketamine

Craven R (2007) Ketamine. *Anaesthesia* 62 (S1): 48–53.
Staroverov D (2010) Ketamine. *Medical Journal of Zambia* 37 (3): 186–192.
Persson J (2010) Wherefore ketamine? *Curr Opin Anaesthesiol* 231: 435–436.
World Federation of Societies of Anesthesiologists (n.d.) Ketamine is a medicine campaign, available at http://www.wfsahq.org/the-campaign, accessed February 2018.

Procurement, transport, and storage

Atkinson RS, Rushman GB, Davies NJH (1993) *Lee's Synopsis of Anaesthesia*, 11th ed. London: Butterworth Heinemann Ltd.
WHO (n.d.) WHO medicines supply, available at: http://www.who.int/medicines/areas/access/supply/en/index1.html, accessed February 2018.

Minimum standards

Merry A et al. (2010) International standards for a safe practice of anaesthesia. *Can J Anaesth* 57 (11): 1027–1034.
WHO (2017) WHO model list of essential medicines March 2017, available at: http://www.who.int/medicines/publications/essentialmedicines/en/

Blood transfusion

Strandenes G et al. (2014) Emergency whole blood use in the field: a simplified protocol for collection and transfusion. *Shock* 41 (S1): 76–83.
Doughty H et al. (2016) A proposed field emergency donor panel questionnaire and triage tool. *Transfusion* 56: S119–S127.
Selo-Ojeme DO et al. (2003) Autotransfusion for ruptured ectopic pregnancy. *Int J Gyn Obstet* 80: 103–110.
WHO (n.d.) WHO recommendations, available at http://www.who.int/bloodsafety, accessed February 2018.

Further reading

Chapter 5

Perioperative Care

Tom Bashford, Wayne Morriss, Clare Roques, Naomi Shamambo, and Matt Wilkes

Preoperative assessment

Preoperative assessment is essential for all patients undergoing surgery. According to a study by the World Health Organization (WHO), inadequate preoperative assessment is a contributing factor in perioperative morbidity and mortality and this is particularly true in low- and middle-income countries (LMICs).

The aims of preoperative assessment are the same the world over:
- Is the patient fit for surgery now?
- Can the patient be made fitter for surgery in the future?
- How urgent is this surgery?
- What resources are required to provide safe surgery, anaesthesia, **and postoperative care**, for this patient, for this operation? Do you have them or can you get them?
- Is there a safer option available?
- Is the potential benefit worth the risks?
- What would be the safest anaesthetic technique?

The assessment is made in a similar fashion to that for a patient in a high-income country (HIC), but with points to consider unique to the low-resource setting.

Considerations

The type of patient
- There are fewer geriatric patients.
- Patients commonly present late and are therefore often very sick needing prolonged resuscitation. Time and the required drugs and fluids may not be readily available.
- Patients may have undiagnosed congenital or acquired pathology, e.g. rheumatic heart disease or diabetes.
- There may be poor documentation of previous diseases and surgeries.
- Patients may need blood and radiological investigations that are not available, take a long time to obtain, or are unaffordable.
- Malnutrition, anaemia, and coincidental infectious and tropical diseases are common.

Most of the surgical procedures required by patients in LMICs will fall into obstetric, trauma, paediatric, or oncology categories.

Treatment so far

Medical facilities may be scarce and expensive. Traditional remedies may have been tried first, so ask about:
- Any herbal medication: establish from local staff the likely effects of such remedies.
- Any traditional cutting/bloodletting: tetanus risk.

Exercise tolerance and functional reserve

The best assessment is to ask what they do for their livelihood, and ask if they have become less active than before or ask about activities they have been requiring assistance to perform.

Airway assessment

Management of the difficult airway is compounded in LMICs, where limited equipment, skilled assistance, and patient condition can all play a role in making the task daunting.

- Patients presenting with head and neck problems may often have advanced disease, which complicates airway management.
- Be aware of coincidental neck masses! A patient presenting for laparotomy for intestinal obstruction may have a huge goitre for which they are not seeking medical attention.
- Airway problems may be well hidden by head scarves, make sure you have checked!
- Is a regional technique possible?
- In some cases, such as facial trauma, an elective surgical airway under local anaesthesia may be the safest option when advanced airway techniques such as fibreoptic intubation are not available.
- See Chapter 6 (p. 93), for further discussion.

Circulation assessment

- Hypovolaemia is a leading cause of anaesthesia-related deaths in LMICs.
  - Is there enough time to resuscitate before theatre or is concurrent resuscitation and surgery required to control haemorrhage? This is more likely in the face of a limited blood supply.
- Undiagnosed hypertension:
  - Can you wait?
  - If you wait, can you treat?

Clinical personnel

- Anaesthesia in most LMICs is provided by a non-physician anaesthetist. Many are highly skilled, however they have their limitations. You may be the only physician anaesthetist in the region.
- The surgeon may not be a trained surgeon (especially in rural areas) but a medical officer or non-physician surgeon, who may also have his or her own limitations.
- You may not have trained people to assist you. You will have some willing hands but they may be untrained. Watch how they do things so you understand their team dynamics before you plunge in and make your own demands.
- Recovery and ward staff training and numbers may be limited.

Equipment and infrastructure

- Donated equipment may be present but is often non-functional. Thus, you may be limited in what you are able to achieve with the limited resources available and your plan needs to take these issues into consideration.
- Laryngoscopes may be out of batteries, electricity supply cut off, or oxygen cylinders empty. It may take a whole day to access these supplies!
- What is the sterile technique and instrument sterility like?

Support services

- Essential lab work may not be available or, if available, may take longer to get results than you have time for.
- If you are adamant that you will only do this procedure when all investigations have been done, you may just increase morbidity and mortality for your patients. Carefully consider:
  - Will the tests change my anaesthetic?
  - Is there any safe alternative to use that doesn't require this test?
  - What are the risks vs benefits?
- Radiology may not be available.
- Blood may not be available or, again, may take longer to source.

Technique: general vs regional anaesthesia

The decision as to whether to use a general anaesthetic or regional technique is dependent on the resources available and the skill set to utilize those resources. For the reasons discussed in the previous section, if a procedure can be done under a regional technique, it is generally safer to do so.

There is often no way of assessing clotting profile or platelet count. The debate is whether to do a spinal or general anaesthetic. Consider:

- Bedside bleeding time can be done to ascertain clotting. If the blood takes more than 7 min to clot, try to avoid doing a spinal.
- A careful physical examination, looking for any ecchymotic patches or any bleeding tendency on cannulation, etc.

To wait or not to wait

If, after assessment, you consider there is a benefit to delaying surgery and optimizing the patient, ensure there is a clear **achievable** plan. Otherwise you may postpone your case today, and still have the same problem a week or indeed a month later.

Occasionally there may be pressure to expedite surgery for non-clinical reasons, e.g.

- Limited availability of specialist surgeons.
- Limited access to a functional operating theatre.

The relative risks and benefits must always be carefully balanced and patient safety made a priority.

To conclude, preoperative assessment in LMICs is not fundamentally different from other settings. Overall, one's clinical acumen comes into greater play and an appreciation of the wider clinical environment is required.

Consent

Introduction

- Informed consent is fundamental to ethical clinical practice and research.
- Consent is based around the fostering of a shared understanding of any proposed intervention, its intended benefits, and possible risks.
- Consent should be a dynamic, mutual process whereby the clinician engages the patient in an understanding about their care.

Consent in LMICs

- Be aware of any guidelines and legal frameworks within the host country or organization(s).
- The principles of consent are global. However, consent approaches and processes formulated in the Western world may not always fit the local context.
- A number of context-specific issues may complicate the obtaining of consent in LMICs (see Table 5.1).
- Obtaining consent that is both appropriate to the clinical situation and the context of the country in which you are working may be difficult and require a deep understanding of the local culture.

Table 5.1 Factors affecting the consent process in LMICs.

Context-specific factor	Example of effect on consent
Language	Can be difficult to convey nuances and subtleties of risk to patient
Power structures	Patients may not feel empowered to challenge treatment plans/ask questions
Religion	May play a larger part in decision making than you expect
Education	Level of formal education or literacy may be different to that assumed
Family dynamics and gender	The head of the family or a male relative may need to give consent for other family members
Age	The age at which a patient is deemed able to make autonomous decisions may vary between settings
Immediacy of need	Patients may present late in the clinical course, limiting time for consent
Access to healthcare	Limited access to alternative (unaffordable) treatments may affect decision making

Consent for research and quality improvement projects

- Issues around consent to medical research, both generally and specifically pertaining to LMICs, have been well explored.
- Implementing a new 'best practice' recommendation in an HIC does not always require consent over and above the usual clinical consent process. Careful consideration of the ethical and consent issues involved in a change to 'best practice' in an LMIC setting, is mandatory, however, particularly if the practice concerned has been imported from an HIC context, is poorly evidence-based for this context, and/or lacks national/local acceptance. Consider:
  - Is explicit consent from local colleagues or patients required before intervening to change practice?
  - Should quality improvement projects require the same standard of consent as research?
  - How do you obtain consent for system-wide interventions?
- Proposed guidelines on quality improvement in LMICs advocate for both a participatory approach and accountability as core elements: consent is central to these two themes.
- It is important to note that exhaustive forms, whether they provide legal protection or not, may not be a reliable indicator that consent is informed.

Use of patient details

- Monitoring, evaluation, and reporting are often a requirement of global health funding bodies—use of patient data in this context raises consent issues.
- The use of identifiable patient details and images in any context requires explicit consent.
- Many agencies have internal protocols pertaining to the gathering and use of such information.

Pain management

Overview

- The WHO estimates that over 80% of the world's population has inadequate access to treatment for pain.
- In LMICs, limited resources frequently result in the treatment of pain being given low priority. However, simple and cheap measures can be used effectively in many situations.
- Beyond the personal suffering of the individual patient, many other consequences of untreated pain are often not fully appreciated by healthcare workers or patients and their families:
  - increased length of hospital stay
  - disability
  - chronic pain
  - economic impact to the family, the healthcare system, and wider society.
- Anaesthesia providers in some LMICs have very little role in the management of pain outside the operating theatre. Postoperative pain is often left to the surgical team and is managed poorly.
- There are potentially huge gains to be made through educational initiatives. This section is based on an educational programme called Essential Pain Management (EPM). EPM is designed for use in low-resource settings but is used worldwide, including in the UK. See 'Further Reading' in this chapter, p. 91.

Managing pain—general principles

EPM uses the acronym RAT: Recognize, Assess, and Treat.

Recognize

- Patients and staff may not report pain for many reasons, including beliefs that treatment will be unnecessary, ineffective, or unobtainable. Cultural reasons may also prevent reporting of pain.
- It is important to actively ask patients if they are in pain and to encourage other staff members to do the same.

Assess

- Assess the severity and type of pain, and other contributory factors.
- Pain scores (e.g. numbers, visual analogue scale) can be useful for assessing severity and the effectiveness of treatment but communication barriers, especially when working through translators, can be problematic. The use of a simple 0–3 pain scale (no pain, mild, moderate or severe pain) may be the most useful.
- The Faces Pain Scale (see Figure 5.1) was developed for the assessment of pain in children but may be useful for any patient when communication is difficult. A printable version and multiple translations are available. Note, however, that you should always try to get the patient to communicate their pain verbally in the first instance.
- The assessment of pain type can be simplified to acute or chronic, cancer or non-cancer, and nociceptive or neuropathic. This helps guide treatment and is a useful classification when teaching others.

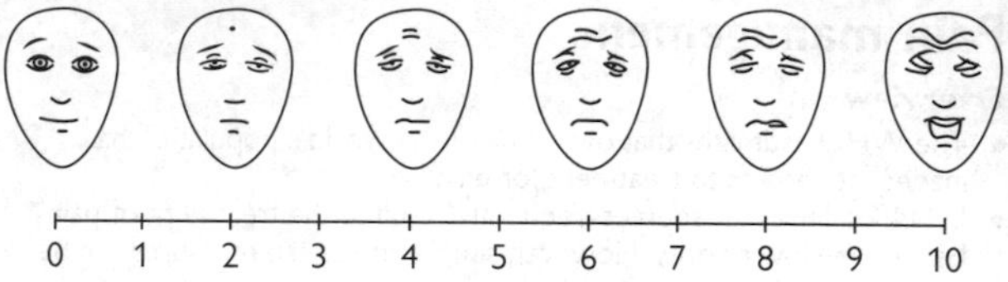

Figure 5.1 Faces Pain Scale.

Hicks CL, von Baeyer CL, Spafford P, van Korlaar I, Goodenough B. Faces Pain Scale—Revised: Towards a Common Metric in Pediatric Pain Measurement. *PAIN* 2001; 93: 73–183. With the instructions and translations as found on the website: http://www.iasp-pain.org/FPSR. This Faces Pain Scale—Revised has been reproduced with permission of the International Association for the Study of Pain® (IASP). The figure may NOT be reproduced for any other purpose without permission from IASP.

- Other factors may contribute to the patient's pain, including anxiety and coexisting illness.

Treat

- Non-pharmacological measures may be particularly important when medications are scarce or when treating some types of non-surgical pain, e.g. chronic cancer or non-cancer pain. Strategies include explanation and reassurance, immobilization of fractures, surgical interventions, and basic physiotherapy.
- For postoperative pain, use simple pharmacotherapy in the following order:
  - local anaesthetic infiltration by the surgeon
  - regular paracetamol (acetaminophen)
  - non-steroidal anti-inflammatory drugs (NSAIDs), codeine, tramadol—if available.
- The use of regional analgesia, e.g. peripheral nerve blocks or spinal, is especially useful in the management of postoperative pain where the availability of medications or trained recovery staff is limited.
- In many resource-poor environments, complex techniques, such as epidural analgesia or nerve plexus infusions, will not be appropriate.
- In general, be very careful about introducing new treatment techniques. You will need to consider factors such as educational requirements, availability of equipment and medications, and management of potential complications. Also, consider who will ensure good governance of novel techniques when you have returned home.
- Patient controlled analgesia (PCA) is often not possible because of a lack of equipment and training.

Pharmacological treatment of acute pain

- The WHO ladder, originally created for the treatment of cancer pain, describes a stepwise approach to treating pain of escalating severity.
- It can be 'reversed' (see Figure 5.2) and used to guide the pharmacological treatment of acute pain. For severe acute pain, start at step 3 of the ladder and move down the steps as the acute pain subsides.
- Encourage the use of regular rather than 'as required' analgesia for the treatment of moderate to severe pain.
- In many hospitals, there are no simple guidelines or protocols for the management of pain. Overseas teams can make a very valuable contribution by helping to develop and implement these documents—contact EPM (see 'Further Reading') for sample protocols.

Opioids

- Morphine and other strong opioids often have low/no availability in LMICs, especially in sub-Saharan Africa, despite inclusion in the WHO's Model List of Essential Medications. Country-level data showing opioid use, broadly reflecting availability, are available.
- Even when available, there may be reluctance to use strong opioids ('opiophobia') because of concerns about side effects and addiction. It is important to try and understand these concerns when treating patients with severe pain.
- Morphine is cheap and very effective for the treatment of acute nociceptive pain and cancer pain. However, in some environments, inadequate staffing and monitoring combined with low knowledge levels may mean that the use of strong opioids for postoperative pain should be restricted to the operating theatre and recovery areas.
- In better-resourced environments, it may be appropriate to use low-dose oral morphine for postoperative patients on the ward.

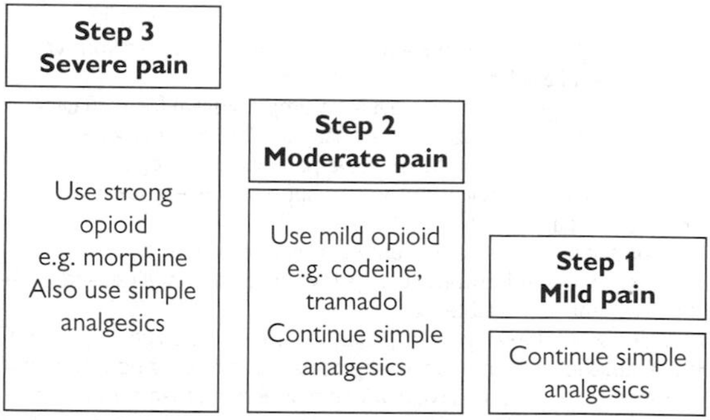

Figure 5.2 Reverse WHO pain ladder for treatment of acute pain.

Adapted with permission from WHO. Cancer pain ladder for adults. https://www.who.int/cancer/palliative/painladder/en.

- Ideally, naloxone should be readily available when strong opioids are used.
- The WHO recommends regular oral morphine for the treatment of cancer pain.
- In some LMICs, pethidine is more easily available than morphine and is seen (incorrectly) as a 'safer morphine'. Other opioids, now less commonly used in HICs, such as pentazocine and buprenorphine, may also be available.

Other analgesic medications

- Ketamine is often more easily available than strong opioids and may be a good option for treating moderate to severe pain in recovery or on the ward, especially in the absence of naloxone and/or adequate safeguards for the use of morphine and strong opioids. See 'Ketamine' in Chapter 4 (p. 56).
- Recent evidence suggests that a low-dose ketamine bolus (e.g. 0.2–0.3 mg/kg IV intra-operatively) may reduce the risk of chronic post-surgical pain in susceptible patients.
- Unfamiliar medications may be available, e.g. metamizole (dipyrone)—a centrally acting cyclo-oxygenase inhibitor with minimal anti-inflammatory effects (typical dose: 500 mg three to four times daily). Always check local protocols before using any unfamiliar drugs.

Treatment of other types of pain

- You may be asked for advice about managing non-surgical pain. Do not underestimate your knowledge in this area—as an anaesthetist you will probably be in a good position to offer helpful advice.
- A good starter question to the local provider is: 'How would you usually manage this problem?' This puts the problem in a local context and can give very useful information about local resources and constraints.

Cancer pain

- There is a high burden of painful cancer in LMICs coupled with very low levels of opioid availability.
- The WHO analgesic ladder provides a simple system for managing cancer pain and emphasizes giving analgesics 'by mouth, by the clock, and by the ladder'. If possible manage patients at home.
- Prescribe adjuvant medications where appropriate, e.g. laxatives, steroids, antispasmodics.
- Neuropathic pain may be present in invasive cancer and should be treated with medications such as low-dose amitriptyline, and anticonvulsants if available.
- There are several examples of palliative care services running in LMICs with established systems for managing pain and running educational programmes. They may have a wider clinical remit than services in HICs and be a valuable source of expertise and local knowledge. More information is available at the International Association for Hospice and Palliative Care (http://www.hospicecare.com).

Chronic non-cancer pain

- Examples include chronic back pain, chronic headache, and arthritis. These types of pain can be very difficult to treat.
- The pain may have nociceptive and neuropathic features.
- Non-pharmacological treatments are likely to be relatively important and, in general, strong opioids should be avoided.
- Antidepressants and anticonvulsants may be helpful.

Neuropathic pain

- This is defined by the International Association for the Study of Pain (IASP) as pain 'caused by a lesion or disease of the somatosensory nervous system'. It is classically described using terms like burning, shooting, pins and needles, or electric shocks.
- Neuropathic pain is underdiagnosed and undertreated, even in high-income settings, so it is important to ask about symptoms.
- Causes include post-amputation pain, spinal cord injury, HIV, chronic post-surgical pain, and diabetes.
- Neuropathic pain can be very difficult to treat and frequently does not respond to standard analgesics.
- The following medications are currently recommended in many HICs specifically for the treatment of neuropathic pain: tricyclic antidepressants (e.g. amitriptyline), serotonin-noradrenaline reuptake inhibitor antidepressants (e.g. duloxetine) and anticonvulsants (e.g. gabapentin and pregabalin), and, in some circumstances, carbamazepine.
- Medication availability is highly likely to be problematic in LMICs, with only amitriptyline and carbamazepine currently included in the WHO's Model List of Essential Medicines.
  - The amitriptyline dose is usually 25 mg at night. Start low, go slow, especially in elderly patients, e.g. start at 10 mg, increase every 2–3 days as tolerated.
  - The carbamazepine dose is 100–200 mg BD PO, increased to 200–400 mg QDS as tolerated.
- Side effects with all of these medications are common but can be minimized by starting at low doses and slowly titrating as tolerated.

Anaesthesia at high altitude

As altitude increases, the percentage of oxygen in the atmosphere remains the same, but the partial pressure falls, reducing oxygen delivery and altering oxygen utilization in the tissues. Altitude illness usually occurs above 2,500 m and rapid ascent is the primary risk factor. *Acclimatization* is adaptation to altitude, and rates vary between individuals. The mountain environment also presents risks of hypothermia and cold injury, dehydration, sunburn, and trauma.

Acute physiological changes

- High altitude increases: minute ventilation, alveolar–arterial gradient, cardiac output, cerebral and pulmonary blood flow, hypoxic pulmonary vasoconstriction, haematocrit (due to reduced plasma volume followed by erythropoiesis and angiogenesis), urine output, and renal bicarbonate excretion.
- There is activation of the acute phase response leading to microcirculatory dysfunction, increased thrombotic events, and catabolism.
- Sleep becomes poor and periodic breathing occurs.
- There are variable effects on cognition, judgement, and memory for both the patient and the treating clinician.

Altitude illnesses

Acute mountain sickness

- Symptoms and signs: headache, dizziness, vomiting, anorexia, fatigue, and sleep disturbance within 36 h of altitude exposure.
- Self-limiting.
- Oxygen saturations are of limited use in acute altitude illness, but trends may help monitor the effects of therapy.
- Treat with descent and oxygen. Consider acetazolamide 250 mg BD PO and dexamethasone 4 mg PO stat dose.

High-altitude cerebral oedema (HACE)

- Ataxia (most important sign, positive Romberg's test—can they stand with feet together and eyes closed).
- Severe headache, vomiting, and confusion.
- Potentially life-threatening, treat with descent, oxygen, and dexamethasone 8 mg IV/IM/PO. Consider acetazolamide 250 mg BD PO.

High-altitude pulmonary oedema (HAPE)

- Dyspnoea at rest, cough, frothy sputum, cyanosis.
- Crepitations may be unilateral or absent and HAPE has been fatally misdiagnosed as pneumonia.
- Potentially life-threatening, avoid any further exertion and treat with descent, oxygen, and nifedipine 20 mg TDS oral. Consider adding acetazolamide, dexamethasone, portable hyperbaric chamber (Gamow bag) or continuous positive airway pressure (CPAP).

- *Do not treat* with morphine and diuretics as you might with other forms of pulmonary oedema.
- HACE and HAPE may coexist and exacerbate one another.

Chronic mountain sickness (Monge's syndrome)
Syndrome of long-term high-altitude residence

- Polycythaemia, dyspnoea, cyanosis, venodilatation, insomnia, dizziness, paraesthesia, confusion. Finger clubbing, right ventricular hypertrophy, raised pulmonary artery pressure, *cor pulmonale*, and congestive cardiac failure.
- Relocate to lower altitude before surgery if possible, encourage smoking cessation and weight loss, consider isovolumetric venesection and acetazolamide 250 mg daily for 3–12 weeks prior to surgery (limited evidence).

Infants born at, or travelling to, high altitude are at risk of pulmonary hypertension, pulmonary oedema, and delayed closure of the ductus arteriosus.

Preoperative care

- Assess altitude status:
  - Unacclimatized.
  - Acclimatized.
  - High-altitude dweller.
- Treat altitude illness:
  - Consider chest radiograph to look for oedema or cardiomegaly.
  - Ask explicitly if patient has been taking dexamethasone (consider perioperative steroid cover).
- Warm to normothermia prior to surgery.
- Monitor blood glucose and fluid status carefully.
- Consider perioperative oxygen supplementation if available.

Intraoperative care

- Preoxygenate (reduced partial pressure of arterial oxygen (PaO_2) and functional residual capacity (FRC)) and humidify gases where possible.
- All patients are at risk of aspiration from delayed gastric emptying.
- Avoid IV injection of air bubbles (there is a higher prevalence of patent foramen ovale at altitude).
- Maintain normothermia.
- Take extra care with pressure areas.

Drugs may have different potencies at high altitude: there is limited evidence, but long-term high-altitude dwellers may require higher doses of propofol and there has been a case report of apnoea with low doses of ketamine. Nitrous oxide is less efficacious at a given percentage compared with administration at sea level.

Regional techniques appear similarly efficacious at altitude as at sea level, though there is a report of increased rates of post-dural puncture headache. Be cautious with any technique that may cause pneumothorax or phrenic nerve palsy.

Coagulation at high altitude is incompletely understood: the overall tendency appears to be prothrombotic.

Postoperative care

- Impaired wound healing.
- Low threshold for thromboprophylaxis.
- Avoid drugs that blunt hypoxic respiratory drive (opioids and benzodiazepines).
- Dexamethasone is a useful antiemetic.

Effects on anaesthetic equipment

- Endotracheal tube (ETT) and laryngeal mask airway (LMA): if anticipating a change in altitude, consider filling cuffs with saline rather than air to avoid barotrauma or dislodgement.
- Capnographs may malfunction at high altitude and should be recalibrated at ambient pressure.
- Ventilators may misreport tidal volumes and tend to under-deliver unless pressure-compensated.
- Bobbin flowmeters deliver more gas than set (i.e. they under-read) at altitude.
- Venturi masks deliver a slightly higher fraction of oxygen.
- Vaporizers—the potency of anaesthetic gases is proportional to their partial pressure. In variable-bypass vaporizers, delivered concentration will increase as barometric pressure falls and partial pressure remains the same, so providing an equipotent anaesthetic at altitude as at sea level (i.e. set the vaporizer percentage the same as at sea level). The Ohmeda Tec 6 (desflurane) vaporizer is an exception, and set percentage needs to be increased with altitude. Most vaporizers have some degree of temperature compensation or buffering, however if the ambient temperature is below their operating range, the set percentage may also need to be increased to achieve equipotent anaesthesia.

Further reading

Preoperative assessment

McQueen K et al. (2015) The bare minimum: the reality of global anaesthesia and patient safety. *World J Surg* 39 (9): 2153–2160.

Bainbridge D et al. (2012) Perioperative and anaesthetic-related mortality in developed and developing countries: a systematic review and meta-analysis. *Lancet* 380 (9847): 1075–8.1

Consent

Swiss commission for research partnerships with developing countries (2012) A guide for transboundary research partnerships: 11 principles: 7 questions. DOI:10.7892/boris.81006

Grady C et al. (2017) Informed consent. *N Engl J Med* 376 (9): 856–857.

Bhutta ZA (2004) Beyond informed consent. *WHO Bull* 82(10): 771–777.

BMA (n.d.) BMA advice, available at: https://www.bma.org.uk/advice/career/going-abroad/volunteering-abroad/gmc-guidance (accessed February 2018).

Pain management

Essential Pain Management: http://www.essentialpainmanagement.org

Faculty of Pain Medicine, Australian and New Zealand College of Anaesthetists (2015) Evidence on pain management, available at: http://www.fpm.anzca.edu.au/documents/apmse4_2015_final (accessed September 2019).

International Association for the Study of Pain: http://www.iasp-pain.org

WHO (n.d.) WHO global atlas on palliative care at the end of life: worldwide provision of palliative care services and barriers to implementation, available at: http//:www.thewhpca.org/resources/global-atlas-on-end-of-life-care (accessed September 2019).

Anaesthesia at high altitude

Johnson C et al. (2015) *Oxford Handbook of Expedition and Wilderness Medicine*, 2nd ed. Oxford: Oxford University Press.

Leissner KB, Mahmood FU (2009) Physiology and pathophysiology at high altitude: considerations for the anesthesiologist. *J Anesth* 23 (4): 543–553.

Luks AM et al. (2014) Wilderness Medical Society practice guidelines for the prevention and treatment of acute altitude illness: 2014 update. *Wilderness Environ Med* 25: S4–S14.

Further reading

Chapter 6

The Difficult Airway

Rachael Craven and Rachel McKendry

Assessment and planning

Airway-related difficulties in the developing world may be more challenging due to limited anaesthetic and airway equipment, advanced pathology, and late presentation of congenital abnormalities. Many difficulties can be navigated with thorough preoperative assessment, planning, and a team-based approach. This being said, it is prudent to consider your resources when undertaking a difficult elective or semi-elective case if the expertise and equipment available do not provide a safe option for anaesthesia and surgery. In these cases the patient should, if possible, be transferred to a suitable centre.

Contributing factors in airway disasters

- Failure to properly assess the airway.
- Poor planning and communication.
- Failure to plan for failure.
- No plan for extubation—one third of airway incidents happen during emergence and recovery.

Airway assessment

- Mallampati score, thyromental distance, jaw protrusion, neck mobility.
- Stridor, voice change, drooling, nutritional status.
- Can the patient lie flat? Are there any symptoms of airway obstruction in any particular positions?
- Examine the oral cavity thoroughly using a light and check nasal passage patency. Check under the tongue for mandibular tori (bony mandibular outgrowths in the floor of the mouth, more commonly seen in East Asian and Inuit populations).
- Ensure that the neck has been examined (including patients wearing head scarves).
- Prior to any difficult airway case the crico-thyroid membrane should be located and marked for potential emergency front of neck access.
- Chest X-ray, if relevant, looking for tracheal deviation.

Planning

- After thorough assessment discuss options with the surgeon. Is a local/regional technique possible?
- Ensure the whole team is aware of airway plans A, B, C, etc. and their role in them, including the surgeon for front of neck access.
- Ensure your equipment for each airway plan is in reaching distance and checked—you will probably not have a trained assistant who understands when you shout for a bougie, alternative blade, etc.
- Ensure you have everything you need for optimal positioning of the patient—ramped position, ear level with sternal notch, head extended on a flexed neck.

Useful techniques

Spontaneous breathing under ketamine

Indications

- Useful in patients requiring short (<45 min) procedures where intubation/oral access/face mask ventilation is expected to be difficult.
- Examples:
    - Cleaning and debridement of facial burns.
    - Incision and drainage of dental/neck abscesses.
    - Release of burns contractures causing limited mouth opening or neck movement to then allow intubation/laryngeal mask airway (LMA) insertion.

Method

- Preoxygenate and give supplemental oxygen throughout.
- An antisialagogue is recommended.
- Use slow titration of ketamine to avoid apnoea.

Troubleshooting

- Airway obstruction and/or apnoea are uncommon but possible; jaw thrust or nasopharyngeal airway may be required.
- Laryngeal reflexes are well preserved so laryngeal spasm is possible, careful suctioning of secretions is needed.
- You must have a plan for loss of the airway.

Spontaneous breathing facemask volatile anaesthesia

Indications

- Useful in patients requiring short (<45 min) procedures where intubation/oral access is expected to be difficult but no problems are anticipated with face mask ventilation.
- Also used to obtain sufficient depth of anaesthesia and suppression of laryngeal reflexes to allow attempt at intubation whilst maintaining spontaneous respiration.

Method

- Co-induction with ketamine or gas induction alone to maintain respiration.
- Spontaneous breathing of volatile to achieve surgical depth of anaesthesia.
- Sevoflurane or halothane are the smoothest agents to use.
- There should be a gradual increase in volatile percentage to avoid apnoea.
- Adequate depth of anaesthesia is gauged by Guedel's eye signs (eyes return to centre, pupils mid-sized), regular respiration, and no toe movement with jaw thrust.
- If the aim is intubation, if a good view is obtained at laryngoscopy, muscle relaxation may be given to aid intubation.

Troubleshooting

- Breath holding during gas induction can occur; this may be less of a problem if ketamine is used for co-induction as the patient passes through the phases of anaesthesia more rapidly.
- Airway obstruction, hypoventilation, and apnoea are more common than with ketamine spontaneous breathing technique so you must be prepared with nasopharyngeal or Guedel airways and to assist ventilation with a bag and mask.

Local anaesthetic topicalization of the airway

Indications

- This allows a variety of awake airway techniques to be performed, such as awake LMA insertion, awake blind nasal intubation, awake direct laryngoscopy, and awake fibreoptic intubation

Method

- Good communication and rapport with the patient is essential.
- The maximum dose of lidocaine via the topical route is 9 mg/kg.
- Use an antisialagogue to dry secretions and aid topicalization.
- For topicalization of the nose:
  - Use 2% lidocaine (4% is better but is rarely found).
  - Spray along the floor of the nose front, middle, and back using an atomizer if possible.
  - Repeat whilst the patient takes a deep breath to help topicalize the glottis.
  - Repeat with ephedrine 0.5% or phenylephrine 0.05% or adrenaline 1:200,000 to vasoconstrict.
  - Mix KY Jelly® with 2% lidocaine and coat a nasopharyngeal airway for nasal dilation and further topicalization.
- For topicalization of the oropharynx:
  - Use a gargle with 2% lidocaine or a spray as for the nose.
- For topicalization of the glottis:
  - Spray 2% lidocaine (as for the nose) at the back of the throat.
  - If a nebulizer is available, then 2% lidocaine may be nebulized to help anaesthetize the entire airway.
- For topicalization of the sub-glottis:
  - Nebulized lidocaine as above.,
  - Or cricothyroid puncture with 22G cannula, then spray 2% lidocaine through the cannula.
- The adequacy of oropharyngeal anaesthesia may be usefully assessed by suctioning the back of the mouth.

Awake LMA insertion

Indications

- For patients with abnormal anterior oral anatomy or decreased mouth opening (sufficient to allow LMA insertion) but a normal glottis, e.g. noma, burns contractures.
- Mask ventilation is expected to be difficult.

Method

- Topicalize the oropharynx and glottis as above.
- Insert an LMA and ensure it is well secured and the airway is unobstructed before the induction of anaesthesia.

Troubleshooting

- A reinforced LMA, if available, usually works best but may need to be guided in with a finger or stylet.

Intubation through LMA

Indications

- For patients with anticipated or unanticipated difficult intubation.
- May be used after awake LMA insertion in anticipated difficult intubation but the subglottis will need to be topicalized as well.

Method

- Place the LMA and ensure a clear airway.
- Pass a bougie through the LMA, feel the 'clicks' of the tracheal rings.
- Remove the LMA leaving the bougie in place.
- Railroad an endotracheal tube (ETT) over the bougie; a laryngoscope or jaw thrust will aid passage through the glottis.
- Alternatively, a well-lubricated size 6.5 ETT will pass through a size 4 iGel™ or Proseal™ LMA.
- If available this can be done under direct vision using a fibreoptic scope.

Troubleshooting

- Jaw thrust and pressure on the LMA may be required, especially with an anterior larynx.
- The LMA classic has bars across its opening that may need to be cut—Proseal™, iGel™, and intubating LMAs are all good options.
- Lubricate the bougie and ETT well.

Blind nasal intubation

Indications

- This is useful in patients where access for a laryngoscope is difficult, e.g. trismus from all causes, anterior oral tumours, etc.
- This is a spontaneously breathing technique that may be performed either under deep inhalational anaesthesia, awake under topical anaesthesia, or under topical anaesthesia with ketamine sedation. For awake and sedated procedures an antisialagogue is recommended.

Method

- Positioning: pillow under occiput so neck is slightly flexed and head slightly extended on neck.
- Give oxygen via the contralateral nostril.
- Use most patent nostril.
- Ensure adequate anaesthesia.
- Instill vasoconstrictors in the nose (e.g. ephedrine 0.5%, phenylephrine 0.05%, adrenaline 1:200,000).
- Gently insert well-lubricated 6.0 or 6.5 endotracheal tube along floor of nose, with the cuff completely deflated.

- Once in the pharynx listen for breath sounds and watch for misting of the tube, or if capnography is available watch the capnography trace.
- Advance the tube on inspiration.
- Further local anaesthetic may be 'sprayed as you go' down the ETT.
- Observe the neck to watch for tube impingement to the right or left of the larynx: if noted, withdraw and rotate tube appropriately.
- Keep the proximal end of the tube pointing towards the contralateral nipple to aid directing the tip of the tube towards the midline.
- Gently advance the tube into the trachea.
- Confirm tube placement.
- If awake, induce anaesthesia and then inflate cuff.

Troubleshooting

Tube going posteriorly into oesophagus

- May be recognized by loss of breath sounds.
- Extend the head further.
- Slowly withdraw the ETT until breath sounds reappear and are maximal.
- Gently inflate the ETT cuff to push the tube away from the posterior pharyngeal wall.
- Pass a nasogastric tube or paediatric bougie down the ETT into the larynx.
- Deflate the ETT cuff.
- Railroad the ETT over the nasogastric tube.

Tube hitting anterior larynx or epiglottis

- Flex the head on the neck.
- In the awake patient ask them to protrude their tongue.
- In the asleep patient perform a jaw thrust.
- Rotate the tube 180°.

Tube going to right or left of larynx

- Withdraw the tube a few centimetres.
- Rotate the ETT in the direction required.
- Manipulate the larynx in the direction required.

Front of neck access

- Should be performed by the person with the most experience—this may be the surgeon or the anaesthetist.
- Depending on the experience of the operator, the safest and quickest option is generally to perform a cricothyrotomy, which, once the airway is secured, may then be converted to a tracheostomy if required.
- Equipment: size 10 scalpel blade, artery forceps or tracheal dilator, bougie, size 6 ETT or tracheostomy tube.

Indications

- May be performed electively as plan A under local anaesthetic in the awake patient or, for those unable to cooperate, it may be performed under ketamine sedation.
- May be performed as a 'plan B' under controlled circumstances where plan A has failed or as an emergency in patients who have lost their airway.

Method

- Position with roll under the shoulders for maximum neck extension.
- Identify the cricothryroid membrane by palpation (Figure 6.1) or by ultrasound (Figure 6.2).
- The most prominent landmark is the thyroid cartilage notch; the membrane is approx. 20 mm caudad to this.
- Infiltrate lidocaine with adrenaline.
- Stabilize the thyroid cartilage.

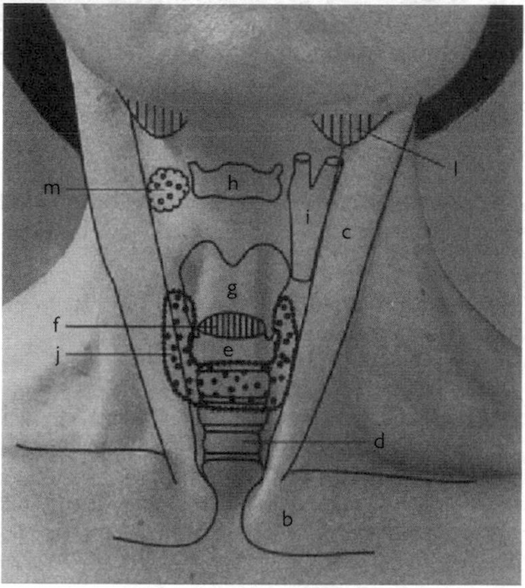

Figure 6.1 Surface anatomy of cricothyroid membrane. (b) clavicle, (c) sternocleidomastoid, (d) trachea, (e) cricoid cartilage, (f) cricothyroid membrane, (g) thyroid cartilage, (h) hyoid, (i) carotid bifurcation, (j) thyroid.

Reproduced from R. Corbridge and N. Steventon. The Neck. In: *Oxford Handbook of ENT and Head and Neck Surgery* (2 ed.). Oxford, UK: Oxford University Press. Copyright © 2009, Oxford University Press.

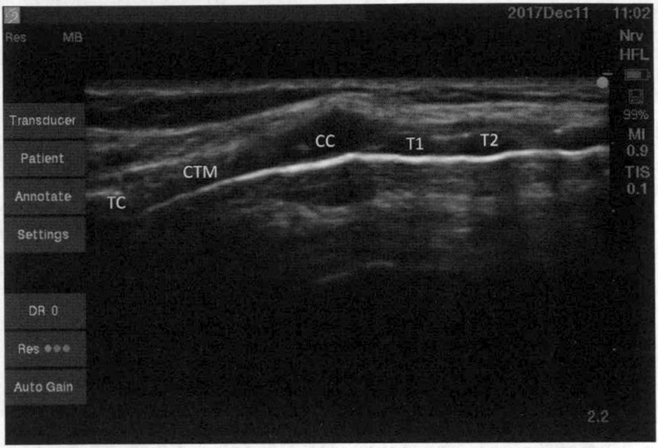

Figure 6.2 Ultrasound anatomy of cricothyroid membrane. Sagittal view. TC thyroid cartilage, CTM cricothyroid membrane, CC cricoid cartilage, T1 tracheal ring 1, T2 tracheal ring 2.

- Make a 4 cm vertical incision through the skin over the cricothyroid; blunt dissect with fingers to the membrane.
- Make a horizontal incision through the membrane, rotate the scalpel through 180°.
- Open the hole with artery forceps alongside the scalpel.
- Insert a bougie.
- Railroad tube.

Tracheostomy care

In many settings experience with tracheostomy care may be low. In general, these patients will need to be nursed in a critical care area allowing a better nurse to patient ratio. As the anaesthetist the supervision and management of these tracheostomies on the ward may be down to you. For emergency management of a tracheostomy, see Figure 6.3.

General nursing care of tracheostomy patients

Monitoring

- The patient should be monitored for any difficulty with respiration and the anaesthetist alerted if necessary.
- The tracheostomy should be checked regularly to make sure it is well secured and that the dressings are clean.
- If the cuff is inflated, ensure that it is not overinflated.

Equipment

- Oxygen and suction with suction catheters should be available.
- If possible, oxygen should be humidified—a heat moisture exchanger (HME) filter can be used.
- A spare tracheostomy tube of the same size and one size smaller should be available, along with a tracheal dilator and bougie should the tracheostomy become dislodged.
- A paediatric face mask should be available to ventilate the stoma in an emergency

Cleaning

- Tracheostomy tubes may become blocked with secretions.
- If available use a tracheostomy inner tube that can be removed and cleaned—this should occur at least every 6 h—using sterile water.

Suctioning

- Clean technique should be used with a new suction catheter each time.
- Frequency will be patient dependent—poor cough, noisy breathing, decreasing saturations, and visible secretions in the tube are all indications for suction.
- Saline nebulizers loosen secretions and aid clearance.

Oral hygiene

- Swallow may be affected and secretions may pool in the mouth.
- Regular oral hygiene is required to reduce aspiration/pneumonia risk.

Tracheostomy change

- The first change should not happen before 7 days to ensure the tract is fully established.
- Tubes should be changed every 10 days or every 28 days if an inner tube is present; it may need changing sooner if there is evidence of blockage.
- Ensure you have a tracheostomy tube of the same size and one size smaller.
- Ensure you have equipment and drugs for emergency reintubation if there is a patent glottis.
- Always use an airway exchange device such as a suction catheter to ensure you do not make a false passage.

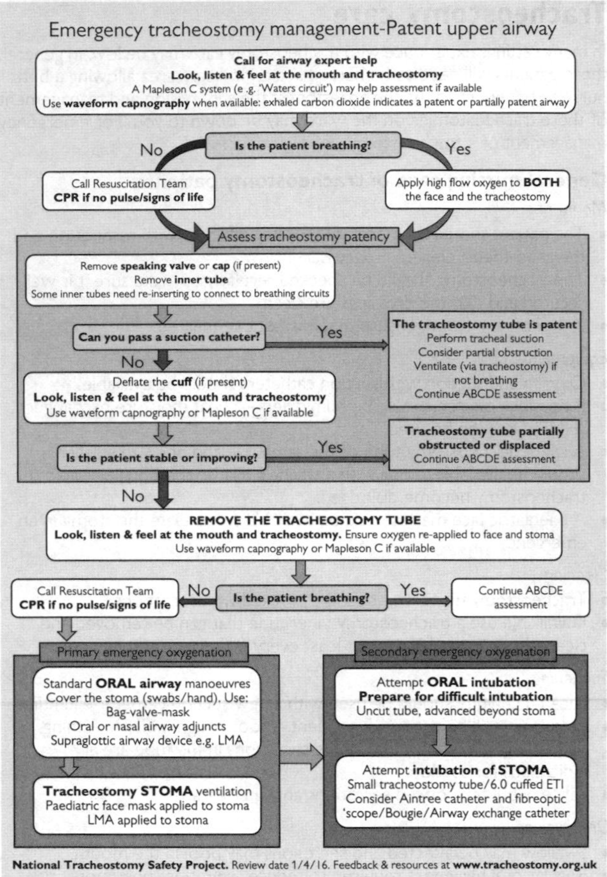

Figure 6.3 Emergency management of the tracheostomy patient with breathing difficulties.

Decannulation

- Can occur when the patient:
  - is able to clear secretions without suction
  - has tolerated the cuff down for 24 h
  - upper airway is patent (they are able to vocalize or breath with the cuff down and trachy tube occluded)
  - is able to swallow secretions.
- Once decannulated, cover the stoma with a clean dressing.
- The stoma will close naturally within 1–2 weeks.

Common pathologies and considerations

Tumours

- Large tumours of the oral cavity (especially the tongue) may make oral intubation impossible. Awake intubation is preferable. Tracheostomy under local anaesthetic should be considered.
- Ameloblastomas are (usually) benign growths of the odontogenic epithelium causing tumours of the lower and upper jaw and localized tissue destruction. These have the potential to become massive. If the mandible is involved, access for a tracheostomy may be challenging.
- Massive facial tumours may involve a significant proportion of the cardiac output. Availability of blood is important in these cases, especially in the paediatric population. If possible, computerized tomography (CT) imaging +/− angiography should be carried out.

Infection

- Noma virus (p. 137) can cause gross deformity of the anterior and superior airway structures, though the pharynx and larynx are usually normal.
    - Bony ankylosis may cause complete trismus, rendering access via the mouth very difficult. Such cases can normally be managed with awake or asleep nasal fibreoptic intubation or blind nasal intubation, or intubation via an LMA if access allows.
    - Bag mask ventilation is normally straightforward in these patients, perhaps assisted by a low body mass index (BMI).

Burns

- Facial burns often present as healed contractures. Restriction of jaw and neck movement may cause problems for intubation.
- Release of contractures under local anaesthetic or under ketamine sedation may be helpful to enable intubation if required.

Thyroid

- Endemic goitres may be very large. Check for retrosternal extension and prepare accordingly.
- Intubation is rarely difficult but the larynx is often deviated to the side.
- Before closure ensure the surgeon checks for venous bleeding using a Valsava manoeuvre and head down tilt, and arterial bleeding by augmenting the blood pressure.

Congenital

- Cleft lip surgery may be operated on under ketamine, local anaesthetic, and nasal oxygen. For cleft palate surgery, the patient should be intubated as bleeding into the airway may occur. See 'Paediatric Surgical Conditions' in Chapter 7 (p. 130).

Management of the unanticipated difficult intubation

- Basic management of the unanticipated difficult airway should not stray far from Difficult Airway Society (DAS) guidelines (Figure 6.4) even in a resource-limited environment.

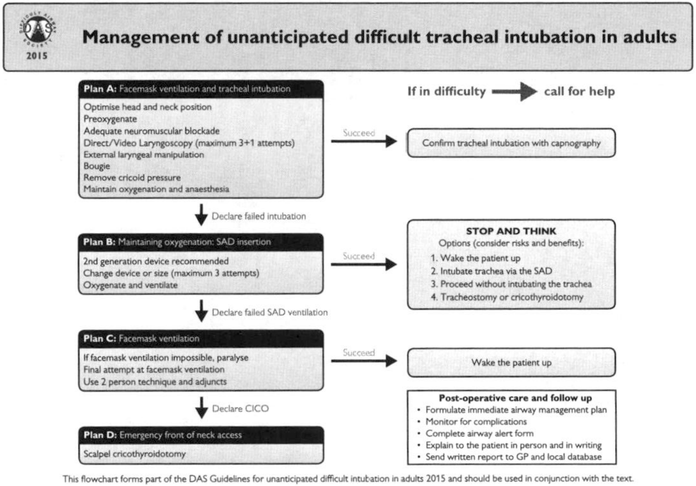

Figure 6.4 Difficult Airway Society 2015 guidelines for management of unanticipated difficult intubation in adults. SAD, supraglottic airway device, e.g. LMA; CICO, cannot intubate cannot oxygenate.

- In 'can't intubate **can** ventilate' scenarios front of neck access may be a safer option in some cases rather than waking the patient up since:
  - Surgery is often urgent.
  - Awake intubation options may be limited.
  - Neuromuscular blocker and reversal agent availability may limit options for the rapid resumption of spontaneous ventilation.

This should be balanced with the risk of tracheostomy and subsequent care and safety of a tracheostomy in your particular hospital setting.

Further Reading

Apfelbaum JL et al. (2013) Practice guidelines for management of the difficult airway: an updated report by the American Society of Anesthesiologists task force on management of the difficult airway. *Anesthesiol* 118: 251–270.

Frerk C et al. (2015) Difficult Airway Society 2015 guidelines for management of unanticipated difficult intubation in adults. *Br J Anaesth*, 115 (6): 827–848.

Coupe M et al. Airway management in reconstructive surgery for noma (cancrum oris). *Anesth Analg* 117 (1): 210–217.

Chapter 7

Paediatric Anaesthesia

Nick Boyd, Ibironke Desalu, Faye Evans, Paul Firth, Sarah Hodges, Mary Nabukenya, Susane Nabulindo and Isabeau Walker[1]

1 Dr Faye Evans and Dr Isabeau Walker are the chapter leads.

Surgical systems for children in LMICs

There are few specialist paediatric surgeons or anaesthetists in LMICs, and even fewer children's hospitals. Up to 50% of the population in many countries is under 14 years, therefore most anaesthetists will manage children as part of their routine practice. This chapter considers general principles of paediatric anaesthesia in LMICs and specific common procedures.

The most common operations for children are for trauma (including burns), general and urological surgical conditions, congenital abnormalities, and infections. Late presentation is common, and most operations are conducted as urgent or emergent procedures. The risk of anaesthesia and surgery in neonates and infants is high. Mortality for conditions expected to have 90% survival in a high-income setting (e.g. abdominal wall defects) may have 90% mortality in LMICs, even in specialist hospitals. It is therefore important to remain realistic about what can be offered in the district hospital, and to always act in the best interests of the child. It can be difficult to accept a child dying in the knowledge that in a high-income country (HIC) they may have survived. Beware of heroic but futile surgery. Alternative choices may include offering a palliative intervention, such as a colostomy under local anaesthesia (LA), or not offering an intervention if the child has complex disease and surgery is likely to be futile.

Visiting teams

Specialist surgical visiting teams frequently provide surgery for children at district and referral hospital levels. It is essential for such teams to work closely with local colleagues, and to assess facilities carefully. Issues to consider include: the requirement for specialist drugs and/or equipment, the impact of the operative caseload on basic supplies such as appropriately sized endotracheal tubes (ETTs) and analgesia, the adequacy of postoperative care (particularly for major surgery), and its location (a paediatric ward generally being preferable to a general surgical ward). Potential pitfalls include proceeding with major surgery in an inappropriate setting, proceeding to operate on an unwell child (rather than optimizing and postponing surgery), and failure to work effectively with local paediatricians and other staff.

Assessment and preparation

Immature anatomy and physiology in neonates and infants increases vulnerability to illness, as well as to surgery and anaesthesia. The following definitions are used throughout this section:

Neonate: first 44 weeks of post-conceptual age
Premature neonate: under 37 weeks gestational age
Infant: 1–12 months old
Low birth weight (LBW): ≤2.5 kg at birth

General assessment

- History: may be scanty. Includes presenting condition, gestational age, birth history, postnatal course and feeding. Ask about wet nappies (renal function, hydration), and for neonates, ask about handling problems (respiratory distress, apnoeas, desaturations).
- Examination:
  - Check for signs of respiratory distress (tachypnoea, tachycardia, noisy breathing, nasal flare, recessions), circulatory compromise (tachypnoea, tachycardia, poor capillary refill, cool peripheries), and oxygen saturation.
  - Airway examination depends on the child's cooperation.
  - Check for clinical signs of anaemia—sclerae or palms. Consider preoperative iron supplements and treatment of common causes of anaemia (malaria, parasites).
- If the child has one congenital abnormality (e.g. cleft), look for other congenital abnormalities, e.g. cardiac anomalies.
- HIV: consider in children with chronic or atypical infections (including TB) or poor nutritional status. Untreated infants may have a high viral load; universal precautions should be used for all patients. A child with known HIV infection requires planned multidisciplinary care, and assessment of current status. Antiretroviral therapy (ART) should be continued perioperatively and meticulous aseptic technique used to protect the child from hospital acquired infection.
- Malnutrition: if possible, consider referral to a nutrition unit. May be due to feeding difficulties such as cleft palate.

Specific issues

The child with a cold

Upper respiratory tract infections (URTIs):

- are common in children
- increase the risk of perioperative complications such as laryngospasm, coughing, wheeze, and pneumonia.

Young children are often exposed to open cooking fires in the home and may have copious secretions, making them even more vulnerable to serious complications.

Consider postponing elective surgery for 2–4 weeks in the following situations, depending on local facilities for postoperative care:

- all infants <1 year

- airway surgery
- major surgery
- fever >38°C, general malaise
- productive cough or wheeze
- oxygen saturation <96% in air.

If surgery needs to proceed in an emergency, the child will need close postoperative monitoring, with a low threshold for antibiotics and oxygen therapy if oxygen saturations are <90%.

Difficult airways in children

Problems may relate to facemask ventilation or intubation or both. Neonates and infants may be more difficult to intubate than older children, compounded by the fact that they have limited oxygen reserves. Watch out for: noisy breathing (inspiratory or expiratory stridor, stertor), wheeze, increased work of breathing, and the child's preferred posture. Take particular note of neck movement and mouth opening, and examine the child in profile to look for micrognathia.

Acquired conditions associated with a difficult airway

- Acute obstruction:
  - infection (epiglottitis, retropharyngeal abscess)
  - foreign body aspiration
  - trauma.
- Chronic obstruction:
  - adenotonsillar hypertrophy
  - haemangioma
  - subglottic stenosis.
- Poor mouth opening or mobility of jaw, neck:
  - temporomandibular joint fusion (infection)
  - burns contractures
  - measles stomatitis
  - ameloblastoma.

Congenital conditions associated with a difficult airway

- Hypoplastic mandible (micrognathia)—difficult intubation:
  - Pierre Robin sequence
  - Treacher Collins
  - hemifacial microsomia (Goldenhar syndrome).
- Midface hypoplasia—difficult bag-mask ventilation (BMV):
  - craniofacial abnormalities, e.g. Apert, Crouzon or Pfeiffer syndrome.
- Macroglossia—difficult BMV **and** potential difficult intubation:
  - Downs syndrome
  - Beckwith–Wiedemann syndrome
  - mucopolysaccharidoses (Hunters, Hurlers).

The child with a murmur

Congenital heart disease is rare, but cardiac murmurs are common, particularly in children with fever or anaemia. Congenital heart disease increases the risk of anaesthesia and surgery. Ideally, a child with a murmur will be investigated. Babies with complex disease are unlikely to survive due to lack of access to corrective or palliative surgery. The most common cardiac conditions seen in older children are:

- Acyanotic conditions ('pink'):
  - atrial septal defect (ASD), ventricular septal defect (VSD), patent ductus arteriosus (PDA)
  - coarctation of the aorta, aortic stenosis, pulmonary stenosis
- Cyanotic conditions ('blue'):
  - tetralogy of Fallot.
- Acquired rheumatic heart disease is common in areas of overcrowding with poor nutrition.

Where referral is not available or surgery is emergent

Clinical differentiators of innocent and pathological murmurs include:

- 'Innocent' heart murmur: asymptomatic, with no other signs or symptoms of heart disease; murmur is quiet, early in systole, and changes with position (softer when standing).
- 'Pathological' heart murmur: murmur is diastolic, pansystolic, or late systolic, loud or continuous, associated with signs and symptoms of cardiac disease:
  - failure to thrive
  - recurrent chest infections
  - reduced exercise tolerance
  - hypertension
  - radiofemoral delay
  - syncope
  - cyanotic episodes.
- The following approach may be helpful in emergency surgery in a child with undiagnosed cardiac disease:
  - Child is breathless, pink, with cardiomegaly. The most likely condition is a left to right shunt causing heart failure with increased work of breathing (ASD, VSD, PDA). Avoid deep halothane anaesthesia and support ventilation during surgery.
  - Young child, 'well', but has always been blue. The most common condition is tetralogy of Fallot, which is associated with reduced pulmonary blood flow. As above, + use high inspired oxygen concentrations, control CO_2, and avoid sympathetic stimulation.
  - Any neonate, or older child with poor function, syncopal episodes, or who has become cyanosed. These cases are very high risk. Only lifesaving surgery should be undertaken. Use a balanced anaesthesia technique with positive pressure ventilation. Ketamine is useful.
  - Give perioperative antibiotic prophylaxis to all cases as indicated for the surgical procedure; consider specific endocarditis prophylaxis in high-risk dental surgery involving suturing or dental infection.

Preoperative investigations

- Weigh all children before surgery. In an emergency, the weight can be estimated using standard growth charts (50th centile), a Broselow tape, or according to standard formulae (see Appendix Table A.8), although these may overestimate the child's weight in some populations.

- Routine investigations are not required before elective surgery in healthy children. A full blood count (+/− malaria screen in endemic areas) may be indicated, particularly before major surgery. Electrolytes and blood cross-match may be required depending on the surgery.
- Blood sugar should always be measured in children with sepsis.

Preoperative instructions

- Ideally, children should be washed and a name band applied prior to surgery. Informed consent should be obtained, the surgical site marked, and a preoperative checklist completed to include weight, allergies, starvation time, and results of preoperative investigations.
- Excessive starvation before surgery increases discomfort for the child, increases the risk of hypovolaemia and hypoglycaemia, particularly in malnourished infants, and makes intravenous (IV) cannulation more difficult. See Table 7.1 for recommended fasting times.

Premedication

Routine sedative premedication is not required. Where a pre-med is indicated for anxiety, the following may be given 30 min prior to surgery (dilute IV midazolam or ketamine solution in juice or paracetamol syrup to hide the bitter taste):

- midazolam 0.5 mg/kg PO
- ketamine 5 mg/kg PO
- atropine 20 μg/kg (to reduce secretions associated with ketamine: may be given PO or can be administered IV at induction).

Neonates should have received vitamin K prior to surgery (in some countries, this is offered routinely at delivery).

Table 7.1 Fasting times in children.

Oral intake	Fasting time (h)
Water	2
Breastmilk	4
Cow's milk, infant formula	6
Food	6

Some centres now recommend a 1-h fasting time for water in children.

Induction and maintenance

Induction

- Parental presence on induction is to be encouraged, but the parent/caregiver may not know what to expect. A member of the theatre team should look after them.
- Prepare and check all equipment, drugs, and fluids before sending for the patient. Double-check drug doses. Identify a member of the theatre team to act as a dedicated assistant.
- Turn air conditioning off, minimize exposure by wrapping the child as far as possible. Warmed IV fluids can be used as warming devices, but must be wrapped to avoid direct skin contact and burns.
- Complete routine sign-in safety checks. Attach monitoring before induction if possible, minimum precordial stethoscope and oximeter.
- Obtain IV access, ideally prior to induction. Keep deadspace in the lines low, avoid airbubbles and make sure all drugs are flushed after administration.

Induction drugs

- Ketamine:
  - Intramuscular (IM): 5 mg/kg. Useful if no IV access, particularly in infants and young children.
  - IV: 1–2 mg/kg over 1 year (not more than 1 mg/kg < 1 year). Particularly useful in high-risk cases. Good perioperative analgesia is provided by 0.25–0.5 mg/kg IV. Emergence may be slow after ketamine anaesthesia, particularly in combination with opioids.
- Propofol IV: 2–3 mg/kg. Add lidocaine 1% (1 mg/kg) to reduce injection pain.
- Thiopental IV: 3–5 mg/kg (2 mg/kg in neonates/sick patients).
- Gas induction:
  - Be sure that the person who will manage the airway while IV access is obtained is appropriately skilled.
  - May be more challenging if using a draw-over system (as effective vaporization of agent depends on the mask–face seal).
  - Sevoflurane in oxygen (cupped hand or clear facemask): incremental induction or induction with 6% inspired concentration, reducing inspired concentration during maintenance. Emergence delirium may be problematic in young children, and is reduced if IV analgesia is used.
  - Halothane in oxygen: smooth induction. Increase concentration incrementally by 0.5% every few breaths. Beware deep halothane anaesthesia in infants or shocked patients, particularly if it takes a long time to obtain IV access. Do not increase inspired halothane above 3% and reduce the inspired concentration to 0.5–0.8% as soon as positive pressure ventilation is used.

Additional tips

- Rapid sequence induction may be indicated for the child with a (possible) full stomach. Ensure your assistant knows how to apply cricoid pressure. Effective preoxygenation can be difficult: modified rapid sequence induction is not uncommon, i.e. gentle positive pressure ventilation with cricoid pressure, prior to intubation.
- Check the position and length of the ETT if the child is intubated. The trachea is short in absolute terms, and uncut ETTs may be used routinely—confirm the ETT is well positioned and secure it carefully. Ketamine may induce copious secretions, affecting tape adhesion.

Maintenance

- A balanced anaesthesia technique is ideal, incorporating simple regional anaesthesia techniques wherever possible to reduce postoperative analgesia requirements on the ward.
- Extreme vigilance is required during the maintenance phase. Small children should be positioned with the arms at the level of the head to allow ready access to the IV line, and to monitor peripheral perfusion and capillary refill easily.
- Halothane-induced arrhythmia is associated with hypercarbia and high levels of endogenous adrenaline. Support ventilation, provide analgesia, and reduce the inspired halothane concentration. Resistant arrhythmias may resolve with magnesium 25 mg/kg IV.

Postoperative care

- Consider recovering children in theatre, particularly if there are limited recovery facilities.
- All neonates require monitoring for postoperative apnoeas; the baby should ideally be monitored in a special care unit. Failing this the baby should remain in a high-care area. Parents may be the most vigilant monitors for apnoea but will also need to sleep.
- Postoperative care facilities should be taken into account when planning the list, including lighting on the ward, oxygen, suction, monitoring, staffing, and power cuts. Special arrangements may be required if IV fluids or IV analgesia are required on the ward.

Equipment for paediatric anaesthesia

The continuous presence of a trained anaesthesia provider is essential.

The following equipment should always be available for children:

Airway equipment

- Facemasks: clear, sizes 0–4. Sizing: should touch the bridge of the nose and extend to below the lower lip.
- Oropharyngeal airways: sizes 000–4. Sized by holding against the side of the face—should reach from incisors to mandibular angle.
- Nasopharyngeal airways: sizes 20–34Fr, or the same size as an uncuffed ETT for that child. Sized from the external auditory meatus to the tip of the nose. Airways that are too long will induce coughing or laryngospasm. A shorter airway may be required if there is a congenital abnormality of the midface.
- Laryngeal mask airways (LMA): sizes 1–4. May be used for maintenance of anaesthesia or as a rescue airway in difficult intubation. See Appendix Table A.9 (p. 339) for LMA size by weight.
- Laryngoscopes: Macintosh sizes 1–3; a straight blade may be helpful for infants and neonates.
- ETTs:
  - Formulae to estimate ETT size are given in Appendix Table A.10 (p. 339).
  - Uncuffed tubes are commonly used below size 5.0, although cuffed tubes are available for all ages; the latter are particularly useful if not all sizes are available as the leak of a small ETT can be reduced by inflating the cuff slightly (if using, check cuff pressure <20 mmHg to minimize post-intubation swelling).
  - Preformed oral RAE (south-facing) tubes are useful in cleft, ear, nose, and throat (ENT), and eye surgery, though they may be too long in some populations.
  - An ETT that is too large will cause post-extubation stridor, but ventilation is impossible if the tube is too small. A high-pressure leak is acceptable around an uncuffed ETT. Routine use of a throat pack to seal the tube introduces unnecessary risk.
  - ETTs are often re-used—if this is common practice, confirm the lumen is clear immediately before use.
- Stylets and bougies: 6, 10, and 14Fr.

Ventilatory equipment and circuits

- Oxygen supply: high-pressure oxygen supplies may be limited. A working oxygen concentrator and back-up oxygen cylinder (size F or G) with appropriate valve and regulator are essential. A back-up power supply is important if relying on oxygen concentrators.
- Self-inflating bag: essential in case of equipment, power, or gas supply failure. Adult and child size (500 ml) bags must be available.
- Anaesthetic breathing systems:
  - Ayre's T-piece with Jackson Rees modification: commonly used for children <20 kg. Used with continuous flow or with fresh gas flow supplied by a draw-over machine or oxygen flowmeter.

- A circle system with adult-sized tubing (and appropriate monitoring) is acceptable for children >20 kg. Paediatric-sized tubing is preferable for children <20 kg.
- Draw-over anaesthesia can be used without modification for children >20 kg, or 15 kg if intermittent positive pressure ventilation (IPPV) is used, although inhalational induction, preoxygenation, and providing continuous positive airway pressure (CPAP) are more difficult. Below these limits, see 'Draw-over Anaesthesia' in Chapter 3 (pp. 40–45). Continuous flow anaesthesia is generally preferred for children <10 kg.

- Ventilation:
  - Use IPPV for children <5 kg and for children 5–10 kg if the procedure is longer than 20 min. Spontaneous ventilation is possible for children >10 kg, depending on the surgery.
  - Mechanical ventilator: if available, must be suitable for children, ideally with pressure-limited ventilation. Usual tidal volumes are 6–8 ml/kg, respiratory rate standard for the age of child and peak airway pressures <20 cmH_2O.
  - Heat and moisture exchanger (HME) filter: size by weight.

Cannulation and fluids

- Cannulae: 24–20G are suitable for most cases.
- Intraosseous (IO) access needle: for fluid resuscitation where IV access is difficult, particularly in shocked children; 19G butterfly needles (babies), large-bore adult cannulae, or a blood transfusion access needle may be used if specialized needles are not available.
- Paediatric burette (100 ml): for children <20 kg. If not available, manual injection of IV fluid using a 20 ml syringe is an option.

Monitoring

(Also see Chapter 2 (p. 21).)

'Highly recommended'

(Minimal standards of monitoring at all levels of hospital.)

- Pulse oximetry.
- Stethoscope (precordial), sphygmomanometer, thermometer.

'Recommended'

(Should be available at district hospital level and above.)

- Paediatric pulse oximeter probe: wrap around, paediatric clip, or ear probe. An adult probe can be used on the foot of infants.
- Automated non-invasive blood pressure monitor with appropriate cuff sizes to fit child.
- Electrocardiogram (ECG).
- Nerve stimulator.
- Glucometer.

Where available, integrated monitors with end-tidal carbon dioxide and agent monitoring are ideal.

Additional equipment

- Warming: consider warm blankets, over or under heating devices.
- Nasogastric (NG) tube: 6Fr-12Fr.

Fluid management in children

General principles of fluid management

Children should take fluids orally whenever possible, and should be given clear fluids up to 2 h preoperatively before elective surgery. Common pitfalls of IV fluid administration include:

- Iatrogenic hyponatraemia: isotonic fluids (e.g. Ringer's lactate, Hartmann's, 0.9% saline) should be used in the perioperative period.
- Excessive volume loading with crystalloids should be avoided in severely anaemic children.
- Neonates, malnourished children, or children suffering prolonged starvation may be at risk from perioperative hypoglycaemia.

Intraoperative fluid management

For losses, a simple approach is to give isotonic fluid boluses of 10–20 ml/kg, reassess clinical signs, and repeat as necessary. Monitor losses and check Hb, base excess, and lactate as able. Consider blood after 60–80 ml/kg IV fluid or reaching a transfusion trigger (Table 7.2). The latter will depend on the patient's age, comorbidities, the presence or absence of chronic anaemia, and the availability of other means of improving oxygen delivery and/or critical care.

- Warm fluids if high volumes or blood are given.
- Glucose-containing maintenance fluid (e.g. Ringer's 1% to –10% glucose) will be required in children at high risk of hypoglycaemia (e.g. neonates, extended fasting period, debilitated, or malnourished children). This should be given as a second infusion.

Blood transfusion

Estimated blood volume varies with age (see Table 7.3).

If the starting haemoglobin is known, the maximum allowable blood loss (MABL) before transfusion is required can be calculated:

$$MABL = \frac{starting\ Hb - trigger\ Hb}{starting\ Hb} \times EBV$$

Table 7.2 Transfusion triggers and patient condition.

Condition	Transfusion trigger	
	Hb (g/l)	Hct (%)
Healthy child	70	21
Severe sepsis	100	30
Cyanotic heart disease	100	30

Hb, haemoglobin Hct, haematocrit.

Table 7.3 Estimated blood volume.

Age	Estimated blood volume (ml/kg)
Premature neonate	100
Neonate	90
Infant	80
Adult	70

- For example, a healthy 20 kg child has a starting Hb of 120 g/l. The estimated blood volume is 1400 ml. Estimated blood loss before transfusion is required is:

$$MABL = \frac{120-70}{120} \times 1400 = 583\,ml$$

In general, minimize donor exposure by avoiding repeated small 'top-up' transfusions, and transfuse as much as possible from each donor unit. As a rough guide, 4 ml/kg packed cells raises the Hb by 10 g/l and 8 ml/kg whole blood raises the Hb by 10 g/l.

Postoperative fluid maintenance

Ideally, children should take fluids orally after surgery. IV fluids may be difficult to manage on the ward.

- Hypotonic IV fluids should be avoided. If the plasma sodium is not known, it is safer to use isotonic fluids postoperatively.
- Children <6 years require glucose in postoperative maintenance fluids, e.g. 5% glucose–Ringer's or 5% glucose–0.9% saline.
  - Make these by replacing 50 ml from a 500 ml bag of Ringer's or 0.9% saline with 50 ml 50% glucose.
- In neonates, a glucose-containing (D10) balanced salt solution should be continued for maintenance fluids in the perioperative period and guided by clinical assessment of fluid balance and plasma sodium levels.
- The Holliday and Segar '4:2:1' formula is used to calculate postoperative fluid volumes in infants and children (usual maximum: 2 l/day for females, 2.5 l/day for males) (see Table 7.4).
- Ongoing nasogastric losses should be replaced millilitre for millilitre with 0.9% saline with potassium chloride 10 mmol/l.

Table 7.4 IV maintenance fluid calculation by weight.

Weight	IV maintenance fluid volume (cumulative)	
	ml/kg/h	ml/kg/day
First 10 kg	4	100
Second 10 kg	2	50
Subsequent 10 kg	1	25

IV, intravenous.

Malnutrition

Causes of malnutrition

- Low energy intake: poor diet, inability to eat properly (e.g. cleft palate), poor absorption (e.g. intestinal worms).
- High energy expenditure: severe or repeated infections (e.g. TB, HIV, recurrent pneumonia), burns.

Classification of malnutrition

The classification of malnutrition severity is summarized in Table 7.5, for children aged 6 months to 5 years.
There are two distinct clinical malnutrition syndromes:

- Marasmus—caused by deficiency in protein and other nutrients. Characterized by severe muscle wasting.
- Kwashiorkor—caused by deficiency of protein despite adequate overall energy intake. Characterized by muscle wasting and peripheral oedema.

Signs of severe malnutrition

- Thin or wasted appearance.
- Peripheral oedema or abdominal swelling (can mask wasting).
- Dehydration (dry skin and mucous membranes, tongue, reduced skin turgor).
- Skin ulceration.
- Loss of appetite.
- Electrolyte abnormalities (particularly low potassium/magnesium).

Principles of refeeding and stabilization

- Admit the child for inpatient care if there is severe malnutrition, medical complications, severe oedema, or poor appetite.
- Treat shock, hypothermia, and hypoglycaemia. Antibiotics if septic.
- Avoid rapid IV fluid resuscitation as this will cause heart failure.
- Use oral or nasogastric (NG) rehydration solutions wherever possible. Ideally a specific Rehydration Solution for Malnutrition (ReSoMal) preparation should be used.
- Give micronutrient supplements, including vitamin A (recommended 5,000 IU daily). Avoid iron supplements for first 2 weeks.

Table 7.5 Severity criteria for acute malnutrition.

Severity of acute malnutrition	Mid-upper arm circumference (cm)	Weight for height Z-score*
None	>13.5	>−1
At risk	12.5–13.4	−2 to −1
Moderate	11.5–12.4	−3 to −2
Severe	<11.5	<−3

*Z-score or SD score: expresses how far from the reference average the measured value is, in standard deviations (SDs). It is found most easily by using a height–weight nomogram.

- Avoid giving high sodium loads; total body sodium is raised even if plasma sodium is low.
- Start refeeding gradually with frequent (every 2–3 h) small oral feeds to reduce the risk of developing refeeding syndrome. For full details of protocols see the World Health Organization (WHO) Pocket Book of Hospital Care for Children ('Further Reading' section).

General principles of anaesthesia

- Identify malnourished patients as early as possible.
- Involve general paediatric or malnutrition services if available.
- Postpone elective surgery to allow controlled refeeding and stabilization of condition for at least 2 weeks.
- For emergency surgery, correct dehydration, hypoglycaemia, significant electrolyte disturbance, and anaemia preoperatively.

Preoperative assessment

- Measure current weight.
- Assess for shock and signs of right heart failure: treat if present.
- Check blood sugar, Hb, electrolytes, renal function, and albumin if available. Treat as necessary.
- Minimize preoperative fasting, using fasting guidelines.
- Consider inserting NG tube pre-op to reduce gastric distension.

Intraoperative management

- Prepare usual equipment but ensure smaller sizes are available.
- High risk of hypothermia: warm theatre, fluids, use HME filter and blankets. Measure temperature intraoperatively if possible.
- Intubation is appropriate for most cases. Consider rapid sequence induction. All malnourished patients are at risk of a full stomach.
- Protect pressure areas and eyes (there is a risk of corneal rupture due to vitamin A deficiency).
- Smaller doses of anaesthetic agents are often required due to low plasma protein binding.
- Higher risk of arrhythmias; avoid deep halothane, catecholamines, and neostigmine if possible.
- Risk of hypoglycaemia; give maintenance fluids with glucose and check blood sugar regularly.

Postoperative management

- Extubate fully awake. Severely malnourished children are at risk of postoperative respiratory failure.
- Keep child warm and observe closely postoperatively.
- Restart oral or NG feeding as soon as possible. If oral or NG feeding is not possible, use continuous maintenance fluids with glucose and monitor for signs of pulmonary oedema.
- Involve paediatric or nutritional services if they are not already involved.

Critical care

There is a significant deficit of critical care services in LMICs. Many causes of critical illness in children are reversible, and application of basic critical care may be lifesaving.

Triage

- All children should be assessed on arrival to the hospital.
- For useful mnemonics, see 'Resuscitation of the Sick Child'.
- Provide emergency treatment before transfer to the critical care unit.

High-dependency unit (HDU) care

The essential aspects of high-dependency care for children may be achievable even in very low-resource settings. For a discussion of appropriate staffing and facilities and equipment, see Chapter 12. Note that appropriately sized equipment for children will be necessary (see 'Equipment for Paediatric Anaesthesia' in this chapter (p. 117–18), and 'Critical Care' in Chapter 2 (pp. 32–35)). Also consider the following.

Dedicated space

- In children's ward, near the nursing station, or a separate unit.

Guidelines

- Written admission and discharge criteria. Always consider family, cultural, and religious preferences.
- Standard guidelines for monitoring and recording essential clinical signs and early warning scores for children.
- Written guidelines for specific emergencies (e.g. hypoxia, dehydration, shock, acute hypoglycaemia, and nursing the unconscious child) and common conditions (e.g. malaria, pneumonia, and post-op care).

Intensive care unit (ICU) care

There should ideally be dedicated ICU facilities for children (which may be within adult ICUs), to provide oxygen therapy, CPAP, positive pressure ventilation, invasive monitoring, and inotropic support. Conventional adult ventilators may be suitable for older children. Specialized ventilators are required for infants and neonates.

Oxygen therapy in children

Oxygen therapy improves outcomes in children with oxygen saturation (SpO_2) <90%.

Nasal prongs

This is the preferred method of oxygen delivery in children <5 years:

- Neonates 0.5–1 l/min.
- Infants 1–2 l/min.
- Older children 1–4 l/min.

If CPAP is not available, a facemask with a reservoir bag can be added to increase the fractional inspired oxygen concentration (FiO_2).

Bubble CPAP

Bubble CPAP is a cost-effective method of delivering oxygen therapy and positive pressure support during spontaneous ventilation.

- Components of bubble CPAP are shown in Figure 7.1:
  - Air compressor, which provides a source of continuous airflow: 5–10 l/min.
  - Oxygen source (piped supply or concentrator), blender, and humidifier.
  - Patient interface (nasal prongs).
  - Expiratory limb placed under water to provide positive pressure. The depth of the tube under water determines the CPAP pressure.
- Indications for bubble CPAP include apnoea of prematurity, respiratory distress syndrome, pneumonia, and postoperative hypoventilation.
- Complications include nasal trauma (relatively common) and pneumothorax (very rare).

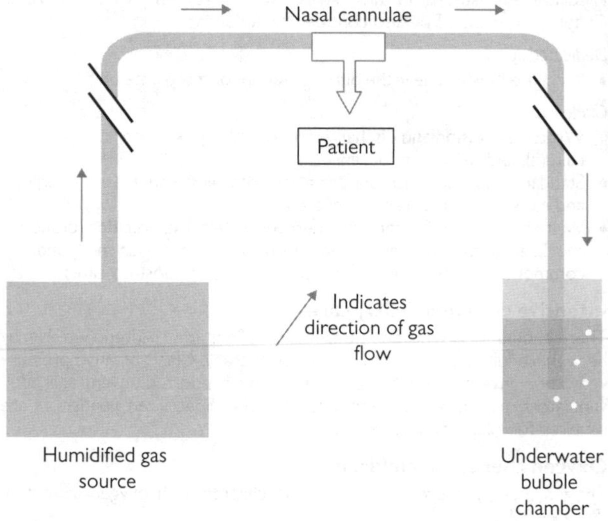

Figure 7.1 Components of a bubble CPAP system.

Paediatric sedation

Sedation may be provided for burns dressings, simple dental procedures, orthopaedic procedures such as fracture manipulation, or drainage of abscess. The goals of paediatric sedation include anxiolysis, amnesia, analgesia, and control of movement/behaviour. Older cooperative teenagers and young infants (<6 months—bundled and fed) may not need sedation for painless procedures. However, many older infants, toddlers, and school-aged children may not cooperate for short procedures.

Assessment

A detailed history and examination should include an airway assessment, other comorbidities, and difficulty with previous procedures. Particular care is required for infants <1 year, American Society of Anesthesiologists (ASA) III and IV, children with special needs, airway problems, or tonsillar hypertrophy/obstructive sleep apnoea (OSA).

Facilities

- Serious complications of sedation include airway compromise, saliva aspiration, laryngospasm, hypoxaemia, apnoea, and cardiac arrest.
- Facilities, personnel, and equipment must be available to manage all complications. The procedure room should be co-located with the operating theatre where these facilities are routinely available.
- A pulse oximeter, oxygen source, bag valve mask, appropriate-sized facemasks, and suction must be available in the procedure room. Emergency airway equipment and drugs must be easily accessible.

Management of sedation

- The child should be fasting as for general anaesthesia (GA).
- At minimum, the child should be monitored by a trained provider with a precordial stethoscope, pulse oximeter, and a finger on the pulse. The proceduralist should not be the sedationist—there should be a second person to monitor the patient.
- Medications administered IV are more predictable.
- Common combinations include: sedative agent (benzodiazepine, ketamine/propofol) +/− analgesic (opioids, paracetamol) +/− LA (see Table 7.6).
- Ideally, reversal agents should be available (flumazenil and naloxone for benzodiazepines and opioids, respectively). NB: the half-life of these agents is shorter than the drugs they reverse.
- Be patient before giving repeated doses; oversedation is more of a problem than undersedation.

Recovery

The child should be monitored by a trained provider until awake.

Table 7.6 Common medications used for paediatric sedation.

Sedative agent	Route	Initial bolus (mg/kg except where stated)	Follow-up dose (mg/kg)	Time to onset (min)	Duration of action (min)
Diazepam	IV	0.1–0.3	–	1–3	15–30
	Rectal	0.2–0.3	–	2–10	15–30
Midazolam	PO	0.5–0.75	–	15–30	60–90
	IV	0.05–0.15	–	2–3	45–60
	Rectal	0.5–0.75	–	10–30	60–90
Pethidine	IV	1–3	–	<5	120–240
	IM	1–3	–	10–15	120–360
Fentanyl	IV	1–5 μg/kg	1–5 μg/kg in 0.5–1.0 μg/kg increments	2–3	30–60
Ketamine (consider adjuvant antisialogogue and benzodiazepine)	PO	5–7	–	5–10	30–60
	IM	3–4	–	2–5	20–40
	IV	1–1.5	Repeat dose at 10 min if sedation not adequate	1–3	10–30
Propofol	IV	2–3	0.5–1	<1	5–10

IV, intravenous; PO, per os; IM, intramuscular.

Pain management in children

As in adults, pain is common but is often poorly managed (see 'Pain Management' in Chapter 5, pp. 83–87). Dedicated pain teams are rare. Inadequate pain relief has significant psychological and physiological consequences, and may have a life-long effect on the child's attitude to healthcare. Common causes of pain in children include:

- Trauma, burns, surgery or infection.
- Sickle cell disease—acute and chronic pain.
- Childhood cancers.

Pain assessment

Age-appropriate pain assessment tools should be used, such as the FLACC (Face Leg Activity Cry Consolability) score, or a faces scale.

Pain should be assessed on a regular basis, and before and after every intervention. Pain management education should include ward nurses.

Pain management strategies

The following principles are widely applicable:

- Aim for a multimodal approach that is adaptable to evolving requirements for analgesia.
- Provide analgesia at regular intervals rather than 'as required', according to age and weight.
- Reduce doses in malnourished children.
- Deliver analgesia by the simplest route; avoid the intramuscular (IM) route if possible. The rectal route is unpredictable for all drugs.
- Avoid codeine in children <12 years. Some ethnic groups have a high proportion of 'fast metabolizers' who are at risk from opioid toxicity with the usual doses of codeine.
- Avoid non-steroidal anti-inflammatory drugs (NSAIDs) in infants <6 months.
- See Appendix Tables A.6 and A.19 for analgesic doses.

For surgery in children, a suitable strategy is:

- Mild pain: paracetamol, NSAIDs, local anaesthetic infiltration.
- Moderate–severe pain: paracetamol, NSAIDs, ketamine, opioids, local anaesthetic (infiltration or regional technique).
- Ketamine is a useful perioperative analgesic drug but is no longer recommended to be given via the caudal route.
- For spinal anaesthesia in children, see 'Neuraxial Blocks' in Chapter 11 (pp. 258–261).

Clonidine and dexmedetomidine IV may be considered as adjuvant agents if available. Facilities to manage patient controlled analgesia (PCA) or continuous epidurals are unlikely to be available at the district hospital level.

Sickle cell disease (SCD) in children

General principles

SCD is an autosomal recessive congenital haemoglobinopathy associated with a gene mutation on the beta globulin of the haemoglobin chain. HbS replaces HbA as the main circulating haemoglobin. It affects approximately 5 million people worldwide, particularly in sub-Saharan Africa, India, Saudi Arabia, and the Mediterranean.

- In the deoxygenated state, HbS forms insoluble fibrils that cause sickling of red blood cells.
- Children with homozygous disease (HbSS) typically present with symptoms from early childhood. High levels of HbF are protective. Children with the heterozygous carrier state sickle cell trait (HbSA) are largely asymptomatic.
- Co-dominant inheritance of HbS with another abnormal haemoglobin can result in symptomatic disease, e.g. HbS and HbC (HbSC) or sickle haemoglobin-thalassaemia (HbS-B thal).
- There is limited capacity to manage SCD in LMICs. Children with severe disease experience high morbidity and early mortality.
- Patients with SCD have increased perioperative mortality.

Clinical presentation of SCD in children

- Chronic haemolytic anaemia.
- Acute painful crises affecting hands, abdomen, or long bones.
- Acute chest syndrome: acute lung injury characterized by new pulmonary infiltrate on chest X-ray, and fever of greater than 38.5°C, tachypnoea, wheezing, and/or cough.
- Stroke: 'watershed' infarcts associated with acute sickling episodes.
- Gram-negative sepsis, particularly urinary tract infection, biliary sepsis, and non-typhi salmonella infection. Repeated sickling leads to splenic infarction and functional asplenia in most patients.
- Progressive vascular disease and end-organ damage to lung, kidney, and brain.

Other features include splenic sequestration crisis, aplastic crisis, adenotonsillar hypertrophy, osteomyelitis, cholelithiasis, priapism, leg ulcers, and avascular necrosis.

Infants in sickle cell endemic regions presenting for surgery with unexplained low Hb should be screened for SCD, particularly in the presence of a positive family history.

Surgery can trigger acute complications such as pain crisis and acute chest syndrome.

Common surgical procedures in children with SCD

- Childhood surgery unrelated to SCD.
- Adenotonsillectomy.
- Cholecystectomy for pigmented gallstones.
- Splenectomy for repeated episodes of splenic sequestration.
- Circumcision for priapism.

Preoperative management

- Assess:
  - Severity of the disease: type and frequency of crises, triggers of crises, transfusion history, frequency of hospitalization.
  - Disease progression including evidence of organ dysfunction (especially lungs, brain, kidneys).
  - Current medications (folic acid, penicillin prophylaxis, +/− hydroxycarbamide to promote HbF production) and compliance.
- Measure:
  - Oxygen saturation as an indicator of lung function.
  - Baseline Hb, particularly if blood loss is anticipated.
  - Further investigations should be guided by type of surgery to be performed and level of suspected organ dysfunction.
- Continue current medications.
- Avoid dehydration—use standard fasting guidelines, encourage free clear fluids up to 1–2 h preoperatively for elective surgery.
- Blood transfusion:
  - May decrease the incidence of perioperative complications: balance possible benefits with potential risks of transfusion.
  - If the decision is taken to transfuse, give a simple top-up transfusion aiming for a haemoglobin level of 10 g/dl.
  - Avoid over-transfusion as this will increase viscosity and may trigger sickling.
  - Ensure blood is available to replace intraoperative losses and provide a top-up transfusion in the event of a sickle crisis.
  - Blood must be sickle negative and screened for malarial parasites in endemic areas.

Intraoperative management

- Well-performed general, regional, or neuraxial anaesthesia are all suitable techniques.
- Prophylactic antibiotics should be given, especially in patients with functional asplenia or who have had splenectomy.
- Use orthopaedic limb tourniquets with caution. Exsanguinate the limb carefully prior to application of the tourniquet.

Postoperative management

- Monitor closely for common postoperative complications: acute painful crisis, acute chest syndrome. Rare: cerebrovascular accident, acute splenic sequestration.
- Good postoperative pain control is essential. Patients may have very high analgesia requirements. Multimodal and regional techniques are ideal.
- Incentive spirometry (or simple versions like blowing up a surgical glove) may reduce atelectasis and associated acute chest syndrome.
- Continue antibiotics.
- Resume regular medications as soon as possible.
- Encourage early mobilization.

Paediatric surgical conditions

Cleft lip and palate repair

Procedure	Repair of defect in upper lip and/or palate
Time	1.5–4 h; occasionally much longer
Pain	Cleft lip + Cleft palate ++
Position	Supine with roll under shoulders, head extended
Blood loss	Cleft lip +; cleft palate ++
Practical techniques	GA with reinforced or (S) RAE ETT, IPPV Cleft lip only: LA/ketamine in selected patients (see 'Perioperative' comments below)

Cleft lip/palate (CLP) is one of the most common congenital abnormalities. Cleft lip +/− palate is usually an isolated abnormality; isolated cleft palate is more likely to occur in association with a syndrome. Cleft lip repair is ideally at 3 months; palate repairs at 9–12 months, before speech development. Delayed repair (>1 year of age) is usual in LMICs, particularly where local facilities are not suitable for prolonged surgery in infants.

Preoperative

- Cleft palate is associated with several syndromes: examine airway anatomy, ask about OSA symptoms, examine cardiac system carefully.
- Consider optimization and timing of surgery:
  - Malnutrition is common in this group and should be addressed.
  - Children with a cardiac murmur suggestive of symptomatic congenital heart disease should be referred (see 'Assessment and Preparation' in this chapter (pp. 111–114)).
  - Airway safety: upper airway obstruction may worsen after palate repair. Consider delaying surgery until 1–2 years old.
  - Infections: respiratory tract infections (RTIs) are common, due to aspiration. Wound dehiscence is more common in children with active infection. Defer for 2–4 weeks if an active RTI is present. Otitis media is common and should be treated prior to surgery.
- A full blood count and malaria screen should be carried out prior to surgery.
- Facilities for cross-match and blood transfusion should be available.
- Pre-med is not required <1 year; use with caution if OSA present.
- Prepare for a difficult airway if suspected.

Perioperative

- In carefully selected patients and with an experienced surgeon and anaesthetist, isolated cleft lip surgery may be done under LA with ketamine sedation and nasal oxygen supplementation.
- For GA:
  - Intubate with south-facing RAE or reinforced tube.
  - A small pack or dental roll in a left-sided cleft palate may prevent the laryngoscope blade displacing into the cleft. This must be removed

    after the child is intubated. Check tube position carefully with the head extended as for surgery.
  - A throat pack will be required and is usually placed/removed by the surgeon. The surgeon will place a mouth gag during surgery (check the ETT is not occluded when the gag is opened).
- Give prophylactic IV antibiotics (e.g. co-amoxiclav 30 mg/kg IV).
- Cleft lip surgery is less painful than cleft palate surgery. Multimodal analgesia including surgical infiltration of LA or an infraorbital block, paracetamol, and ibuprofen is ideal. Opioids may be required for palate surgery but are usually not necessary for lip surgery.
- Dexamethasone 0.25 mg/kg IV reduces postoperative airway oedema. If intubation has been difficult with multiple attempts, or the tongue is oedematous, consider continuing dexamethasone 0.1–0.5 mg/kg IV × 3 doses postoperatively.
- Tranexamic acid 10 mg/kg IV is useful if there has been a lot of bleeding.

Postoperative
- Consider whether a nasopharyngeal airway (NPA) is required (if high risk for airway obstruction after extubation); if so, use the same size as the ETT. Surgical placement is usual.
- Suction early under direct vision to avoid damage to the repair.
- Remove the throat pack.
- Extubate awake.

Ward care
- Patients at high risk for postoperative airway obstruction or with an NPA *in situ* (which requires regular suctioning) should be cared for in an HDU. All patients must be monitored closely postoperatively and should not be sent to the ward until the airway is safe.
- The nurse should be given clear instructions when to call for help, e.g. if the breathing is noisy, if the SpO_2 is <94%, or if there is a lot of bleeding, particularly if the child is swallowing a lot.
- Discuss feeding protocols for both cleft lip and palate repair with the surgeon. Ideally, the child should be encouraged to feed and take a soft diet as early as possible. Try to prevent babies putting their fingers, fists, or anything hard in their mouth.
- Oral analgesia should suffice postoperatively (regular paracetamol + ibuprofen, +/− oral morphine).
- Mothers are often in a rush to feed their child and will need to be encouraged to follow postoperative protocols and to go slowly, particularly in restricting the child to a soft diet.

Fracture management

Limb fractures are common injuries of childhood. Closed reduction is suitable for most simple fractures. Percutaneous 'pinning' may be required to maintain reduction. Open reduction with internal fixation may be necessary if it is not possible to perform closed reduction or pinning.

Preoperative

- Fractures with neurovascular compromise (supracondylar injuries are particularly commonly associated with this complication) and open fractures are surgical emergencies; most other surgery can be delayed for an appropriate fasting period.
- A careful history and examination should be carried out to exclude associated injuries.
- Confirm the last oral intake before injury to help guide airway management. Pain and opioid analgesics delay stomach emptying. If in doubt, assume a full stomach.

Perioperative

- Consider GA with a secure airway with rapid sequence induction/awake extubation if there is potentially a full stomach. Muscle relaxation may assist fracture reduction.
- Ketamine may be used as a sole anaesthetic/analgesic for selected cases.
- Regional anaesthesia (axillary block, caudal) provides excellent intra- and post-analgesia for suitable cases. A superficial cervical plexus block may be useful for clavicle fractures.

Postoperative

- Careful postoperative monitoring of distal extremities for capillary refill time should be carried out, especially when a regional block has been used and if the cast has not been split.

Hernia repair

Procedure	Repair of hernia (inguinal, umbilical most common)
Time	30–90 min
Pain	+
Position	Supine
Blood loss	+
Practical techniques	GA with ETT + IPPV +/− rapid sequence induction (RSI) GA with LMA, spontaneous ventilation (SV) in older children Analgesia: caudal/ilioinguinal/infiltration block

Preoperative

- This is one of the most common procedures in paediatric surgery.
- It can be an emergency (incarceration) or elective procedure. Umbilical hernias have a lower risk of incarceration and usually do not require surgical treatment until about 5 years.
- Incarceration is more common in infants, and in LMICs, due to delayed presentation. The child may be unwell, hypovolemic, and may need preoperative fluid resuscitation.
- Consider placing an NG tube preoperatively. Laboratory investigations are not usually required for uncomplicated elective cases.

Perioperative

- Elective:
  - >5 kg: inhalational or intravenous induction with LMA or facemask for maintenance. If using a draw-over system, see 'Draw-over Anaesthesia' in Chapter 3 (pp. 40–45) for more guidance.
  - <5 kg: intubation preferable.
  - Spinal anaesthesia without additional sedation may be considered in preterm neonates at risk of postoperative apnoeas.
- Emergency (e.g. incarcerated hernia):
  - A modified RSI with intubation.
- Use positive pressure ventilation if the child is intubated.
- Analgesia options include:
  - Caudal block: see 'Neuraxial Blocks' in Chapter 11 (pp. 258–261).
  - Ilioinguinal/iliohypogastric block.
  - Local infiltration by the surgeon.

Postoperative

- Oral analgesia with regular paracetamol +/− NSAID.
- For routine elective cases, the patient may be managed as a day case given certain prerequisites: the parent/carer is literate, has access to a phone and transport, lives in good housing conditions, with water and electricity, close to the hospital.
- Take-home analgesia will need to be supplied to the family, with clear instructions on how to use it. Liquid paracetamol must be clearly labelled with the dose and supplied in a child-proof bottle.

Inhaled foreign body (FB)

Procedure	Retrieval of FB using laryngoscopy/bronchoscopy
Time	15 min – unknown
Pain	+
Position	Supine with roll under shoulders
Blood loss	+
Practical techniques	GA + SV (preferred) or IPPV +/− muscle relaxation

General considerations

- Commonest among children aged 6 months to 4 years.
- Leading cause of accidental death in children <1 year.
- Presentation:
  - Often acute after a witnessed choking event, which is followed by cough, dyspnoea, wheezing.
  - Stridor implies a FB in the laryngeal inlet and is an ominous sign.
- Most FBs that pass the subglottic region become lodged in the distal airway, with equal probability in right or left main bronchus.
- Often presents late in LMICs with complications such as pneumonia, lung collapse/consolidation, empyema.
- The airway is shared with the surgeon; good communication between the surgeon and anaesthetist is critical.

Preoperative

- Most FBs are located in the distal airway and removal can proceed as a semi-elective procedure. The child should be appropriately fasted and a chest X-ray performed.
- Rarely, the child may present in extremis following a witnessed choking episode.
  - A supraglottic FB may be dislodged using standard emergency manoeuvres for choking (sit child up, assist the child to cough, chest thrusts, back slaps).
  - A tracheal FB is a surgical emergency and the child must be taken to theatre immediately, irrespective of fasting status.
- Anticipate the possibility of complete airway obstruction. Plan for an emergency rigid bronchoscopy, advancement of the FB into the mainstem bronchus, tracheostomy, thoracotomy.
- Consider deferring IV access until after the child is asleep to minimize distress, if appropriate assistance is available.
- Sedative premedication is not usually indicated; parental presence is helpful.
- Atropine 20 μg/kg PO/IV may help reduce airway secretions and will help to make topical lidocaine applied during the procedure more effective.

Perioperative

- Aim for a smooth, calm induction with minimal air swallowing.
- Preoxygenation by facemask is helpful, but may be difficult.
- SV is often recommended; however, the choice of SV or IPPV will depend on:
  - Adequacy of the child's respiratory function: in the presence of pneumonia or other impairment, SV may not be adequate for oxygenation.
  - Surgical technique: IPPV may interrupt the surgical procedure or be difficult with a bronchoscope *in situ*.
  - Location of the FB: high-pressure IPPV could push it more distally.
- Inhalational induction should be carried out using halothane or sevoflurane in fractional inspired oxygen concentration (FiO_2) 1.0, or IV induction with propofol (if SV is not required).
- Apply topical lidocaine to the airway (maximum dose of lidocaine 3 mg/kg) under direct vision.
  - Beware accidental overdose of lidocaine if using 4% lidocaine spray.
  - If IPPV is planned, paralysis using suxamethonium assists with topicalization.
- The anaesthetist will require access to the anaesthetic machine and the airway; this may be achieved by turning the operating table 90°.
- Ideally a bronchoscopy should be performed by the surgeon with a rigid bronchoscope with an Ayre's T-piece attached to the side arm for insufflation of oxygen +/− volatile. Flexible bronchoscopy may assist with localization of the FB, but is not essential.
- Volatile anaesthetic or total intravenous anaesthesia (TIVA) is appropriate for maintenance; choice may depend on whether SV or IPPV is indicated.
- Following removal of the FB, the tracheobronchial tree should be suctioned and re-examined for evidence of distal fragments or mucosal trauma. The child may be intubated to assist with tracheobronchial toilet prior to extubation.
- Potential complications include laryngeal oedema, bronchospasm, pneumothorax, tracheal/bronchial rupture, death.

Postoperative

- Monitor the child until fully awake; consider prolonged recovery in the theatre suite until the child is stable.
- Chest X-ray to rule out pneumothorax, pneumomediastinum.
- Consider dexamethasone (0.25–0.5 mg/kg IV) if concerned about postoperative airway oedema.
- Antibiotics may be required.

Intussusception

Procedure	Laparotomy +/− bowel resection and anastomosis
Time	2–3 h
Pain	+++
Position	Supine
Blood loss	++ to +++ if bowel necrosis
Practical techniques	GA, ETT, IPPV with RSI

Intussusception is the invagination and telescoping of one loop of bowel into another, most commonly at the ileocecal junction. This causes bowel oedema, and subsequent intestinal obstruction. If unattended, it leads to bowel ischaemia, necrosis, perforation, and peritonitis.

- Commonest cause of intestinal obstruction in children between 3 months and 2 years.
- Presentation: paroxysmal abdominal pain, bloody mucoid (redcurrant jelly) stool, sausage-shaped mass in the right iliac fossa. Symptoms/signs of intestinal obstruction and peritonitis may be present.
- Barium enema may be therapeutic as well as diagnostic if available. It is contraindicated in late cases (may lead to bowel perforation).

Preoperative

- Diagnosis based on history, examination, +/− abdominal ultrasound.
- Fluid resuscitate if shocked and ensure wide-bore IV access early.
- As available: full blood count, electrolytes, liver function tests, blood group, and cross-match.
- Insert a nasogastric tube to decompress the stomach and a urinary catheter to assess adequacy of fluid management.

Intraoperative

- GA with rapid/modified RSI. Ketamine is a useful induction agent.
- Be prepared to give fluid bolus(es) +/− adrenaline (1 μg/kg IV).
- Reduction of the intussusceptum may lead to release of vasodilatory toxins, which may result in sudden profound hypotension. If this occurs, tell the surgeon and give an immediate bolus of fluid 10–20 ml/kg. Use vasopressors early if required.
- Monitor blood loss and replace as necessary.

Postoperative

- Most children can be extubated and return to the general ward.
- Continue intravenous fluids until oral intake is established.
- Multimodal analgesia for pain control including: paracetamol (IV, PO, PR) and small doses of IV opioids. Local anaesthetic wound infiltration is helpful.
- ICU/HDU admission may be required depending on the patient's stability and the level of care available on the postoperative ward.

Noma (cancrum oris)

Procedure	Simple flap to complex microsurgery. Repeat procedures are common
Time	Variable
Pain	+++ (operative +/− donor sites)
Position	Supine
Blood loss	Variable
Practical techniques	GA, ETT, IPPV +/− regional for donor site Anticipate difficult airway/intubation.

General considerations

- Noma is a debilitating childhood disease of chronic poverty and malnutrition with necrotizing gangrene and massive tissue loss. Severe facial scarring and deformity require reconstruction. Stigmatization results in delayed presentation.
- Ankylosis between the mandible and maxilla may cause absolute trismus.

Preoperative

- Examine for features of chronic malnutrition.
- Complete airway assessment must be performed. Anticipate difficult airway management. Previous surgical notes are helpful but airway issues may have changed. Counsel, consent, and prepare for a possible tracheostomy.
- Discuss positioning with surgical team with respect to donor site.
- Ensure adequate blood for transfusion.

Perioperative

- Airway management:
  - Prepare for difficult intubation.
  - Inhalational induction is preferable. Maintain SV until ability to ventilate is confirmed.
  - If mask ventilation is difficult due to facial deformities consider applying gauze to fill in facial defects, using a nasopharyngeal airway or an LMA (though anaesthesia must be deep enough).
  - The tracheal tube should be well secured preferably by stitching.
  - The route of intubation (nasal vs oral) depends on the site of the defect and the procedure planned. A throat pack should be inserted.
- Anticipate prolonged surgery: ensure temperature conservation, adequate monitoring, and consider the potential need for blood transfusion.
- Consider LA or a nerve block to the donor site.

Postoperative

- Patients are commonly kept intubated and should be managed in a HDU/ICU setting.
- NG feeding may be required for 2–4 weeks after the surgery with nutrition supplementation, as for patients with extensive burns.

Pyloric stenosis

Procedure	Open pyloromyotomy: splitting muscle of pylorus down to mucosa
Time	30–60 min
Pain	+
Position	Supine
Blood loss	+
Practical techniques	GA, ETT, IPPV +/− RSI

General considerations

- Pathological thickening of pyloric muscle leading to high-grade gastric outlet obstruction.
- Presentation:
  - Projectile non-bilious vomiting immediately after feeds: the baby is hungry and eager to feed again.
  - Usually at 2–5 weeks old, but can present up to 3 months old with severe failure to thrive, dehydration, and pre-renal failure.
- <10% have associated congenital abnormalities.
- This is a medical, not a surgical emergency. Loss of gastric fluid containing hydrogen ions, chloride, sodium, and potassium leads to the classical hypochloraemic, hypokalemic metabolic alkalosis. The plasma sodium may be low (or high in severe dehydration).

Preoperative

- The baby must be rehydrated and electrolyte abnormalities corrected prior to surgery, particularly metabolic alkalosis.
- An NG tube should be placed to decompress the stomach and the baby kept nil by mouth.
- If the baby is shocked, start with 10–20 ml/kg 0.9% saline bolus.
- Otherwise, rehydrate slowly with isotonic fluids at the normal maintenance rate (5% glucose, 0.9% saline, 4 ml/kg/h IV).
- Rehydration may take 24–48 h if severe.
- Once the baby is producing wet nappies, consider adding KCl 10–20 mmol to each 500 ml bag of fluid. Monitor electrolytes if able.
- Assess the baby clinically—they should be alert, with warm peripheries, good capillary refill, good pulse rate and strength, with good urine output (wet nappies), and moist mucous membranes.
- If available, desirable laboratory test parameters include: bicarbonate <30 mmol/l, potassium >3 mmol/l, sodium in normal range.

Perioperative

- Prior to induction, empty the stomach by aspirating on the NG tube with the baby in different positions (right and left lateral positions as well as supine).
- Modified RSI or inhalational induction can be used as the baby is nil by mouth and the stomach has been emptied.
- Intubation and IPPV are required.

- Wound infection is common: give antibiotics prior to skin incision (guided by local protocols).
- The surgeon may ask for air to be injected down the NG tube to check the integrity of the mucosa.
- Use opioids with care (risk of postoperative apnoea: consider 1 μg/kg fentanyl IV after the patient is awake and extubated).
- Local anaesthetic infiltration of the wound is ideal.
- This operation is sometimes performed under LA (with or without adjunctive ketamine boluses).

Postoperative

- Reverse neuromuscular blocking agents and extubate fully awake.
- Monitor the child in theatre until certain there is no risk of apnoea.
- Remove the NG tube at the end of surgery.
- Continue to monitor closely for postoperative apnoeas.
- Oral feeds can be usually started 4 h postoperatively; continue IV fluids until tolerating oral intake.
- Give paracetamol PO/PR.

Tropical abscess (pyogenic amoebic liver abscess)

Procedure	Drainage of abscess (percutaneous or open)
Time	Variable
Pain	++
Position	Supine
Blood loss	Variable
Practical techniques	GA, ETT, IPPV +/− RSI

General considerations

- Tropical abscess describes an inflammatory space-occupying lesion of the liver common in tropical and subtropical zones. There is usually a solitary lesion in the right lobe.

Preoperative

- Also see 'Resuscitation of the Sick Child' section on pp. 143–155. Children may present with sepsis, acute abdomen, peritonitis.
- Evaluate for associated medical conditions such as SCD, congenital or acquired immunosuppression.
- Blood investigations may reveal anaemia, leucocytosis, elevated liver enzymes, and serum bilirubin.
- Chest X-ray may reveal elevated hemidiaphragm, pleural effusion, empyema, and atelectasis.
- Initiate broad-spectrum antibiotics and metronidazole early.
- Percutaneous drainage is indicated if the volume of the abscess is large, if there is a lack of clinical improvement after 48 72 h of medical treatment, or evidence of liver failure.
- Open surgical drainage is reserved for ruptured abscess, multiloculated abscess, presence of ascites, or failed percutaneous drainage.

Perioperative

- Standard monitoring and urinary output for open surgical procedures.
- RSI is indicated. Ensure adequate preoxygenation. Ketamine is preferred if the child is acutely ill.
- Ensure adequate fluid resuscitation especially if jaundice is present.
- Minimize the use of drugs with hepatic metabolism or excretion.
- Fentanyl and paracetamol should be used for analgesia. If the child is haemodynamically unstable, us sub-anaesthetic doses of ketamine and local infiltration with local anaesthetic.
- Extubate awake in the left lateral position.

Postoperative

- Admit to HDU if available.
- Continue fluid resuscitation and antibiotic therapy.

Typhoid perforation

Procedure	Exploratory laparotomy + proceed (simple repair of perforations, bowel resection +/− anastomosis, stoma formation)
Time	2–3 h
Pain	+++
Position	Supine
Blood loss	+++
Practical techniques	GA, ETT, IPPV, RSI

General considerations

- Perforation is the most serious complication of typhoid fever, predominantly affects children (50% of cases), and has a high mortality.
- The presentation of typhoid includes:
  - Systemic symptoms: step-wise fever (rises and falls each day, but overall trend is rising) or no fever, malaise, relative bradycardia, headache.
  - Abdominal symptoms: pain and distension, headache, constipation, later may develop diarrhoea.
  - Truncal 'rose spots' are rare in reality.
- Diagnosis of typhoid intestinal perforation requires a high index of suspicion in endemic areas. Diagnostic tests may not be readily available or are non-specific (Widal test).
- Typhoid is often misdiagnosed as malaria and children may therefore present late with complications such as perforation and severe sepsis. This poses significant challenges, especially where paediatric critical care services may be limited.
- While corticosteroids have been found to reduce mortality in typhoid enteritis, their benefit in cases of perforation is not proven.

Preoperative

- Assess for signs of shock and resuscitate as required prior to urgent surgery, with IV crystalloid boluses titrated to response, +/− blood.
- As available: check full blood count, electrolytes, renal, and liver function. Send blood for group and cross-match. Anaemia is common and there may be electrolyte abnormalities.
- Insert an NG tube and urethral catheter.
- Start broad-spectrum IV antibiotics immediately, effective against Gram-negative and anaerobic bacteria.
  - Refer to local guidelines but a typical regimen would be ciprofloxacin (or a third-generation cephalosporin) and metronidazole.
  - Gentamicin is useful if that is all that is available.
- This is an infectious disease—the patient should be isolated and staff should use barrier protection including gloves and aprons.

Perioperative

- Typhoid perforations can be challenging to manage surgically: discuss the plan with the surgeon and prepare accordingly.
- Aspirate NG tube and perform an RSI/modified RSI. Ketamine is the anaesthetic drug of choice, but be careful if sympathetic stimulation is already at maximum.
- Be prepared for significant hypotension at induction. Have fluids and a rescue dose of adrenaline prepared (inotropic dose—1 μg/kg, i.e. 0.1ml/kg 1:100,000 adrenaline).
- Use blood according to the haematocrit measurement in theatre, if available. If not, consider giving blood after 40–60 ml/kg of crystalloid has been administered.
- Local anaesthetic blocks (e.g. transversus abdominis plane or rectus sheath blocks) are ideal, or the surgeon can provide local infiltration under direct vision. Avoid spinal or caudal anaesthesia in the presence of sepsis.
- Keep the patient warm using all available techniques. Do not forget to warm fluids.
- Inotropic support may be necessary if the patient remains hypotensive despite adequate fluid resuscitation. See 'Cardiovascular Support' in Chapter 12 (pp. 271–272).

Postoperative management

- Depends on local resources, the operation, and the child's condition.
- It may be possible to extubate some children, but the majority will benefit from continued support of ventilation, possibly with inotropic support. Ideally, the child should return to an HDU to be closely monitored.
- Urine output is a useful indicator of adequate fluid replacement.
- Continue intravenous antibiotics.
- Use multimodal analgesia for pain control including: paracetamol (IV, PO, PR) and small doses of IV opioids such as morphine.

Ventriculoperitoneal shunt

Procedure	Placement of a ventriculoperitoneal shunt for hydrocephalus (congenital or acquired). Endoscopic third ventriculostomy technique (ETV) also possible
Time	2–3 h
Pain	+
Position	Supine, head turned to contralateral side
Blood loss	+
Practical techniques	GA, ETT, IPPV, +/− RSI

Preoperative

- Peak ages of presentation are neonatal and 2–4 years old.
- Normal intracranial pressure (ICP) in neonate is 2–4 mmHg. Compliant infant skull allows compensation if hydrocephalus is gradual; untreated, the head may become very large with 'sunsetting' eyes.
- Examine for signs of raised ICP.
  - May be vague (e.g. irritability, poor feeding).
  - Classic signs (hypertension, bradycardia, reduced conscious level) occur late.
  - If symptomatic, surgical intervention may be urgent.
- Consider other congenital abnormalities (e.g. cardiac).
- Request haemoglobin and coagulation tests, if available.

Perioperative

- If the head is massively enlarged, place the baby on folded towels so that the occiput remains on the bed and the neck is in a neutral position. Intubation should not be difficult in this position.
- Use IV or inhalational induction, depending on the clinical situation.
- Use an oral ETT, ideally reinforced to reduce kinking. Secure the tube carefully.
- Use IPPV to achieve normocarbia. Hypercarbia increases cerebral blood flow and ICP. Hypocarbia can cause regional brain ischaemia.
- There is a high risk of intraoperative hypothermia. Warming and temperature monitoring is ideal.
- Prophylactic antibiotics are usually required.
- Painful phases of the operation are the incision and tunnelling of the shunt. Short-acting opioids such as fentanyl (1–3 μg/kg) or remifentanil (1 μg/kg) are ideal if available.
- Local anaesthetic infiltration should be carried out by the surgical team.
- Paracetamol and NSAIDs should be used unless contraindicated. Avoid NSAIDs if the patient is <6 months old.

Postoperative

- Extubate fully awake (and lateral if there are concerns about aspiration).
- Oral analgesia.

Wilms' tumour (nephroblastoma)

Procedure	Partial/radical nephrectomy
Time	3–4 h
Pain	+++
Position	Supine
Blood loss	++ to +++
Practical techniques	GA, ETT, IPPV. +/– caudal analgesia

Preoperative

- This is the commonest abdominal tumour in childhood: mean age at presentation 3.5 years; 10% have syndromic associations. Some syndromes are associated with macroglossia, hypotonia, hyperinsulinism, or congenital heart diseases.
- Clinical presentation is non-specific: late presentation with a huge mass may be seen, often following bleeding into the tumour.
- Check blood pressure (BP): 50% of patients are hypertensive.
- Anaemia may be present as a result of occult haematuria. Check renal function if possible.
- Review imaging if available to exclude tumour in the inferior vena cava (IVC) (if present, right atrial thrombus may also exist—refer for echo if available).
- Prepare for major haemorrhage. Group and cross-match blood.
- Children may have received chemotherapy including:
  - dactinomycin (impairs hepatic and hemopoietic function increasing risk of coagulopathy)
  - vincristine (syndrome of inappropriate ADH secretion, SIADH)
  - doxorubicin (acute cardiomyopathy).

Perioperative

- Inhalational or IV induction. Consider RSI with large tumours that could be obstructing gastric outflow. Head up positioning may help.
- Obtain adequate (2× wide-bore) IV access in the upper limbs; there may be massive haemorrhage from the IVC.
- Invasive BP monitoring is ideal if available: BP may be labile due to tumour handling (hypertension) or bleeding (hypotension).
- Muscle relaxation will be required.
- Analgesia: caudal if no contraindications, +/− IV opiates as required.
- Maintain normothermia for prompt recovery from anaesthesia.

Postoperative

- Patients may require HDU care postoperatively.
- There is a high risk of secondary haemorrhage because of the vascular nature of the dissection.
- Postoperative ventilation may be required in cases of prolonged surgery, massive blood loss, tumour embolization, or significant atelectasis.

Neonatal surgical conditions

Gastroschisis and exomphalos

Procedure	Primary closure (small defects) Silo placement and staged closure (larger defects)
Time	2–3 h
Pain	++
Position	Supine
Blood loss	++
Practical techniques	GA, ETT, IPPV

General principles

- Gastroschisis and exomphalos are abdominal wall defects associated with herniation of the abdominal contents.
  - Exomphalos: the intestine herniates into the umbilical cord and is covered in a sac; the defect may be small (exompaholos minor), allowing single stage closure. Exomphalos major usually requires staged reduction of the bowel using a protective silo. Other anomalies are common (intestinal atresias, cardiac, chromosomal).
  - Gastroschisis: the defect is lateral to the cord, and there is no covering sac. The bowel is exposed to amniotic fluid *in utero* and is thickened and covered in an abnormal 'peel'; staged closure is usual and most patients require several weeks of total parenteral nutrition until gut motility improves. If TPN not available, IVF with glucose can be used to support nutrition.
- Antenatal diagnosis of these defects is rare in LMICs. Diagnosis is made at birth, and late presentation is usual.
- Mortality for exomphalos major and gastroschisis is very high in LMICs.

Preoperative

- These are neonatal surgical emergencies; there is a risk of fluid loss from the exposed bowel, sepsis, bowel obstruction, and bowel ischaemia.
- Initial management involves covering the exposed bowel with wet gauzes. This can be further covered by a cling film or sterile polythene paper to reduce fluid and heat loss by evaporation.
- Assess fluid status and treat as necessary.
- Also assess severity/presence of: hypothermia, gastrointestinal (GI) obstruction, sepsis, gut infarction, metabolic acidosis.
- If the baby is in good condition and there is potential for survival, the child should be transferred to a specialist centre. It may be better to offer palliative care and for the child to remain with the mother.

Perioperative

- Naso or orogastric tube should be placed (if not already present).
- Use modified rapid sequence IV induction.
- Use careful positive pressure ventilation with low peak inspiratory pressures to avoid gut distension.

- Central venous access is ideal, particularly in gastroschisis, as the child will require total parenteral nutrition postoperatively. If available, consider an arterial line.
- The child is at risk of abdominal compartment syndrome following reduction of the bowel, which may also affect lung compliance and airway pressures.
- Assess changes in lung compliance during reduction of the abdominal contents; let the surgeons know if inspiratory pressures exceed 30 cmH_2O. Primary closure should be abandoned in this situation, and a silo fashioned to allow for staged reduction.

Postoperative

- Postoperative ventilation for 48–72 h is usual.
- Monitor for respiratory compromise, abdominal compartment syndrome, renal failure, infection, hypothermia, and coagulopathy.

Imperforate anus

Procedure	Colostomy, anoplasty, or posterior anorectoplasty (PSARP)
Time	2–3 h
Pain	Colostomy: + Anoplasty/PSARP: +++
Position	Colostomy: supine Anoplasty/PSARP: prone (slight jack-knife)
Blood loss	Colostomy/anoplasty: + PSARP: ++
Practical techniques	GA, ETT, IPPV, +/− caudal

General considerations

- Usually identified upon first examination or within 24 h when newborn is observed to have abdominal distension and fails to pass meconium.
- Type of surgery:
  - Low anorectal malformation (ARM): perineal anoplasty (or colostomy in remote settings).
  - High ARM: initial colostomy in the newborn period, followed by PSARP when the child is 3–6 months.
- Presentation may be delayed in LMICs and the child may present with severe abdominal distension, electrolyte derangement, dehydration, sepsis, and acidosis.
  - These children will benefit from an initial colostomy before definitive surgery.
- This is specialist surgery; a colostomy may be performed in a rural setting, but the child should be transferred to a referral hospital for more major procedures.

Preoperative

- Associated with congenital abnormalities, e.g. VACTERL (vertebral, anal, cardiac, tracheal, oesophagus, renal, and limbs) syndrome.
  - Detailed physical examination is mandatory.
  - Any cardiac murmur should be investigated before proceeding with anaesthesia.
- Patients should be NPO and given IV maintenance fluids.
- Monitor neonates closely for hypoglycaemia. Glucose is required in maintenance fluids.
- If abdominal distension is present, site an NG tube preoperatively.
- Urinalysis may help to determine the presence of a rectourinary fistula +/− infection. If suspected, give broad-spectrum antibiotics.
- Bowel prep for anoplasty/PSARP may cause an electrolyte imbalance.
- Serious consideration should be given to doing a colostomy under LA in rural settings where anaesthesia expertise and/or facilities are lacking.

Perioperative

- Inhalational or IV induction (for IV induction ketamine preferable; or low-dose thiopental/propofol).
- Standard monitoring should include temperature and urinary output.
- Maintain normothermia.
- Maintain anaesthesia with inhalational agents in air–oxygen mixture if air is available. Avoid nitrous oxide (bowel distension).
- Administration of muscle relaxant provides better operating conditions for the surgeon; however, if administered, this should be reversed prior to extubation.
- Anticipate increased fluid requirements due to insensible losses and third space losses with bowel manipulation.
- Analgesia:
  - A single caudal injection with preservative-free bupivacaine can provide good analgesia. It is important to exclude a lower spine defect before embarking on caudal injection.
  - Local infiltration of the incision site at the end of surgery can help to reduce the need for opioid analgesics postoperatively.
  - If required and available, titrate small doses of opioid to effect.

Postoperative

- Usually extubated at the end of the procedure.
- Ensure 10% glucose is provided in maintenance fluid until oral feeding has been established.

Note

- Similar principles may apply to defunctioning surgery for Hirschsprung's disease.

Myelomeningocele

Procedure	Repair of myelomeningocele
Time	1–2 h
Pain	++
Position	Prone
Blood loss	Variable
Practical techniques	GA, ETT, IPPV

General considerations

- Can occur at any site along the spinal cord but it is most common in the lumbar and lumbosacral regions.
- About 70% of patients with myelomeningocele also have hydrocephalus and Chiari II malformations.
- Associated with multiple congenital abnormalities including hydrocephalus.
- Cognitive development is normal in the majority of patients.
- Patients can develop latex allergy due to repeated exposure (surgery or bladder catheterization).

Preoperative

- Initially after birth, exposed neural tissue should be covered with sterile, saline-soaked gauze. The infant should be positioned on their abdomen to reduce trauma to exposed neural tissue.
- Primary closure should be performed within 48 h of birth to reduce the risk of rupture and infection. Delay in closure increases the likelihood of progressive neural damage.
- A ventriculo-peritoneal (VP) shunt is frequently inserted at the time of surgery in patients with co-existing hydrocephalus.
- If the neural sac is ruptured, there is cerebrospinal fluid (CSF) leakage, which can result in hypothermia and infection. The neonate is at risk of becoming acutely septic.
- Careful assessment of volume status is required.

Perioperative

- Positioning:
  - For induction and intubation, avoid pressure on the neuroplaque. Employ a 'doughnut' or towel rolls for the defect to sit in; consider a lateral position if experienced.
  - For surgery: prone positioning. Avoid excessive head rotation (can be associated with Arnold-Chiari malformation).
  - Reconfirm the ETT position after every change in patient position: accidental extubation/endobronchial intubation is not uncommon.
  - Protect all pressure points meticulously.
- Inhalational or intravenous induction. An armoured ETT is preferred. IPPV is mandatory. Avoid high FiO_2, especially if the baby is premature.

- Surgical blood loss can be difficult to measure and can be considerable. The surgical site may be infiltrated with local anaesthetic and adrenaline by the surgeon to help maintain haemostasis (of particular relevance if you expect to use halothane).
- Heat loss during surgery can be difficult to control especially as autonomic control below abnormality may be defective. Wrapping the head and keeping the baby covered at all times will help reduce heat loss.
- There is a high risk of hypoglycaemia: ensure glucose maintenance is given throughout the case.

Postoperative
- Extubate patient fully awake, supine.
- Monitor closely postoperatively for apnoea, desaturation, bradycardia. An HDU bed should be used if available.

Oesophageal atresia and tracheo-oesophageal fistula

Procedure	Thoracotomy +/− rigid bronchoscopy +/− gastrostomy
Time	Variable
Pain	+++
Position	Left lateral (axillary roll)
Blood loss	+
Practical techniques	GA, ETT, gentle IPPV. Caudal or LA by surgeon

General considerations

- Arises from incomplete separation of the oesophagus from the laryngotracheal tube. Oesphogeal atresia (OA) with distal tracheo-oesophageal fistula (TOF) is the most common (type C—see Figure 7.2).
- Presentation:
  - Antenatally: may be suspected if polyhydramnios is present.
  - Postnatally: bubbling and choking on feeds.
  - Late diagnosis at 1 week old is common in LMICs, by which time the child will have suffered repeated aspiration episodes.
- The diagnosis is confirmed on chest X-ray with typical coiling of an NG tube in the proximal oesophageal pouch.
- Mortality is high in LMICs. Specific risk factors include congenital heart disease, birth weight <1.5 kg and late presentation.
- Surgical options:
  - A staged repair may be preferred in some anatomical cases or where neonatal support is limited.
  - Oesophagostomy reduces aspiration of saliva, and gastrostomy allows feeding, followed by repair of the OA at a later date.
  - Ideally the fistula should be ligated at this stage as otherwise the child is at risk of aspiration.

Preoperative

- Many have associated congenital anomalies, e.g. cardiac, gastrointestinal, musculoskeletal and central nervous system anomalies. Surgery should only be attempted in a referral hospital with experience.

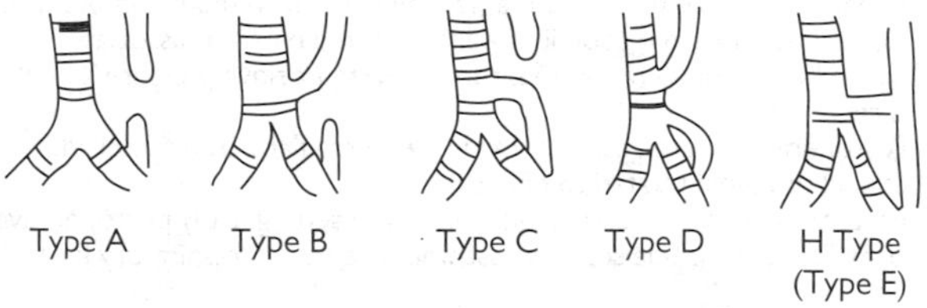

Figure 7.2 Gross's classification of oesophageal atresia.

Data from Gross, RE. *The Surgery of Infancy and Childhood*. Philadelphia, WB Saunders; 1953.

- Patient should be kept in semi-upright position and nil by mouth. A suction catheter should be placed on continuous gentle suction in the oesophageal pouch to prevent aspiration of secretions.

Perioperative

- Inhalational or IV induction in oxygen can be used, according to preference; paralyse the baby and provide gentle IPPV.
- The surgeon may want to perform a rigid bronchoscopy to check for the position of the fistula or the presence of a proximal fistula.
- Intubation and ventilation:
  - The main anaesthetic concern prior to ligation of the fistula is to position the ETT so that the child is ventilated effectively, and gastric distension is minimized.
  - The fistula is in the posterior wall of the trachea, proximal to the carina.
  - Therefore, the ETT should be placed distal to the fistula with the bevel facing anteriorly. It can be placed in the right main bronchus and gently withdrawn until the tip of the tube is just above the carina and bilateral air entry is obtained.
- Intraoperative issues:
  - If there is marked gastric insufflation (more likely with associated small bowel atresia), the stomach may be decompressed through the airway by disconnecting the ETT briefly. Notify the surgeon and proceed with thoracotomy and ligation of the fistula urgently. Avoid the temptation to perform an emergency gastrostomy in this situation as it may then become impossible to ventilate the baby.
  - The anaesthetist must work closely with the surgeon during lung retraction; the surgeon may need to allow intermittent ventilation of both lungs if the SpO_2 falls <90%.
  - A transanastomotic nasogastric tube ('TAT tube') is passed during repair of the oesophagus; this is important to maintain oesophageal patency, reduce fistula formation, and allow feeding. It must be securely fixed and labelled, and must <u>not</u> be removed.
- Analgesia can be provided by a caudal epidural catheter advanced to the thoracic region; or (more commonly in the low-resource setting) titrated opiates with surgical LA infiltration, +/− single shot caudal.

Postoperative management

- It may be possible to extubate a healthy neonate without comorbidities for straightforward ligation immediately. If the baby has associated comorbidities or has aspirated, support with positive pressure 24–48 h is required.
- Postoperatively, analgesia is provided with regular paracetamol and careful IV opioid titrated to effect.
- Postoperative care should be in a high-care setting: early postoperative complications include sepsis, anastomotic leak, and respiratory failure.

Resuscitation of the sick child

For emergency calculations and reference values, see Appendix Tables A.6–A.10 (p. 338). For drug doses, see Appendix Tables A.11–A.19 (p. 339).

A structured approach to the sick child

The child should be assessed in a structured manner treating each symptom in order as it is identified:

A: Airway

- Look for: signs of noisy breathing/airway obstruction.
- Common causes include: inhaled FB, dental abscess, croup, epiglottitis, tracheitis, retropharyngeal abscess.
- Treatment options:
  - If unconscious, use simple airway opening techniques (chin lift, jaw thrust). If conscious, do not distress the child further until simple treatment is started.
  - Consider giving adrenaline nebulizer (5 ml 1:1,000 adrenaline with oxygen), antibiotics (e.g. epiglottitis), and steroids (e.g. croup).

B: Breathing

- Look for signs of increased work of breathing (tracheal tug, intercostal or subcostal recession, nasal flaring, grunting).
- Measure respiratory rate (RR). This is a sensitive sign of illness. Causes of a high RR include pneumonia, sepsis, and dehydration.
- Listen to the chest using a stethoscope. Children with pneumonia can present late with established consolidation.
- Measure peripheral oxygen saturation. Treat with oxygen if saturations <92%.
- Treatment options:
  - Start antibiotics immediately if there are signs of sepsis or pneumonia.
  - Give oxygen using an oxygen concentrator or cylinder.

C: Circulation

- Look for signs of hypovolaemia and shock (see Table 7.7).
- Treatment options:
  - Gain IV access and take blood (cross-match and blood tests, if available). If IV access is difficult and the child is severely shocked, consider intraosseous (IO) access.
  - Consider 10–20 ml/kg bolus of IV fluid for severe shock. Isotonic solutions such as 0.9% saline, Hartmann's, or Ringer's lactate are suitable.
  - Use rapid fluid resuscitation with caution in children with sepsis, particularly if there are no ICU facilities or the child is severely anaemic. Slow rehydration may be more appropriate, particularly if the child has been unwell for some days.
  - Start maintenance fluid using the 4-2-1 formula (see Table 7.4).
  - Start antibiotics if there are concerns about infection or sepsis.

Table 7.7 Signs of shock in children.

Early (compensated)	Late (decompensated)
Tachycardia	Persisting tachycardia or bradycardia
Normal blood pressure	Hypotension
Tachypnoea	Poor capillary refill*
Mildly delayed capillary refill	Altered mental status (poor cerebral perfusion)
Weak peripheral pulses	Irregular breathing pattern/apnoeic episodes
Cool extremities	Poor muscle tone
Fussy, unsettled child	Decreased urine output

*capillary refill should be <2 s. Check nail beds in dark-skinned children.

D: Disability

- Measure blood glucose.
- Check conscious level using the AVPU (alert, verbal, pain, unresponsive) scale. Check pupils, posture.
- Causes of reduced conscious level may be:
  - non-neurological (e.g. hypovolaemia, sepsis)
  - neurological (e.g. meningitis, cerebral malaria, hydrocephalus, head injury).
- Treatment options:
  - Treat low blood glucose (<3 mmol/l) with a bolus of 2 ml/kg of 10% glucose.
  - Start treatment for low conscious level according to the likely cause.

E: Exposure

- Measure temperature.
- Look for rash, bruising, or other injuries. Examine abdomen for signs of tenderness and for enlarged liver, which may suggest heart failure.

Trauma

Consider in addition to the above:

- **Stop catastrophic haemorrhage immediately**: may require direct pressure or a tourniquet on the affected limb.
- Airway: assess 'airway with C-spine control'. Minimize neck movement using a collar, head blocks, and tape. An alert child who moves their own neck without pain has a low risk of neck injury.
- Breathing: look for signs of chest trauma (pneumo/haemothorax, rib fractures). Request a chest radiograph if possible. Young children have an elastic rib cage; rib fractures are a sign of severe trauma.
- Circulation: large-bore IV access and request blood urgently in haemorrhage. Transfuse with warmed blood early and observe for a response. Whole blood is ideal (in boluses of 10 ml/kg). Packed red cells are also suitable (boluses of 10 ml/kg) but clotting factors (e.g.

fresh frozen plasma) and platelets should also be given. Give tranexamic acid early, if available (15 mg/kg IV).
- Disability: assess for signs of head injury. Look for visible head trauma, palpable depressed skull fractures, bruising behind the ear (Battle's sign), bleeding from the ear canal or CSF leak. Management of head trauma can be challenging in low-resource environments and will depend on local services available. If intubation and ventilation is required the patient may need to be transferred to a facility with an ICU. Neurosurgical intervention is likely to be limited.
- Imaging: plain radiographs of the chest and pelvis may be helpful. If available, a computerized tomography (CT) scan may be appropriate, particularly in head injury.
- Urgent surgical intervention: this may be required to control haemorrhage or to stabilize fractures. Minor procedures may be possible under ketamine sedation. If a general anaesthetic is required:
  - Consider C-spine precautions intraoperatively.
  - Ensure blood is available and transfuse early.
  - Manage as an emergency and consider RSI.
  - Positive pressure ventilation may cause a simple pneumothorax to tension. Ensure you have the appropriate equipment available to manage this.
  - Keep the patient warm throughout.
- See Chapter 9 (p. 197).

Emergency triage, assessment, and treatment (ETAT)

The WHO developed the ETAT course based on the principles of advanced paediatric life support (APLS), modified for LMICs. ETAT defines emergency signs and priority signs to assist with the process of emergency treatment and triage.

ETAT emergency signs 'ABCD'

Problems with (A)irway, (B)reathing, (C)irculation/(C)oma/(C)onvulsion, or with (D)ehydration mandate immediate treatment.

ETAT priority signs '3 TPR-MOB'

These cases need to be at the front of the queue for assessment and rapid attention:
- Tiny baby: any sick child aged under 2 months.
- Temperature: child is very hot.
- Trauma or other urgent surgical condition.
- Pallor (severe)—look at palm of hand.
- Poisoning.
- Pain (severe).
- Respiratory distress.
- Restless, continuously irritable, or lethargic.
- Referral (urgent, from another facility).
- Malnutrition: visible severe wasting.
- Oedema of both feet.
- Burns.

Further reading

Allman K, Wilson I. (2016) *Oxford Handbook of Anaesthesia*, 4th ed. Oxford: Oxford University Press.

Cote C, Lerman J, Anderson B. (2013) *A Practice of Anesthesia for Infants and Children*, 5th ed. Philadelphia, PA: Elsevier.

Holtzman R, Mancuso T, Polaner D. (2015) *A Practical Approach to Pediatric Anesthesia*, 2nd ed. Philadelphia, PA: Lippincott Williams and Wilkins.

Homer R, Walker I, Bell G. (2015) Paediatric Anaesthesia and Critical Care (Special Edition). *Update in Anaesthesia* 30 (1).

James I, Walker I (2013) *Core Topics in Paediatric Anaesthesia*. Cambridge: Cambridge University Press.

Maitland K et al. (2011) Mortality after fluid bolus in African children with severe infection. *NEJM* 364: 2483–2495.

Kopf A, Patel NB (2010) *Guide to Pain Management in Low Resource Settings*. Seattle, WA: IASP. Available at: https://www.iasp-pain.org/files/Content/ContentFolders/Publications2/FreeBooks/Guide_to_Pain_Management_in_Low-Resource_Settings.pdf (accessed February 2018).

World Health Organization (2005) *Emergency Triage and Assessment (ETAT+) Course*. Geneva: World Health Organization. Available at: http://www.who.int/maternal_child_adolescent/documents/9241546875/en (accessed September 2019).

World Health Organization (2013) *Updates on the Management of Severe Acute Malnutrition in Infants and Children*. Geneva: World Health Organization. Available at: http://www.who.int/nutrition/publications/guidelines/updates_management (accessed September 2019).

World Health Organization (2016) *Oxygen Therapy for Children: A Manual for Health Workers*. Geneva: World Health Organization. Available at: http://apps.who.int/iris/bitstream/10665/204584/1/9789241549554_eng.pdf?ua=1 (accessed September 2019).

Chapter 8

Obstetrics and Gynaecology

Rachel Collis, Rebecca Jones, and Sarah O'Neill

Preoperative assessment

Key points

- Certain pregnancy-associated conditions rarely seen in well-resourced countries are more commonly encountered in low- and middle-income countries (LMICs), e.g. severe eclampsia, uterine rupture, life-threatening anaemia.
- In LMICs, desirable investigations, equipment, and drugs may be unavailable—inevitably some assumptions and compromises will have to be made in planning safe care.

Urgency of delivery

The urgency of the procedure to be undertaken is a key initial question—some form of categorization can help to prioritize, even if these systems are not formally recognized in many countries.

- The Royal College of Obstetricians and Gynaecologists categorizes Caesarean sections (CSs) into four levels of urgency (see Table 8.1). The following should be noted:
- Categories 1–4 represent a continuous spectrum of risk: delivery should be carried out with an urgency that is appropriate to the risk to the baby but takes into account the safety of the mother.
- Consequently, the suggested decision-to-delivery interval (DDI) time is a guide only—a 'Cat. 1' may need delivery quicker than 30 min; a 'Cat. 2' may not need delivery within 1 h.
- The foetus should be monitored throughout if feasible: urgency may change at any time prior to the start of surgery.
- This system can be used for other obstetric interventions, not just Caesarean deliveries.

Past medical history

Cardiovascular

Structural heart disease

- Congenital heart disease and some types of acquired problems such as rheumatic heart disease are much more common in LMICs.

Table 8.1 Urgency of delivery for Caesarean section.

Category	Definition	Suggested decision-to-delivery interval
1	Immediate threat to life of woman or foetus	Delivery within 30 min
2	Maternal or foetal compromise needing early delivery	Delivery within 1 h
3	No immediate threat to life of woman or foetus but requires early delivery	Delivery within 24 h
4	Delivery at a time to suit the woman and maternity services	n/a

Data from RCoG Good practice guide No. 11. Classification of urgency of Caesarean section.

Hypertension
- Pre-existing hypertension is more common in LMIC populations, often untreated and is associated with early onset pre-eclamptic toxaemia (PET) syndrome and renal impairment in pregnancy.

Anaemia
- Symptoms of anaemia will be exacerbated by pregnancy.
- Anaemia is more common and more severe in LMICs due to:
  - chronic bacterial infections, e.g. osteomyelitis
  - parasitic infections, e.g. hookworm, malaria
  - malnutrition.

Respiratory
- Severe (untreated) asthma and tuberculosis are common in many LMICs. The condition may deteriorate during pregnancy, though asthma can also improve.

Neurological
- Exacerbation of epilepsy is common and needs to be differentiated from other causes of grand mal convulsions such as eclampsia.

Endocrine
- Diabetes is often poorly controlled without access to specialist services. There is an increased risk of hypo- or hyperglycaemic crises in pregnancy and worsening of secondary complications of diabetes.

Infectious diseases
- The condition of mothers with chronic infections such as HIV and hepatitis can deteriorate in pregnancy.
- Malaria is a serious and potentially life-threatening infection in pregnancy. It is more likely to present atypically, e.g. hypoglycaemia, pulmonary oedema, cerebral malaria. There is an increased risk of developing clotting abnormalities.

Obstetric history

Gravidity (G) and parity (P)
- G: the number of pregnancies.
- P: the number of births.
  - P0: expect long labour; possibility of obstructed labour with subsequent high risk of uterine atony.
  - P4 and above: expect short or 'precipitous' labour; high risk of uterine atony and postpartum haemorrhage (PPH).

Previous mode of delivery
- Previous CS with history of obstructed labour will make CS more likely.
- Prolonged labour with a uterine scar increases the risk of uterine rupture in labour.
- In any patient with previous CS or uterine surgery, try to ascertain the placental position—low anterior placenta with previous CS increases the risk of placenta accreta and severe PPH.

Twins
- Increased incidence of PET and gestational diabetes.

- Increased risk of malpresentation of the foetuses leading to difficult delivery and PPH.

Placenta praevia or abruption

There is a risk of obstetric haemorrhage. See 'Obstetric Haemorrhage' (pp. 179–84).

Medical problems associated with pregnancy

Gestational diabetes

- May be diagnosed late, is associated with poor glucose control in the mother, and leads to:
  - Increased risk of foetal macrosomia, leading to difficult vaginal delivery.
  - Polyhydramnios, leading to an increased risk of premature labour, cord prolapse, and sudden stillbirth.
- Insulin is often not available (difficult to transport and store).
- The requirement for hypoglycaemic medication drops immediately after delivery, with a significant risk of hypoglycaemia to the mother (metformin is safe whilst fasting pre-CS).
- The baby is also at high risk of hypoglycaemia post-delivery.

Pre-eclampsia/eclampsia

See 'Pre-eclampsia and Eclampsia' (pp. 185–8).

Sepsis

- Sepsis derived from the genital tract is termed puerperal sepsis and can be rapidly fatal for mother and baby.
- All forms of sepsis are more common in pregnancy and a high index of suspicion is required to identify and rapidly treat cases.
- Common causes are chorioamnionitis, urosepsis, pneumonia, and wound infections (Caesarean site or perineum).

Antepartum haemorrhage

- Ask: how recently and how much? Loss may be concealed.
- The foetus is usually affected by maternal hypovolaemia (tachycardia or bradycardia) before the mother shows signs of hypovolaemia herself.

Medication and allergies

- Current medication.
- Recent heparin? Ideally allow the following time interval prior to spinal or epidural anaesthesia:
  - Prophylactic low molecular weight heparin—12 h.
  - Treatment dose low molecular weight heparin—24 h from last dose, even if given in divided doses.
  - Unfractionated heparin—4 h.
- Allergies—can be difficult to ascertain the cause of past reactions if there are any language difficulties.

Fasting and reflux risk

- Elective cases (Cat. 4) should be fasted as per normal guidelines.
- Gastric acid prophylaxis should ideally be given to pregnant women from 18 weeks' gestation to 48 h post-delivery.

- H2 receptor antagonists should be prescribed regularly for women in labour at high risk of needing to go to theatre (very aspirational):
  - Oral ranitidine 150 mg, every 12 h (onset 1–3 h, duration 10–12 h).
  - Intravenous (slowly) ranitidine 50 mg, every 8 h (onset 30 min, duration 6–8 h).
- Give sodium citrate 30 ml 0.3 M prior to emergency anaesthesia if available. If not available (very likely)—do not give a particulate antacid and accept that none is given.

Investigations

The ideal standard

- Haemoglobin, platelet count, and blood typing ('group and save') as a minimum in all women.
- If haemorrhage is likely, request cross-matched blood to be available.
- Urine dipstick for protein to check for PET.
- If sepsis or PET suspected: white cell count, electrolytes, and creatinine. NB: white cell count (WCC) is normally raised in labour (see Table 8.2).
- + Liver function tests (LFTs) in suspected PET only.
- + Coagulation tests if severe PET, ongoing haemorrhage, or malaria.
- Electrocardiogram (ECG) if cardiac disease suspected. In pregnancy, normal variants include:
  - More ectopics than normal.
  - A degree of left axis deviation.
  - Small Q wave in lead III.
  - Slight ST-segment depression and T-wave inversion in the inferior and lateral leads.

Low-resource environments

- You may not have access to any laboratory tests at all or the ability to transfuse blood.
- You will have to rely on clinical history and examination.
- Without blood, the surgical approach may need to be modified, e.g. earlier recourse to hysterectomy in severe PPH.
- Being unable to test platelets and clotting function makes decision making harder, particularly in patients with PET.

Table 8.2 Normal laboratory values in pregnancy.

Investigation	Normal range in third trimester (↑ or ↓)
Haemoglobin	95–150 g/l (↓)
White cells	6–16 × 10^9/l (↑) (transiently higher in labour mean 17 × 10^9/l)
Creatinine	35–80 µm/l (0.4–0.9 mg/l) (↓)
Platelets	150–430 × 10^9/l (↑)
Fibrinogen	3.7–6.2 g/l (↑)

Arrows indicate the direction of change of values in pregnancy from non-pregnant values.

Data from Abbassi-Ghanavati M, Greer LG, Cunningham FG. Pregnancy and laboratory studies: a reference table for clinicians. *Obstet Gynecol.* 2009 Dec; 114(6): 1326–31. PMID: 19935037.

- In low-resource settings, without any lab tests, and in the absence of major bleeding, the risk of a single-shot spinal is almost always lower than that of a general anaesthetic for mothers with PET.
- In any patient with clinical evidence of coagulopathy (bleeding from the cannula site, bruising), regional anaesthesia should be avoided if another option is safely available.

When to operate—special considerations

Transfers

- When working in low-resource settings it is sometimes possible to transfer women to another centre rather than proceed yourself. There are usually risks involved (see 'Patient Transfer' in Chapter 9 (pp. 223–5). Involve the patient in all discussions before initiating a transfer.
- Only facilitate the transfer of a woman to another centre if:
    - She is willing.
    - Time allows.
    - It is logistically safe to do so. (How will they travel? Who will accompany them?)
    - A better level of care is accessible, not just available. (NB: paying for healthcare in expensive facilities does not always guarantee a better level of care.)
    - The mother/foetus may derive benefit from a higher level of care.

Caesarean sections

- The decision to perform a CS should be made by the woman herself in consultation with the medical team caring for her.
- Following a CS it is generally advised that future deliveries should take place in or near a health facility (risk of uterine rupture, especially in prolonged labour). However, in many LMICs this may be/become difficult for financial, geographical, and/or political reasons.
- Consequently, the woman's predicted access to future obstetric care may subtly shift the bar for her choosing to undergo a CS (or not).

Analgesia in labour

Introduction

- Attitudes to labour pain vary. However, worldwide there is a vast unmet need for analgesia in labouring women.
- Pain is often greater in nulliparous women, those undergoing induction of labour, or with foetal malposition. It is also greater in the supine position than upright or lateral.
- The gold standard technique for pain control in labour is epidural analgesia. However, this is not practical in most LMIC hospitals due to lack of staffing, training, monitoring, equipment, and drugs.

Pain relief options commonly available in LMICs

- A supportive lay adult known to the mother (effective in reducing anxiety, pain, and complications).
- Massage, positioning, relaxation, and water bath.
- Paracetamol in early labour.
- Opioids—may be available in limited supply. Note can cause neonatal respiratory depression.
  - pethidine (meperidine): 50–100 mg intramuscular (IM)
  - morphine: 5–10 mg IM
  - tramadol: 50–100 mg IM
  - meptazinol (partial μ receptor agonist): 75–100 mg IM.
- Pudendal or paracervical block—consider for analgesia in second stage, e.g. for instrumental delivery or episiotomy.
- Perineal local anaesthesia infiltration (prior to episiotomy).

Pain relief options sometimes available in LMICs

- Entonox® (high cost in LMICs).
- Inhalational anaesthesia, e.g. 0.7% isoflurane for second stage.
- Neuraxial techniques, e.g. epidural, low-dose spinal.

Analgesics contraindicated in labour

- Non-steroidal anti-inflammatory drugs (NSAIDs)—risk of closure of foetal ductus arteriosus *in utero*.
- Codeine—risk of respiratory depression in neonate (dihydro-codeine acceptable but unlikely to be available).

Mitral stenosis (MS) in obstetrics

Introduction

- Whilst other causes of MS exist, it is commonly related to rheumatic heart disease, which has a higher incidence and often an accelerated course in LMICs compared with high-income countries (HICs).
- MS is often unmasked in pregnancy due to the cardiovascular changes that occur:
  - Cardiac output (CO) normally begins to increase from around 5 l/min at week 5 of gestation to a peak at week 20–24 of 7.5 l/min.
  - CO rises further during labour, especially during contractions, to approximately 10–11 l/min.
  - Following delivery, blood from the vasculature of the contracting uterus is released into the venous system. This represents an 'auto-transfusion' of up to 500 ml.
  - CO starts to fall within the first 48 h but takes several weeks to return to pre-pregnancy levels.

Presentation

- Patients with MS cannot increase their CO to the required degree and therefore develop congestive cardiac failure, pulmonary hypertension, and left atrial enlargement.
- This commonly presents with dyspnoea on minimal exertion, palpitations, cough, chest pain, haemoptysis, or even stroke.
- It may present for the first time in pregnancy, labour, or postpartum.

Signs

- Atrial arrhythmias, most commonly atrial fibrillation (AF): a sign of severe disease.
- Mid-diastolic murmur, often with a thrill.
- Heart failure (tachypnoea, tachycardia, orthopnoea, desaturation, pulmonary crepitations, hypotension, peripheral oedema).

Investigations

- Echocardiogram if available:
  - normal mitral valve area: 4–6 cm^2
  - mild stenosis: 1.5–2.5 cm^2
  - moderate stenosis: 1–1.5 cm^2
  - critical stenosis: <1 cm^2.
- Chest X-ray: may show cardiomegaly, pulmonary oedema, and signs of enlarged left atrium, e.g. double right heart border and a splayed subcarinal angle >120°.
- ECG: may show bifid P wave in lead II (P mitrale) and/or AF.

Management during pregnancy

- Avoid tachycardia (aim for a heart rate of 70–90 beats/min) using beta-blockers to increase time for diastolic filling.
- If there is AF:
  - First line beta-blockers, second line digoxin.

- Avoid amiodarone unless no alternative—increases risk of foetal goitre.
- Consider synchronized electrical cardioversion (if in AF for more than 48 h, exclude cardiac thrombus first if possible).
- Consider thromboprophylaxis.

- If there is heart failure despite rate control: diuretics.
- If there is pulmonary oedema: admit to hospital for intravenous (IV) diuretics.
- If symptoms are persistent despite medical therapy: consider percutaneous mitral valvuloplasty or valve replacement during pregnancy—but this is unlikely to be an option in most LMICs.
- Avoid exertion but also avoid bed rest.
- Keep Hb >9 g/dl (iron, folic acid).
- Make an early plan for management during labour.

Management of labour

- Give oxygen.
- Monitor frequently if possible, e.g. 30-min vital signs—unlikely to have invasive blood pressure (BP) monitoring.
- The patient should be in lateral position, upright or left tilt, not supine or lithotomy.
- Carry out careful fluid management: secure IV access but no IV fluids, allow oral fluids and treat hypovolaemia—administer small IV boluses if there is hypotension, e.g. 200 ml and re-assess.
- Good labour analgesia should be provided as early as possible, e.g. epidural if available or opiates if not.

Labour epidural

- Often lack of equipment and training means an intermittent bolus dose given by an anaesthetist is only available technique.
- 0.5% Bupivacaine is usually available but would cause too much hypotension when given for labour analgesia—dilute with 0.9% saline to make 0.1% bupivacaine with fentanyl 2 μg/ml or 0.125% bupivacaine if no fentanyl is available.
- Administer an initial epidural test dose of 3 ml then 10 ml every 30–60 min until comfortable. Alternatively, an infusion may be run at 8–12 ml/h.
- In low-resource settings care is rarely 1:1. Therefore depending on circumstances the anaesthetist might need to provide as close as possible to 1:1 care themselves until the epidural is removed.
- Ensure that the obstetrician and midwife are aware that the patient may not feel contractions, so they will need to be palpated.
- Once the cervix is fully dilated, delivery should be delayed for at least 1 h (if the patient and foetus are stable) to allow for descent of the foetal head. Avoid pushing if possible and aim for passive 'lift out' of the foetus with ventouse or forceps.

Anaesthesia for operative procedures

- Relatively fixed CO, so aim to avoid tachycardia, maintain sinus rhythm, and normovolaemia and aim for normal to high systemic vascular resistance.

- Choices are usually between combined spinal-epidural (CSE), epidural, General anaesthesia (GA) with increased opiate/reduced induction agent, or, rarely, local infiltration.
- Ketamine is best avoided due to tachycardia.
- A single-shot spinal best avoided unless the mitral valve is known to be only mildly stenosed (valve area >1.5 cm^2). However, this may often be the only option available and should be managed with aggressive use of a vasoconstrictor.
- Antibiotic endocarditis prophylaxis is frequently given but is probably not needed unless there is infection at the site of surgery, e.g. chorioamnionitis. Ampicillin and gentamicin are commonly recommended. Check local guidelines.

Post-delivery

- Uterotonics: avoid bolus IV syntocinon—give a slow infusion e.g. 5 units over 20 min. Avoid ergometrine (increases saturated vapour pressure).
- Misoprostol is relatively contraindicated in women with underlying cardiac disease due to potential hypotension but in practice this is not usually a problem.
- There should be early consideration of surgical techniques for haemostasis.
- Ensure careful fluid balance and avoid rapid fluid boluses. A degree of blood loss is usually well tolerated as it offsets the potentially harmful effect of the post-delivery auto-transfusion (up to 500 ml).
- If IV fluid required give slow IV infusions, e.g. 1 l every 12 h or slower.
- The patient should be closely monitored for the first 2 h postpartum—this is a high risk period for heart failure.
- Keep the patient as an inpatient for a minimum of 2 days but try to mobilize her as soon as possible if stable.
- Before discharge: ensure follow-up arrangements, contraceptive advice, and consider mitral valve surgery 6 months postpartum.

Spinal anaesthesia

Key points

- Where spinal anaesthesia can be safely performed, it is the method of choice for CS in most situations. It can also be used for perineal suturing, evacuation of retained placenta, and forceps delivery.
- It should be avoided in patients with known bleeding disorders (including those on anticoagulant therapy, unless sufficient time has elapsed)—see 'Contraindications' (p. 167).
- Strict asepsis should be used when performing spinal anaesthesia.
- Ideally, equipment to undertake GA should be available in case conversion to GA is required.
- The ability to monitor pulse, BP, and ECG should also be available although only some (or occasionally none) of these things may be available in certain settings.
- Some form of vasoconstrictor drug to treat hypotension is mandatory: if none is available then do not attempt spinal anaesthesia; consider ketamine anaesthesia instead (see 'Ketamine for Caesarean Section' (pp. 175–6).
- Patients should have identical preoperative preparation as for GA, including aspiration prophylaxis.
- Following spinal anaesthesia, the mother should be placed in a left-tilted (15°) or pelvis-wedged position (visible displacement of uterus) to reduce the effects of aortocaval compression.

Contraindications to spinal anaesthesia

These must be weighed against the relative risk of GA in your context, which may be greater than you are used to.

Relative

- Uncorrected hypovolaemia (beware concealed haemorrhage).
- Cardiac valve stenosis.
- Coagulopathy or thrombocytopenia (aim international normalized ratio (INR) <1.4, platelets $>75 \times 10^9$/l, preferably within last 2 h in the case of PET). Note: If platelets are between 50 and 75×10^9/l, a spinal may still be a reasonable option if there are relative contraindications to GA.
- Localized sepsis at the intended injection site or major untreated systemic infection.
- Patients suspected of having raised intracranial pressure.

Absolute

- Maternal refusal.
- Lack of vasoconstrictors, e.g. ephedrine, adrenaline, phenylephrine.

Performing the spinal

- Sterile gown and drapes may not be available without exhausting supplies. Often, the sterile paper of the gloves is used as the sterile field to work from and a sterile gauze to feel for the iliac crest (L3–4).
- Insertion should be performed below the L2–3 intervertebral space.
- Spinal introducer needles are often not available—either use a spinal needle without an introducer (prick the skin first to avoid skin plugging

the spinal needle, not an issue if your spinal needle has an inner stylet) or use a 16G hypodermic needle as an introducer.

- The spread of the local anaesthetic block will depend primarily on:
  - the amount (mg) of drug administered
  - whether the local anaesthetic used is more or less dense than cerebrospinal fluid (CSF) and the position of the patient following insertion
  - barbotage: the local anaesthetic is part injected and then CSF drawn back into the syringe mixing it with the drug remaining in the syringe, then re-injected—this practice increases the spread of local anaesthetic.

Aortocaval compression

- The sympathetic nervous system maintains vascular tone—spinal block produces vasodilatation and a tendency to hypotension.
- Effect is greater in the supine pregnant patient due to compression of the vena cava (and aorta) by the gravid uterus.
- A fall in venous return can lead to severe and sudden maternal hypotension and even cardiac arrest.
- To counteract this, the mother should never be placed flat on her back but either tilted to the left (ideally 15° or more) or a sandbag placed under the right hip with visible uterine displacement.

Preventing hypotension post-spinal

- At least moderate dehydration due to long labours and delays in admission to hospital is common in LMICs, so loading with IV fluid is usually sensible.
- Hypotension is common—a large-bore (16G) intravenous cannula should be placed and attached to a free-running fluid infusion.
- A vasoconstrictor drug should be pre-prepared ready to administer and treat maternal hypotension and/or bradycardia.
- If the mother develops hypotension (more than a 20% systolic drop from the pre-spinal level) or the symptoms of feeling faint, lethargy, or nausea prior to measuring the BP, then administer a vasopressor and increase uterine displacement if possible.
- Table 8.3 shows vasopressor drugs that can be titrated to effect to correct hypotension. Some, e.g. metaraminol, may cause bradycardia (heart rate <50). If necessary, bradycardias can be treated with:
  - glycopyrronium—200 µg bolus
  - atropine—200 µg bolus.
- Note adrenaline is often the only vasopressor available in LMICs.
- Some of the drugs in Table 8.3 can also be given by infusion—see the Appendix.

Choice of drug for spinal anaesthesia

- It is absolutely imperative that only sterile drugs are used and in a formulation that is not neurotoxic (preservative free).
- A number of local anaesthetic drugs can be safely used and choice will depend on local availability and practice. Suggested doses are outlined

in Table 8.4. Always discuss normal dosing regimens with local staff and heed advice.
- The dose should be reduced by around 40–50% when only a perineal block is required, e.g. for perineal suturing.
- Multi-patient dosing from one vial should be avoided.

Spinal opioids

- Will improve the quality of the anaesthesia, may prolong the duration of block, and provide postoperative analgesia after the effect of the local anaesthesia has worn off.
  - Fentanyl—10–25 μg. Duration up to 4 h.
  - Morphine—100 μg. Duration over 24 h.
- Should not be used if appropriate postoperative care is not available—remember they are desirable, not essential, for the CS.
- Fentanyl is the safest option for enhancing intraoperative block with minimal postoperative effect.
- It is essential that the formulation of opiate used is suitable for injection into the spinal space and is free of preservatives—most morphine formulations contain preservative and are not safe for intra-thecal use.

Testing the block

- The block can be tested using temperature, e.g. with ice, pin prick using a blunt needle, or light touch.
- Prior to commencing CS a bilateral sensory block from T4 (nipple) to cold or T6 (xiphisternum) to pin prick is required. Inferiorly, the block should extend to S1 bilaterally with a dense motor block of both legs.
- The light touch element, which can be tested with a finger or gauze, should be blocked to T8.
- The lower extent can be tested by stimulating the sole of the foot or the back of the calf; however, it is unusual not to get a good sacral block with a spinal.
- A useful confirmation of good sensory block is to firmly pinch the patient just below the umbilicus. It is acceptable to feel some sensation but it should not be detected as a sharp pinch.

Suboptimal block

- Depending on the drug used, spinal anaesthesia is usually achieved within 10 min. If not adequate within 15 min, another course of action is required.

Complete failure

- Can be managed by a repeat spinal attempt with the same dose if there is no urgency for delivery.

Options for a partial but inadequate block

- If unilateral: turn the mother onto the inadequate side for 5 min.
- If the block is dense but of inadequate height (common if the baby is premature or small): with the mother in the supine (wedged or tilted) position bring both of her legs into the foetal position and hold her there for 3 min or put the bed in the Trendelenburg position for a few minutes.
- If neither of the above is effective, options include:

Table 8.3 Vasoconstrictors for treating post-spinal hypotension.

Drug	Concentration	Bolus dose
Ephedrine	3–5 mg/ml	1 ml
Adrenaline	5 µg/ml	1 ml
Phenylephrine	25 µg/ml	1 ml
Noradrenaline	5 µg/ml	1 ml
Metaraminol	0.5 mg/ml	1 ml
Methoxamine	2 mg/ml	1 ml

Table 8.4 Local anaesthetic doses for spinal anaesthesia.

Local anaesthetic	Concentration	Dose for Caesarean section	Duration
Bupivacaine (Hyper- or isobaric)	0.5%	2–2.5 ml	–3 h
Lidocaine	2%	3–4 ml	30–45 min
Lidocaine	5%	1.2–1.6 ml	60–90 min
Cinchocaine (heavy)	0.5%	2–3 ml	2–3 h
Tetracaine	1%	0.7–1.1 ml	2–3 h
Tetracaine	0.5%	1.5–2.5 ml	2–3 h
Pethidine (meperidine)	50 mg/ml	1.5 ml	

Note pethidine has opioid and local anaesthetic properties and can be used as a sole agent.

- Repeat the spinal with 50% of original dose but ensure that when placing the mother back into the supine position her shoulders are raised from the mid-thoracic dermatomes (pillow or folded blanket) to prevent a high block.
- Supplement with ketamine.
- Proceed to GA if safe to do so.

Pain during the procedure

- This is more common if intrathecal opiates are not used.
- Options include:
  - Mild pain: intravenous ketamine bolus doses of 10 mg increments up to 0.5 mg/kg or intravenous opiate in small doses, e.g. fentanyl in 25 µg increments after clamping of the cord—neonatal resuscitation may be suboptimal and neonatal naloxone is unlikely to be available.
  - If closing the abdominal wall, the surgeon can give local anaesthetic infiltration to incision site.
  - Convert to GA. Intubate if possible or convert to ketamine with spontaneously breathing technique.

Spinal anaesthesia for other procedures

Perineal repair

- Low spinal block involving just the sacral roots is required. In addition to a lower volume of local anaesthetic solution, spread can be restricted by using hyperbaric solution and keeping the patient sat up after spinal injection for 5 min.

Removal of retained placenta

- Requires a block of uterine innervation. To ensure a dense block of the uterus, it is best to aim to achieve a block to around T8. Intrathecal fentanyl if available is very beneficial.

Forceps delivery

- Requires perineal and uterine anaesthesia, therefore a block to T8.
- Confirm with the surgeon whether the trial of instrumental delivery may proceed straight to CS if vaginal delivery fails, in which case a high sensory block to T4 is required from the outset.

Postoperative

- Observations are required, ideally hourly for at least 4 h (higher frequency if unstable) and every 4 h for the remainder of 24 h.
- Position in the lateral position or propped up, if not hypotensive, to allow breastfeeding.
- Depending on the drug used, full motor power and sensation usually return within 6 h. Following return of function early mobilization should be encouraged.
- Oral fluid and food should be encouraged early unless there is concern about massive haemorrhage or reduced conscious level (prolonged post-CS fasting is common in some countries).
- Many institutions place a urinary catheter at the time of surgery and leave it in place for 12–24 h after the operation. If a catheter is not left in place, monitor closely for any signs of urinary retention (lower abdominal pain/discomfort, unpassed urine).
- Check that the neonate is placed on the mother's skin to prevent neonatal hypothermia and encourage early breastfeeding.
- Post-dural puncture headache: more likely to occur with Quincke needles (up to 25% rate with 25G). Epidural blood patch is not commonly performed as there is an increased risk of sepsis in LMICs. Manage conservatively with simple analgesia and fluids.

General anaesthesia

Key points

- Intubation protects against the high risk of aspiration in obstetric patients and is mandated when expertise and equipment allow.
- Positioning must be optimized for both intubation and uterine displacement.
- Extubation should be delayed until the mother is awake, breathing normally, and protective airway reflexes have returned.
- This is a description of an ideal GA technique for an emergency CS—it will certainly need to be modified and compromises made where resources are limited.

Anaesthetic technique

Pre-anaesthetic

- Check your equipment (see Chapter 2) and prepare drugs. Ensure you have a means to tilt the pelvis.
- Place essential equipment, drugs, and airway equipment nearby, i.e. within easy reaching distance—there is usually no anaesthetic assistant to pass you things.
- Difficult airway equipment is frequently limited in LMICs. Supraglottic airways and bougies may not be readily available—take this into account when making a failed intubation plan.
- Give antacid. See 'Fasting and Reflux Risk' (pp. 160–1).

Position

- Obstetric patients should be anaesthetized and intubated in the ramped position. Place a single pillow under the head to improve head extension and either tilt the table 15° to the left or place a support under the right hip to displace the uterus.

Pre-oxygenate

- Give O_2 via a nasal cannula and leave it on until the patient is intubated.
- Ideal pre-oxygenation (100% oxygen for 3 min) uses a lot of oxygen. If using cylinder oxygen consider the pros and cons of pre-oxygenating in this manner. Alternatives include:
  - Three vital capacity breaths from 100% oxygen.
  - An oxygen concentrator running at 4 l/min through a draw-over system with an oxygen reservoir can provide a fractional inspired oxygen concentration (FiO_2) of up to 0.6 to an adult with normal minute ventilation—this can be used to provide reasonable pre-oxygenation. Modern draw-over systems with a reservoir bag may provide an even higher FiO_2.
  - Use an oxygen concentrator to fill a reservoir (e.g. a large plastic bin bag) with oxygen. This can then be attached to the breathing circuit for pre-oxygenation. Note that when the reservoir has been used up, the bag must be removed or it may occlude the breathing system.

Induction of anaesthesia

- Is classically performed with a rapid sequence induction technique.
- Between giving the muscle relaxant and intubating, gently ventilate the patient if oxygen saturation (SpO_2) is starting to fall.

Management of difficult or failed intubation

- A locally agreed failed intubation algorithm must be in place.
- Laryngeal mask airways are increasingly used to rescue a failed intubation and the risk of aspiration seems to be small. If not available then maintain oxygenation with Guedel airway and hand mask/bag ventilation.
- Consider waking the mother up depending on the adequacy of maternal oxygenation and the urgency of the CS.

Maintenance of anaesthesia

- Ventilate the lungs with oxygen and nitrous oxide or air if available or an air/O_2 mixture.
- Use 0.75–1 minimum alveolar concentration (MAC) of a volatile agent. Remember that the wash-in of halothane is much slower than, for instance, sevoflurane. Therefore, use overpressure, i.e. 2% of halothane.
- Ventilate the lungs to an end-tidal carbon dioxide of 4.0 kPa, or at a tidal volume of 7 ml/kg and a frequency of 12–14 breaths/min. Add positive end expiratory pressure (PEEP) if possible.
- After delivery of the baby give uterotonics. See Table 8.5.
- Antibiotic prophylaxis, e.g. co-amoxiclav 1.2 g IV, should be given prior to induction but in an emergency can be given after delivery.
- If the mother starts to breathe after the suxamethonium has worn off, a small dose of a non-depolarizing muscle relaxant can be given if respiratory effort is interfering with surgery.
- Give analgesia after delivery of the baby, e.g. diclofenac 50–100 mg per rectum if there is no major haemorrhage or other contraindication, plus paracetamol orally or rectally.
- IV or IM opiates can be given after the cord is clamped, e.g. pethidine 50–100 mg or morphine 5–10 mg.
- Alternatively, ketamine can be given, 0.5 mg/kg slowly IV.
- Infiltrate the incision with local anaesthetic.

Recovery from anaesthesia

- Extubate in the sitting position or left lateral head-down.
- Give reversal if supplies allow, e.g. neostigmine 2.5 mg with atropine 600 μg.
- Nerve stimulators are often not available. Adequate power should be assessed clinically, e.g. the ability to lift the head off the bed for 5 s, protrude the tongue, and squeeze a hand.

Modifications

Hypertension or cardiac valve stenosis

- Induction of anaesthesia should be modified in the presence of hypertensive diseases of pregnancy to avoid the hypertensive and tachycardic (detrimental in valve stenoses) response to laryngoscopy and intubation.
- Options include:
  - lidocaine 1.5 mg/kg IV
  - alfentanil 10–20 μg/kg IV

 - fentanyl 1–2 μg/kg IV
 - magnesium sulfate 1–2 g IV
 - labetalol 5 mg IV
 - hydralazine 5–10 mg IV over 5 min (NB: risk of tachycardia).
- If an opioid is used, there is a risk of neonatal respiratory depression requiring ventilation/naloxone after delivery.

Magnesium sulfate
- In patients being treated with magnesium, the dose of non-depolarizing relaxant should be reduced by 50%. The normal dose of suxamethonium should be used.

Monitoring
- In the absence of ECG, capnography, and/or pulse oximetry, monitoring will consist of manual palpation of a peripheral pulse and non-invasive BP recordings.
- It is useful for somebody else to monitor the patient's pulse during induction. Adequacy of chest expansion and colour of the mucous membranes should be assessed regularly during the procedure.

Unavailability of suxamethonium
- If suxamethonium is unavailable, tracheal intubation can be facilitated with a non-depolarizing agent. Options for modified rapid sequence induction without suxamethonium are outlined in 'Absent Drugs and Work-arounds', Chapter 4 (pp. 65–6).

Ketamine for Caesarean section

Key points

- Ketamine is widely used in LMICs for CS.
- It has a wide margin of safety.
- It provides analgesia, anaesthesia, maintenance of sympathetic tone, and uterine tone.
- It is especially useful in patients who are shocked.

Contraindications

- As well as general contraindications to ketamine (see 'Ketamine' in Chapter 4, (pp. 56–60) there are some particular considerations in pregnancy.
  - Pregnancy is a relative contraindication in itself unless ketamine is being used to facilitate delivery of the foetus—increased uterine tone can cause foetal hypoxia.
  - Hypertensive disease of pregnancy, e.g. pre-eclampsia, even if well-controlled, can lead to marked hypertension—ketamine is best avoided unless there is no alternative.
  - Cardiac disease. Certain cardiac lesions, e.g. ischaemic cardiac disease or stenotic valve lesions, may decompensate in the presence of a ketamine-induced tachycardia.

Equipment

- Ideally all the normal equipment required for safe GA in pregnancy should be available. In practice, the decision to perform a CS under ketamine often indicates that resources are very limited.
- Some means to ventilate the patient, e.g. bag, valve, mask, is essential however—patients often become transiently apnoeic and desaturate quickly in pregnancy.
- Supplemental oxygen is not absolutely essential as ketamine does not depress ventilation but it would be advisable only to proceed without oxygen in an absolute emergency. Ventilation would need to be supported in the case of any desaturation.
- Restraints for a non-paralysed patient (e.g. leg strap, bandages for arms) may be required.

Doses and techniques

Induction

- Pre-oxygenate and position as normal.
- Give 1 mg/kg IV (with higher doses babies come out very 'flat'). Inject slowly as rapid injection may cause transient apnoea.
- If the patient is very shocked consider reducing the dose to 0.5 mg/kg.
- Ketamine has a slower onset than other IV agents, wait until the patient is not responding to verbal commands or painful stimulus, e.g. pinch, before proceeding. The induction dose will last about 15 min.
- Gently ventilate if the patient becomes apnoeic—it will be transient.
- Atropine 10–20 μg/kg at induction to reduce salivation is an option. It is relatively contraindicated in a patient who is already tachycardic or pyrexial (reduces sweating). Note it is not essential in an emergency, and can be given later on if required.

- This can be followed by either a spontaneously breathing technique or intubation. Intubate if circumstances allow.
- Diazepam is advised 0.1 mg/kg IV (5 mg is usually sufficient) and, if available, fentanyl or morphine after cord clamping to reduce emergence phenomenon. Although, if breathing is shallow in spontaneous breathing technique, wait until breathing deepens.

Maintenance (intubated and/or spontaneously breathing patients)
- intermittent slow boluses: 0.5 mg/kg every 15 min or
- ketamine infusion: see 'Ketamine' in Chapter 4 (pp. 56–60).

Ketamine anaesthesia with spontaneously breathing patient

- Laryngeal reflexes and pharyngeal tone are relatively preserved, eyes may stay open, and nystagmus commonly occurs (no need to tape eyelids).
- The patient may have involuntary movements during surgery, so it is common practice to restrain the patient's limbs.
- Apply supplemental oxygen via a nasal cannula or face mask; chin lift or jaw thrust may be required.
- Regular, gentle suction of pharyngeal secretions is often required.
- Consider adjuncts (paracetamol, NSAIDs, LA infiltration, opioids).
- Stop giving ketamine 15 min before the end of surgery. Place the patient in the lateral position post-op until awake.

Problems with ketamine

- Apnoea—rare with ketamine, but can happen if an IV bolus dose is given fast. Gently ventilate until breathing resumes.
- Laryngospasm may occur, either because anaesthesia is relatively light or because of secretions on the vocal cords. Open the airway, use gentle suction, and apply positive pressure if possible. If the patient is still breathing, deepen anaesthesia with ketamine. If they are not breathing, attempt gentle ventilation. If there is complete airway obstruction despite normal airway manoeuvres, give a small dose of muscle relaxant.
- Hypertension: maximum response is within a few minutes of injection and can occur in non-hypertensive patients. Options for management are reducing the rate/dose of ketamine maintenance, giving a small dose of supplemental diazepam or opioid, switching to another anaesthetic agent, or, if there are no risk factors, doing nothing.
- Tachycardia is very common with ketamine. If the patient's heart rate >120 beats/min, check whether the ketamine maintenance dose needs to be reduced and check for hypovolaemia.
- Signs of shock can be masked as BP will likely be maintained, and tachycardia is often attributed to ketamine.
- Vomiting: intraoperatively but more commonly postoperatively. Caution: antiemetics available in many LMICs are also sedative.
- Postoperative agitation or psychosis: occasionally a second dose of diazepam, e.g. 2 mg IV, may be required.
- Placental transfer of ketamine may cause neonatal respiratory depression (respiratory depression is more commonly seen in small babies compared with adults following ketamine), hence limiting the initial dose to 1 mg/kg. Give diazepam and opioids after cord clamping so that this does not contribute.

Local infiltration for Caesarean section

LA infiltration for Caesarean delivery is rarely performed due to the wide availability of regional anaesthesia and the increasing safety of GA. However, it can be used as a safe alternative in situations where both regional and GA are contraindicated or difficult to perform.

Indications

- The patient is not suitable for clinical reasons for either regional or GA, e.g. severe kyphoscoliosis or patient with low Glasgow coma score in a hospital with no intensive care unit (ICU) facility.
- Where there has been failure of both regional and GA.
- Lack of anaesthetic expertise.
- Lack of adequate anaesthetic equipment (spinal needles, anaesthetic machine, gas supply, etc.).

Advantages

- Avoidance of haemodynamic changes associated with GA or neuraxial anaesthesia.
- Avoidance of respiratory depression, reduction in conscious level, and changes in uterine tone associated with general anaesthetic drugs.
- Avoidance of neonatal drug exposure.
- Surgeon can deliver the local anaesthetic and perform the CS.

Disadvantages

- Time consuming unless the surgeon is experienced.
- Requires multiple LA injections.
- There is a risk of LA toxicity for the mother and the baby.
- There is a risk of uterine perforation (when infiltrating LA).

Preparation

- Warn the patient that some painful sensation as well as touch and pressure may be experienced.
- An experienced surgeon is preferred—minimal retraction will minimize pain.
- Standard monitoring, large-bore IV access, and fluid infusion. Left lateral tilt position until baby is delivered.
- Drugs and equipment for resuscitation must be available prior to commencing the procedure.
- An anaesthetist should be present if possible to aid analgesia with other analgesics if required, e.g. entonox if available or incremental opioids (preferably after clamping of the cord):
    - fentanyl 25 μg IV
    - pethidine 25 mg IV
    - morphine 2–5 mg IV.

Technique

- Suggested LA preparation—7 mg/kg lidocaine 0.25–0.5% with 5 μg/ml adrenaline.
- Note the maximum dose of adrenaline is 500 μm.
- For a 70 kg patient, the maximum dose would be:
  - lidocaine 100 ml 0.5% with adrenaline 5 μg/ml (1:200,000) or
  - lidocaine 200 ml 0.25% with adrenaline 2.5 μg/ml (1:400,000).
- Procaine 0.5–1% (15 mg/kg) is an alternative though is less commonly available and has a slightly higher risk of allergic reaction.
- A 100–120 mm needle is used to infiltrate under the skin. The abdominal wall, during pregnancy, may become very thin—extreme care must be taken to avoid uterine perforation during infiltration.
- Initial deposition of LA depends on incision.

Pfannenstiel incision

- Infiltrate LA along the incision line.

Midline incision

- A field block of the lower abdominal wall with multiple injections is required. It is more time consuming and associated with a greater degree of discomfort than the Pfannenstiel approach:
  - Infiltrate LA from the umbilicus down to the symphysis pubis in the midline.
  - Then, starting 4 cm lateral to either side of the umbilicus, infiltrate LA caudally in two lines down to the mons pubis.

Post-skin incision

- Once the skin is incised, the rectus sheath is infiltrated. Infiltration of subcutaneous fat is not required as it has few nerve endings.
- The parietal peritoneum is anaesthetized by injecting 10 ml of LA under the linea alba.
- Once the parietal peritoneum is opened, spray 10 ml of LA into the peritoneal cavity.
- Finally infiltrate 5–7 ml of LA into the visceral peritoneum of the lower segment of the uterus. This also helps to separate the peritoneum from the lower segment.
- Before delivery of the head, warn the mother about the risk of experiencing pain, especially if the head is engaged.
- Further injection of LA may be required during closure or use a small dose of ketamine as sedation.

Obstetric haemorrhage

Key points

- Haemorrhage (antepartum haemorrhage (APH) and PPH) is the leading cause of maternal mortality in LMICs.
- Major haemorrhage can be defined as blood loss >1500 ml ('massive' >2,500 ml), continuing blood loss of 150 ml/h, or a transfusion requirement of 4 units of red cells or more.
- Patients are likely to arrive late and possibly in shock.
- Uterine rupture is more common as a cause of APH.
- Pre-existing anaemia is common and a smaller amount of blood loss may be very significant.
- Hypothermia must be treated aggressively.
- In APH, concealed bleeding can be hard to quantify.
- Diagnosis of the cause of major haemorrhage can be remembered by thinking of the four Ts:
  - Tone, i.e. poor uterine tone.
  - Trauma, e.g. laceration to the birth canal.
  - Tissue, e.g. retained placenta.
  - Thrombin, i.e. coagulation disorders.
- Specialist techniques of balloon tamponade or B-Lynch suture are effective in persistent uterine atony.
- Early hysterectomy may be indicated/should be considered when there is a shortage of blood products.
- Coagulation failure is common if the haemorrhage is associated with placental abruption, severe PET, sepsis, or intrauterine death.

Initial assessment

- All patients with more than 1,000 ml blood loss or who appear shocked should be rapidly assessed.
- Careful examination (vital signs, pallor, peripheral temperature, capillary refill) is the most helpful way of assessing the degree of shock.
- Weigh swabs and subtract the dry weight to help measure blood loss.
- Note hypotension is a late sign of hypovolaemia in the peripartum period—up to 40% of the circulating volume (1,500–2,000 ml) can be lost before hypotension ensues.
- Earlier presenting signs include tachycardia, prolonged capillary refill time, foetal distress, and postural hypotension.
- Catheterize and monitor urine output—this guides fluid resuscitation and an empty bladder also improves uterine tone.

'Tone': uterine atony

- Uterine atony contributes to approximately 70% of PPH, and is more likely in: multiple pregnancy, foetal macrosomia, polyhydramnios, prolonged labour, oxytocin augmentation of labour, grand multiparity, precipitous labour, chorioamnionitis, inhalational anaesthesia, and magnesium administration.

Management

- Physical methods: bimanual compression of uterus and/or intrauterine balloon.
- Pharmacological options: uterotonics should be administered in a step-wise approach (see Table 8.5).
- Surgical management options include brace suture, B-Lynch suture, internal iliac artery ligation, and hysterectomy.

Trauma

- Traumatic PPH may be due to CS, uterine rupture, assisted vaginal delivery, perineal tears, and episiotomy, and accounts for about 40% of PPH.
- Early identification of the cause and surgical control is the mainstay of management.

Tissue

- Retained placenta or membranes is a potent cause of resistant atony. If the placenta is retained for more than 30 min, it should be manually evacuated as there is an increased haemorrhage risk. This often requires anaesthesia.
- Manual vaginal evacuation is a technique performed in LMICs for retained placenta (as well as ERPC). It is normally performed with oral analgesia +/− paracervical block.

Thrombin (coagulopathy)

- Dilutional coagulopathy will develop after approx. 2.5–3 l of ongoing bleeding from any cause.
- Early coagulopathy, even before PPH is identified, can occur in abruption, severe PET, severe sepsis, and amniotic fluid embolus.
- Give tranexamic acid early if possible (see below) and, if several units of stored blood have been given, consider giving calcium gluconate 10 ml 10% over 10 min after every 4 units of blood.
- It is much easier to prevent by early identification and halting of blood loss, giving blood early (fresh whole blood if possible), and keeping the patient warm.
- Once coagulopathy is established early recourse to hysterectomy can be lifesaving.

Fluid resuscitation and blood products

Tranexamic acid

- Has been conclusively shown to improve PPH outcomes in LMIC settings whatever the cause of the bleeding.
- As soon as PPH is identified 1 g IV should be given and repeated after 30 min if bleeding has not stopped.
- There is no benefit if tranexamic acid is given more than 3 h after the start of the PPH.

Table 8.5 Uterotonics.

	Uterotonic	Side effects	Cardiac disease
First line	Oxytocin*: 5 units slow IV or IM, repeated once. Infusion: 40 units in 500 ml over 4 h—can give after bolus doses	Tachycardia Hypotension Arrhythmia	Give very slowly IV, e.g. over 10–20 min, or IM
Second line	Ergometrine*: 250–500 µg IM or very slowly IV. Oxytocin 5 units and ergometrine 500 µg available as a combination given IM	Hypertension (avoid in PET) Nausea/vomiting—very common (give antiemetic)	Avoid
Third line (synthetic prostaglandins)	Carboprost: 250 µg IM or intramyometrially. Repeat every 15 min to a maximum of 2 mg (eight doses)	Bronchospasm (avoid in asthma) Caution in women with severe renal or hepatic disease	Avoid
	Or alternative Misoprostol: 600–1,000 µg rectally or sublingually—commonly available in LMICs	Diarrhoea Abdominal pain Pyrexia	Theoretical risk of hypotension. Rarely a problem in practice

*The World Health Organization (WHO) recommends keeping most of the supply of oxytocin and ergometrine in a fridge and away from light. A small supply can be kept out of the fridge, but the drugs lose efficacy after 2 weeks out of the fridge at 40°C or 4 weeks out of the fridge at 30°C. Misoprostol may be the only uterotonic available due to it not requiring refrigeration and being cheap and easy to store.

IV, intravenous; IM, intramuscular; PET, pre-eclamptic toxaemia; LMIC, low- and middle-income country.

Data from Hogerzeil HV, Walker GJA, de Goeje MJ. Stability of Injectable Oxytocics in Tropical Climates: Results of Field Surveys and Simulation Studies on Ergometrine, Methylergometrine and Oxytocin - EDM Research Series No. 008. WHO 1993; and Joint Formulary Committee. British National Formulary (online) London: BMJ Group and Pharmaceutical Press <http://www.medicinescomplete.com> [Accessed on 1/7/2017]

Crystalloids

- The minimum volume required to maintain maternal cardiovascular parameters should be used. Excessive volumes will cause dilutional coagulopathy and pulmonary oedema.
- For women of 40 50 kg, usually no more than 2 l crystalloid should be given before blood is infused.

Red blood cells

Also see 'Blood Transfusion' in Chapter 4 (pp. 70–4)

- Cross-matched fresh whole blood is ideal if safely available.
- If stored red blood cells are used these should be warmed to body temperature before administration if time allows (hold against your body or immerse in warm water bath. Keep blood <43°C to avoid haemolysis).
- Stored whole blood contains very few active platelets and less clotting factors than fresh whole blood but in practice, some platelets will aggregate to help blood to clot.
- Ideally the mother should be transfused to a haemoglobin (Hb) of 70 g/l although otherwise healthy women can tolerate a Hb of 60 g/l or even lower.

Platelets

- Most pregnant women do not need a platelet transfusion during PPH unless: total blood loss exceeds 5 l, there has been severe abruption with consumptive disseminated intravascular coagulation (DIC), or if she is thrombocytopenic prior to delivery.

Clotting factors

- Not usually available and the use of whole blood could be the only source of clotting factors. Recent research has shown that pregnant women develop fibrinogen deficiency before other clotting factor deficiencies. Fibrinogen concentrate or cryoprecipitate, if available, are ideal.

Anaesthesia/theatre

- Regional anaesthesia is safe for most cases of PPH if hypovolaemia has been corrected.
- If bleeding is rapid, more than 30% of circulating blood volume has been lost, or there is ongoing bleeding, then a GA may be safer.
- GA is usually a better option if surgery may be prolonged, e.g. PPH in placenta praevia, uterine rupture, or a hysterectomy is required.

Continuing care

- All mothers where the bleeding has been estimated >1500 ml are best cared for in a high-dependency environment. This may be on the normal ward but with more frequent observations.
- Hourly observations should be made for at least 6 h.
- Postoperative ventilation should be considered if there is ongoing bleeding, hypothermia, severe oliguria/anuria, pulmonary oedema, or poorly corrected metabolic acidosis.

Major PPH: special circumstances

Placenta praevia/accreta

- Placenta praevia (PP) is a placenta that partially or entirely covers the cervix necessitating delivery of the foetus by CS.
- Anterior PP is associated with more blood loss as the placenta is cut before the delivery of the baby but both posterior and anterior PP are associated with PPH because the lower segment contacts poorly and does not respond well to uterotonics.
- Balloon tamponade or brace sutures can be helpful.
- Placenta accreta occurs when there is placentation in a previous uterine scar. Subsequently there is no natural plane for uterine separation.
- The placenta can sometimes be cut away but if the bleeding is severe, if the abnormal placental tissue is extensive, or if it's invading other pelvic organs (percreta), then a hysterectomy is required.
- In patients who have had previous CS or uterine surgery, identify the placental site (if ultrasound available). If anterior, prepare for potential sudden major blood loss and make a plan for transfusion.

Uterine rupture

- Uterine rupture is associated with previous CS, uterine surgery, or uterine perforation associated with termination of pregnancy (which may have been illegal, therefore not mentioned during the history).
- Remember that uterine rupture can also occur without previous surgery—it is more common in LMICs due to the much higher incidence of prolonged obstructed labour.
- It is rapidly fatal for the baby and associated with major concealed haemorrhage. Foetal demise, maternal cardiovascular compromise, and a distended tense abdomen are the only findings.
- Uterine rupture through a previous CS scar may be associated with less bleeding than rupture through the body of the uterus as the old scar is relatively avascular.
- In all cases the mother will require an urgent laparotomy, which must not be delayed as the cause of the haemorrhage is traumatic and will not improve until surgically treated.
- Uterine rupture may be treated with hysterectomy or, in some circumstances, with uterine repair. In the latter case, further pregnancies are possible.

Placental abruption

- Premature separation of the placenta—leads to foetal demise.
- Is associated with PET and can be very difficult to treat as the mother may have severe hypertension as well as major haemorrhage.
- Bleeding occurs between the placenta and the uterus. A clot forms causing localized consumption of fibrinogen and platelets.
- The mother can seem stable as blood loss is usually not severe at this stage. Major PPH then occurs after delivery (vaginal or Caesarean) due to coagulation deficiency.
- If the baby is still alive then Caesarean delivery should be performed. This usually indicates that the abruption is small or early in its development and severe coagulation problems are unusual.

- If the baby is dead, delivery should be expedited to reduce the time over which consumption occurs. This can be vaginal delivery, which is probably safer. There should be early consideration of clotting factor replacement prior to delivery to prevent major PPH.

Ectopic pregnancy

- The classic triad of symptoms of ectopic pregnancy is amenorrhoea, vaginal bleeding, and abdominal pain.
- Significant bleeding usually only occurs when the ectopic has ruptured. Many present with pain only and the patient is cardiovascularly stable.
- Patients may be relatively stable with minimal bleeding or may present with life-threatening haemorrhage.
- Resuscitate and prepare for GA (rapid sequence induction (RSI)) with possibility of significant blood loss.
- Pfannenstiel or midline incision.
- Ketamine is a useful agent if there is haemodynamic instability.
- Spinal anaesthesia is possible for a very stable patient but the risks related to hypovolaemia are high if there is any suggestion of instability.
- If any form of cell salvage is available, use it.

Pre-eclampsia and eclampsia

Definition

- PET is new hypertension presenting after 20 weeks' gestation with significant proteinuria.
- Significant proteinuria is defined as an automated reagent-strip device showing 1+ protein. Hypertension is defined as a diastolic BP of 90–99 mmHg and/or a systolic BP 140–149 mmHg.
- Severe PET is defined as either:
  - severe hypertension and proteinuria with a diastolic BP of 110 mmHg or greater and/or systolic BP 160 mmHg or greater (with or without biochemical and/or haematological impairment)
    or
  - mild or moderate hypertension with biochemical and/or haematological impairment.
- HELLP syndrome is haemolysis, elevated liver enzymes and low platelet count and is classified as severe PET. The mother may not be hypertensive and may not have all three problems.
- Renal impairment is common in PET (the upper normal range of creatinine in pregnancy is about 70 μmol/l) and deteriorating renal function usually indicates severe disease.
- Evidence of pulmonary oedema is associated with cardiac impairment in PET: it requires urgent treatment of the pulmonary oedema with diuretics and delivery as soon as the mother is stabilized.

Management

- Severe pre-eclampsia will ultimately require delivery but the mother should be stabilized as much as possible first. The aims of management are:
  - control of hypertension
  - prevention of seizures
  - careful fluid balance
  - treatment of pulmonary oedema.
- Drugs for the management of hypertension are outlined in Table 8.6 aiming for BP <150/110 mmHg.

Eclampsia

- Is pre-eclampsia with generalized seizures. The ultimate treatment is delivery but this is not an absolute emergency and the mother should be stabilized first.
- Eclampsia can present postpartum, although it is rare after 48 h postpartum; it is not necessarily associated with severe hypertension.

Treatment of seizures

- Left lateral position, support airway, give oxygen. Many seizures will be self-limiting.

Table 8.6 Drugs used in the treatment of hypertension in pregnancy.

Drug	Dose and route	Comments
Methyldopa	PO: 250 mg 8–12 hourly	Slow onset of action. Useful for outpatient treatment in mild PET
Nifedipine (modified release if available)	PO: 5 mg, repeated once	Useful for one-off treatment of severe hypertension. Caution if patient is on magnesium
Labetalol	200 mg PO 12 hourly 5–10 mg IV every 5 min to max 200 mg Hypertensive emergency: 50 mg IV over 10 min repeated up to 200 mg	Not in severe asthma May cause neonatal hypoglycaemia
Hydralazine	5–10 mg IV over 5 min every 30 min to max. 40 mg	Can cause sudden drop in blood pressure, tachycardia, headache, flushing, and/or vomiting

PO, per oram; PET, pre-eclamptic toxaemia; IV, intravenous.

Table 8.7 Magnesium for treatment and prevention of eclampsia.

Protocol	Treatment regime
No infusion pump protocol	Loading dose: 4 g IV slow bolus over 5–15 min. This should ideally be diluted by at least 50% with water for injection or 0.9% saline Immediately followed by maintenance dose: 10 g IM (5 g in each buttock) followed by 5 g every 4 h (change sides with each injection). Continue for 24 h If IM contraindicated (coagulopathy) put 12 g magnesium into 1,000 ml IV fluid attached to a paediatric burette set. Give 85 ml over each hour (approx. seven drops every 5 s). This must be closely observed so that too much is not given too fast. Lidocaine can reduce pain of injection
Infusion pump protocol	Loading dose of 4 g by IV infusion in 100 ml of 0.9% sodium chloride run over 15–20 min Then maintenance dose: 1 g/h by continuous pump infusion for 24 h

IV, intravenous; IM, intramuscular.

- Magnesium is the mainstay of treatment. In most countries it is given IM. In HICs it is usually given as an IV infusion. All options are outlined in Table 8.7.
- A 5 g/10ml ampoule = approx. 20 mmol of magnesium.
- Other drugs, e.g. diazepam, may be used to terminate seizures if magnesium is unavailable but benzodiazepines have a greater respiratory depressant effect on mother and baby.
- Eclampsia is the commonest cause of seizures in this context but consider others, e.g. cerebral malaria, meningitis, or hypoglycaemia.
- Patients with eclampsia should have vital signs including respiratory rate (RR) measured every 30 min once they are stable.
- Monitor for magnesium toxicity every 4 h (exercise particular caution if there is renal impairment):
  - BP
  - RR
  - patellar reflex
  - urine output.
- If RR is <10 or patellar reflex disappears, do not give any further $MgSO_4$ and administer CaGluconate over 10 min.
- Restart magnesium at half the previous rate once the symptoms of toxicity have resolved.
- In the case of break through convulsions, administer an extra bolus of $MgSO_4$; 1 g IV if mother weighs <70 kg, 2 g if mother weighs >70 kg.

Delivery

- Once the seizure is resolved, control BP, check platelets, clotting.
- Vaginal delivery may be possible if the mother's condition is stable but a deteriorating mother may need urgent delivery by CS.

Spinal anaesthesia

- Spinal anaesthesia is usually the technique of choice even in the absence of any blood tests for platelets and clotting.
- Do not use more than 500 ml of IV fluid as a pre-load.
- Do not use prophylactic vasopressors—treat if BP falls only.

General anaesthesia

- If there is clinical or laboratory evidence of coagulopathy or thrombocytopenia (<80 × 10^9/l) or reduced conscious level, then GA may be considered if it is safe in the context.
- Intubation may be difficult due to soft tissue oedema—have smaller endotracheal tubes to hand.
- Avoid ketamine.
- Attenuate the hypertensive response to laryngoscopy and extubation. See 'General Anaesthesia' (pp. 172–4) for drug options.

Considerations for both spinal and general anaesthesia

- Exercise caution with vasopressors (increased sensitivity).

- Conversely, hypotension resistant to vasopressors can be seen if the mother is on $MgSO_4$ but this is usually well tolerated by the mother.
- Ergometrine and NSAIDs are contraindicated.
- There should be close post-op monitoring for the first 24 h (in a high-dependency unit (HDU) if available).
- Ensure careful fluid balance: there is a high risk of developing pulmonary oedema, which is difficult to manage in low-resource settings, but renal impairment is also a risk. It is probably better to err on the side of dryness.
    - Restrict fluid intake to 1 ml/kg/h.
    - Use a urinary catheter and aim for no more than 0.5 ml/kg/h urine.
    - Carry out regular clinical assessment of fluid status. The patient may require IV furosemide.
- If PET and PPH, give small fluid boluses with regular reassessment and give blood early.

Non-obstetric surgery in the obstetric patient

Summary

- There is increased risk of miscarriage (especially if the patient has peritonitis), premature labour, intrauterine growth retardation, and early infant death.
- Avoid all but emergency surgery.
- Anaesthetic agents do not appear to have teratogenic effects.
- Where possible, avoid the first trimester to allow for completion of foetal organogenesis (widely recommended but not evidence based).
- Delay elective surgery until at least 6 weeks postpartum.
- Document US scan/doppler of foetus pre- and post-op.
- If the foetus is dead, beware coagulopathy.
- Consider regional anaesthesia if possible. For GA see 'General Anaesthesia' in this chapter (pp. 172–4).
- Thromboprophylaxis should be strongly considered and NSAIDs avoided (there is a risk of premature closure of the ductus arteriosus).

Specific considerations

- Consider RSI and aspiration prophylaxis from 16 weeks until 48 h postpartum.
- Aortocaval compression is a hazard from about 20 weeks onwards.
- Exercise caution with ketamine (increases uterine tone).
- Pregnancy is associated with lower anaesthetic requirements. MAC is reduced by 30% as early as 8–12 weeks' gestation.
- Avoid hypovolaemia and anaemia. Aggressively treat haemorrhage.
- In the third trimester, if the foetus is of viable age for the context and major surgery is required, consider delivery by CS first. Where possible, surgery should be delayed 48 h to allow steroid therapy to enhance foetal lung maturation. Consider regional anaesthesia for the CS then converting to a GA if required. Anaesthesia post-delivery should be tailored to surgical requirements, with the precaution that volatile agents should be discontinued or used only in small doses (<0.5 MAC) along with oxytocics to minimize the risk of uterine atony and haemorrhage.

Evacuation of retained products of conception (ERPC) and abortion

Key points

- ERPC may be indicated after incomplete miscarriage or following an unsafe abortion. A planned surgical abortion is usually known as a surgical termination of pregnancy (STOP) but has the same anaesthetic considerations.
- Usually done at 6–12 weeks' gestation. It may be later in which case aspiration risk must be considered (16 weeks onwards). There is also greater potential for blood loss after the first trimester.
- There may have been significant blood loss preoperatively, which may be ongoing (greater in LMICs due to late presentation).
- If the patient is not bleeding, they can usually wait until they are fasted for 6 h until surgery.
- General or spinal anaesthesia are both reasonable choices, remembering the increased aspiration risk later in pregnancy.
- Remember that high concentrations of volatile anaesthetic will cause uterine relaxation and potentially worsen bleeding.
- A uterotonic agent may be requested. See Table 8.5.
- Misoprostol may be given preoperatively.
- Antibiotics are not routinely indicated but should be given if appropriate, for example in the case of sepsis after unsafe abortion.

Ethical considerations

- The legality and cultural acceptance of abortions varies widely. It is important to familiarize yourself with the situation in the country in which you are working.
- The rate of abortion in a country is not directly related to its legal status. In countries with restrictive abortion laws women will largely seek and undergo unsafe abortions.
- Legality is not the only barrier to safe abortion services. Lack of trained providers and adequately resourced healthcare facilities in LMICs is a factor in many settings.
- Complications of unsafe abortions include haemorrhage, genital tract trauma, uterine perforation, and sepsis.
- According to the World Health Organization (WHO), abortion accounts for 8% of maternal mortality worldwide.

Female genital mutilation (FGM)

Key points

- FGM, also known as female genital cutting, refers to procedures that intentionally alter the female genital tract for non-medical reasons. It is a traditional practice in parts of Africa, the Middle East, and Asia.
- FGM is recognized internationally as a violation of the human rights of girls and women.
- Sometimes there is pressure upon health professionals to perform FGM as it is perceived as being safer when performed in a healthcare environment. However, international agencies such as the WHO and United Nations (UN) are clear that healthcare providers should not perform any type of FGM in any setting.
- There are different types of FGM:
  - Type 1: clitoridectomy.
  - Type 2: excision of the clitoris and labia minora.
  - Type 3: infibulation: narrowing of the vaginal opening by creation of a covering seal. The seal is created by repositioning the labia minora or majora.
  - Type 4: all other harmful procedures to female genitalia for non-medical purposes, e.g. incising, scraping, cauterization.

Complications

- Immediate—bleeding, pain, infection.
- Longer term—pain, chronic infection, difficulty menstruating, obstetric complications, and psychiatric sequelae.
- Obstetric complications include increased risk of:
  - prolonged labour, instrumental delivery, CS and PPH
  - genital tract trauma.
- Deinfibulation may be required to facilitate safe delivery. Many women/families may then request reinfibulation. This would be considered by the WHO as supporting the practice of FGM and should not be done.

Obstetric fistulae

Key points

- Vesicovaginal fistula refers to an abnormal connection between the genital tract and the urinary tract. Communication between the rectum and genital tract also occurs and is termed rectovaginal fistula.
- In industrialized nations these fistulae are rare, and usually arise as a complication of pelvic surgery or radiotherapy.
- They are more common in LMICs, where they almost always occur as a result of pressure necrosis during prolonged obstructed labour, reflecting a lack of timely access to quality obstetric care.
- For this reason, vesicovaginal and rectovaginal fistulae in this setting are often collectively known as obstetric fistulae.
- Ureterovaginal fistulae can occur after CS or emergency hysterectomy and a small proportion of these fistulae occur as the result of trauma and sexual violence.
- Urine leak, infection, and offensive odour lead to social isolation.
- Around 85–95% of obstetric fistulae can be successfully closed with reconstructive surgery.

Surgical repair

- The patients may be malnourished and in renal failure (as they drink little to try to leak less). Both can lead to anaemia.
- The majority are repaired vaginally. More complex fistulae (and ureterovaginal fistulae) may require an abdominal approach. Some rectal fistulae may require a temporary colostomy.
- Spinal anaesthesia is usually the technique of choice. A single-shot spinal is often adequate for 3 h of perineal surgery.
- It may take 30 min to many hours so plan for supplementation of anaesthesia in case of the spinal wearing off.
- CSE anaesthesia may be more suitable for complex cases if available, otherwise GA may be needed.
- The surgeon may request an intraoperative diuretic to help identify the ureters if they cannot see any urine flow, e.g. 10 mg IV furosemide.
- A catheter usually left *in situ* for at least 1 week. High oral fluid intake, e.g. 4–5 l/day is required to reduce catheter blockage and reduce infection risk.
- Future pregnancies will require a CS if possible—women should be advised to travel to stay near a health centre towards the end of future pregnancies.

Neonatal resuscitation

Five to ten per cent of neonates need help at birth, ranging from tactile stimulation to chest compressions or drug administration. In low-resource settings the anaesthetist is frequently the only person in a position to perform neonatal resuscitation.

Key differences from other age groups

- Babies are born wet, so need to be dried quickly and warmed to avoid hypothermia (important even in hot climates).
- Fluid-filled lungs must be cleared.
- Initially resuscitate with air, not oxygen.

Resuscitation—baby crying

- If breathing is regular give the baby to the mother. Keep the baby warm. Delayed cord clamping is recommended (minimum 1 min after delivery).

Resuscitation—baby not crying

Dry, warm, and stimulate the baby

- This will stimulate breathing in most neonates.

Airway

- Position the head neutral: a folded towel under the shoulders may help.
- Suction only if indicated: see notes below.

Breathing

- Effective ventilation within 1 min of birth is a priority.
- If breathing is inadequate, irregular, or gasping, institute ventilation.
- Inflation breaths may be given; however, most guidelines developed in LMICs do not include them, simply advising effective ventilation at a rate of 30–50/min for 30–60 s before re-assessing the baby.
- Keep ventilating until the baby is breathing well on its own.

Circulation

- After 30–60 s of good chest movement with ventilation, assess heart rate (stethoscope/umbilical pulse). Normal: 110–160 beats/min.
- If the heart rate is <60 beats/min, chest compressions are required.
- Perform three compressions for each ventilation breath (3:1 ratio).
- Compressions can be done most effectively by a second person encircling the chest with their hands and pushing on the middle of sternum with both thumbs or use two fingers finger finger breadth below the nipple line. Compress one third of the antero-posterior diameter of the chest at a rate of 100 compressions/min.
- Recheck the heart rate every 30 s and stop CPR if the heart rate is >60 beats/min.

Drugs

- If drugs are required, the outlook is likely to be poor.
- Consider drugs if the baby does not respond to CPR. They can be given via the umbilical vein (the largest vessel in the umbilical cord) or via the intraosseous route.

- Adrenaline: 10 μg/kg IV bolus (0.1 ml/kg of 1:10,000 solution). If this is not effective, a dose of up to 30 μg/kg (0.3 ml/kg of 1:10,000 solution) may be tried.
- Glucose (10%): 2.5 ml/kg IV bolus (250 mg/kg) should be considered if there has been no response to other drugs.
- If there is a clear history of blood loss from the infant: give 10 ml/kg of 0.9% sodium chloride over 10–20 s and repeat if needed.

Notes

- Air versus oxygen:
  - Outcomes are as good for babies over 32 weeks' gestation if initially resuscitated with air rather than oxygen.
  - Add oxygen: for pre-term babies under 32 weeks gestational age (ideally FiO_2 0.3), or if a neonate remains cyanosed, cardiac compressions are required or SpO_2 are lower than predicted. Note that preductal SpO2, measured on the right hand, will normally be only 60–65% at 1 min, and 80–85% at 5 min after delivery.
- Suction:
  - Is indicated for visible secretions in the nose and mouth of an apnoeic neonate.
  - Is indicated in a neonate born with meconium-stained amniotic fluid, who is apnoeic: in this case, gently suction the trachea under direct laryngoscopy using a small Yankauer sucker or 12–14 Fr suction catheter (or a 2.0–4.0 mm internal diameter endotracheal tube if nothing else is available).
  - Is no longer recommended intrapartum, or for babies breathing spontaneously, or where the amniotic fluid is clear.
  - Beware bradycardia as a result of suction: if detected, stop.
- Resuscitation of neonates with no detectable CO is usually stopped if there is no output at 10 min or if the heart rate is still <60 beats/min at 10–15 min.
- If the heart rate is >60 beats/min but the neonate does not breathe, this is challenging. Ensure the neonate is kept warm. If recent opiate has been administered to the mother preceding birth, try intramuscular naloxone: 200 μg in a full-term baby or 60 μg/kg if the baby is thought to be <3 kg). The practicality of performing prolonged ventilation in your particular setting should be weighed against stopping resuscitation.
- Continuous positive airway pressure (CPAP) can be applied to neonates following initial resuscitation. Systems specifically designed for low-resource settings are available (see http://www.diamedica.co.uk) but a simple set-up can be used if required. Carefully insert a small suction catheter into one nostril and tape to the baby's cheek (use neonatal nasal cannulae if available). Attach to an oxygen concentrator and run at 1–2 l/min—be aware that without any humidification this will be very drying if used for a prolonged period of time.

Equipment for neonatal resuscitation

See 'Operating Theatre' in Chapter 2 (p. 29).

Hysterectomy

Key points

- One of the most commonly performed operations worldwide.
- Indications include menorrhagia, prolapse, malignancy, and intractable postpartum haemorrhage.
- Cancer of the uterine cervix is more common in LMICs compared with HICs. Cancer of the uterine body and ovaries is less common.
- Most countries of the world do not have effective screening programmes to identify and treat early-stage cervical disease.
- Patients may present with advanced pathologies, especially those from remote and rural areas.

Pre-op assessment

- Anaemia may be severe, renal function impaired (if there is extensive intra-abdominal disease), and nutrition poor.
- In severe disease (massive fibroids, advance malignancy) surgery may be very high risk with a chance of significant blood loss. Referral to a specialist centre may be the best option.
- In cases of advanced malignancy, decision for surgery (risks vs likely benefit) should be carefully discussed with patient.

Surgery

- The length of the surgery is variable—discuss with the surgeon.
- Spinal and general analgesia are both an option. Note a higher block will be required for a midline than for a Pfannenstiel incision.
- Abdominal field blocks are useful for post-op pain relief. Rectus sheath blocks can be done by the surgeon at the time of surgery or simply infiltration of the wound with LA.
- Spinal opioids may be useful for post-op pain relief if the recovery facility can support this.
- Postoperative nausea and vomiting is common.

Further reading

Clyburn P, Collis R (2010) *Obstetric Anaesthesia for Developing Countries*. Oxford: Oxford University Press.

Clyburn P, Collis R, Harries S (2008) *Oxford Specialist Handbook in Obstetric Anaesthesia*. Oxford: Oxford University Press.

Fortescue C, Wee MYK. (2005) Analgesia in labour: non-regional techniques. *Contin Educ Anaesth Crit Care Pain* 5 (1): 9–13.

Jones L et al. (2012) Pain management for women in labour: an overview of systematic reviews. *Cochrane Database of Systematic Reviews* 3. Art. No.: CD009234. doi: 10.1002/14651858.CD009234.pub2

Walton N, Melachuri V (2006) Anaesthesia for non-obstetric surgery during pregnancy. *Contin Educ Anaesth Crit Care Pain* 6 (2): 83–85.

WHO (2012a) *Guidelines on Basic Newborn Resuscitation*. Geneva: World Health Organization.

WHO (2012b) *Perioperative Recommendations for the Prevention and Treatment of Postpartum Haemorrhage*. Geneva: World Health Organization.

WHO (2016): *Guidelines on the Management of Health Complications from Female Genital Mutilation*. Geneva: World Health Organization.

Chapter 9

Trauma

Sarah Hodges, Sanja Janjanin, Judith Kendell, Nur Lubis, David Nott, and Nelson Olim[1]

1 Dr Nur Lubis is the chapter lead.

Damage control resuscitation and surgery

Trauma is the biggest contributor to mortality in low- and middle-income countries (LMICs) and can cause significant disability in settings where there is poor provision for the disabled. Often there is a lack of pre-hospital care, including an ambulance service, so patients present late and with minimal intervention. Many of the severely injured never make it to a healthcare facility. However, by following the basic principles of trauma management we can save lives and limbs and limit disability even without a wealth of resources. There are interventions that are simple, affordable and adaptable to the resource-poor setting.

The initial management of the trauma patient should always be based on a team approach with clear roles assigned by the team leader. With limited numbers of staff, the team members might need to undertake more than one role.

Primary survey: (c)ABC

- Catastrophic haemorrhage must be addressed first and external haemorrhage controlled.
- Airway, breathing, and reassessment of circulation are then addressed.
- The time between injury and surgery should be minimized for patients in need of surgical control of bleeding.

Principles of damage control resuscitation

- Early prevention of the lethal trauma triad of acidosis, coagulopathy, and hypothermia.
- Use of permissive hypotension (except in traumatic brain injury).
- Avoidance of aggressive fluid administration to prevent dilutional coagulopathy and diffuse tissue oedema whilst aiming at adequate organ perfusion and oxygen delivery.

The main challenges are due to delayed arrival of casualties, no or limited availability of blood, and limited equipment/diagnostic tools.

Control of massive life-threatening limb bleeding

- Apply direct pressure on a compressible site.
- Apply a tourniquet—the duration should be monitored as prolonged use can lead to complications (2 h is often considered as a limit).
- Reduce and splint fractures.
- For pelvic fractures apply a pelvic binder (may be improvised using bed sheets).
- Limit patient movement and log rolls to avoid disrupting clots.
- Give tranexamic acid: 1 g intravenous (IV) infused over 10 min **within 3 h** of injury, followed by a further infusion of 1 g over 8 h. Outside the 3-h time limit it is not useful and may be harmful.

Restricted volume replacement
- Target a systolic blood pressure of 80–90 mmHg until the bleeding is controlled (except in head trauma).
- Giving crystalloids not colloids for fluid resuscitation is currently recommended.
- Aim for a haemoglobin (Hb) of 70–90 g/l. Fresh whole blood is ideal as it is warm and has red cells, platelets, and clotting factors, even 1 unit may be very beneficial.
- Cell salvage from a haemothorax can be used in the field hospital (see 'Blood and Transfusion' in Chapter 4, p. 73).
- Consider calcium replacement in massive transfusion (1 g calcium gluconate or 0.3 g calcium chloride per 1–2 units transfused; gluconate is preferred as it is less irritant to veins). It is essential for the coagulation cascade and improves systemic vascular resistance and cardiac contractility.
- Be aware of the potential for hyperkalaemia in massive transfusion and monitor for electrocardiogram (ECG) changes if no lab measurement is possible.

Avoid hypothermia
- Warm the patient by covering (e.g. space blanket), remove wet clothes, give warm fluid, increase the ambient temperature if possible, pack warmed bags of fluid in the groin and axillae—take care to avoid burning).

Other
- Monitor blood pressure (BP), heart rate (HR), temperature, level of consciousness, and urine output.
- If available do a FAST (Focused Assessment with Sonography for Trauma) scan.
- If available do point of care Hb, coagulation, electrolytes, lactate, and bicarbonate measurement.

Damage control surgery

Active haemorrhagic shock that is not controllable by direct compression requires a combination of damage control resuscitation and surgery.

The goals of the abbreviated (damage control) surgery are to:
- control haemorrhage and prevent the trauma triad of death: hypothermia, acidosis, and coagulopathy
- curtail sepsis
- maintain oxygenation to vital organs concentrating on treating the physiology.

The surgery should be as fast as possible, ideally not taking longer than 1 h, time should not be wasted on stoma formation or any other non-essential elements at this stage. After a period of physiological improvement, which may take up to 48 h, the patient returns to theatre for completion of surgery—stoma formation, fixation of fractures, etc.

Damage control laparotomy

Pre-induction set-up

- Warm operating theatre, remove all wet or blood soaked sheets and clothes, warm fluids.
- Ensure blood is available if possible, ideally fresh whole blood. Consider cell salvage techniques (see 'Blood and Transfusion' in Chapter 4, pp. 72–4).
- Large-bore IV access × 2 with fluid in pressure bags.
- Ensure antibiotics and antitetanus have been given.
- Patient position supine, T shape with arms out.
- Prep and drape patient from neck (thoracotomy may be needed) to knees before induction.
- An assistant should be briefed to help with induction.

Induction

- Preoxygenation and rapid sequence induction with ketamine.
- Be prepared for sudden hypotension with loss of abdominal muscle tone at induction or massive haemorrhage at release of tamponade with incision.

Maintenance

- Maintain anaesthesia with ketamine (or volatile agent if no longer shocked).
- Gain haemodynamic stability and **communicate with the surgeon**; vasopressor infusion may be helpful until control is gained.

Surgical procedure

- A long midline incision should be made.
- The small bowel should be exteriorized and each abdominal quadrant packed to stem haemorrhage.
- Most massive bleeding comes from the liver, spleen, and major vessels, e.g. aorta, inferior vena cava, and their branches.
- If stability cannot be gained consider retroperitoneal or intrathoracic bleeding.
- Sepsis control is achieved by primary closure of any small bowel perforation; severely damaged bowel is resected and tied off.
- The abdomen should be left open with packs in place. Skin closure if possible or a Bogota bag.
- The aim is purely haemorrhage and sepsis control, and definitive procedures such as stoma formation should not be performed if they will prolong surgery.
- The patient will need to return to theatre in 48 h for removal of the packs, definitive surgery, and closure of the abdomen.

Extubation and postoperative management

- Ensure the abdominal closure is not too tight especially if postoperative ventilation is not going to be possible.
- If extubation is going to be necessary, then ask the surgeon to perform a rectus sheath block.

- Ensure a urinary catheter and nasogastric (NG) tube have been inserted.
- Ideally the patient should be ventilated on the intensive care unit (ICU) with correction of cardiovascular parameters, hypothermia, coagulation, and acidaemia.
- If ICU care is not available, then aim for at least a period of warming and stabilization ventilated in theatre prior to extubation.
- Main postoperative problems are:
  - Respiratory: due to splinting from the diaphragm and systemic inflammatory response; may be helped by continuous positive airway pressure (CPAP) or non-invasive ventilation (NIV) (see 'Respiratory Support' in Chapter 12, pp. 266–8).
  - Coagulopathy: warm the patient; give fresh whole blood and calcium; carry out a tranexamic acid infusion (if within 3 h of injury).
  - Sepsis: ensure antibiotics are given on admission or as soon as possible after. Some injuries will require ongoing prophylaxis.
  - Renal failure: ensure an adequate BP especially in the presence of intra-abdominal hypertension, monitor unrine output.
  - Nutrition: start oral or enteral feeding as soon as gut integrity allows (see 'Nutrition' in Chapter 12, pp. 264–5).
- If a splenectomy has been performed do not forget penicillin prophylaxis and immunization for meningitis and pneumonia if available (increased risk of severe infections); in malaria-endemic areas the patient should be warned of increased susceptibility to malaria.

Thoracic trauma and chest drains

Immediately life-threatening thoracic trauma

There are five immediately life-threatening thoracic traumas that should be picked up and managed in the primary survey (see Table 9.1). They will present with varying degrees of shock and shortness of breath.

Pulmonary contusion

This occurs in up to 20% of blunt trauma to the chest, developing over the course of 24 h. The injury to lung parenchyma causes oedema and blood to collect in alveolar spaces thus impairing lung function.

The presence of blood components in the lung causes an inflammatory reaction.

- A total of 50–60% of patients with significant pulmonary contusions will develop bilateral acute respiratory distress syndrome (ARDS) needing mechanical ventilation. CPAP or NIV may be helpful.
- Be cautious with fluid management: aim to keep the patient as fluid restricted as possible, as contused lungs are unable to handle a fluid overload.

Table 9.1 Life-threatening thoracic trauma management.

	Classical findings	Management
Tension pneumothorax	JVD, tracheal deviation, absent ipsilateral breath sounds and hyper-resonance	Needle decompression and immediate chest drain
Massive haemothorax	Ipsilateral decreased breath sounds and dullness	Chest drain (immediate output ≥1.5 l or ongoing output of ≥200 ml/h is an indication for surgical intervention*)
Open pneumothorax	Sucking chest wound	Three-sided adhesive dressing, chest drain, closure
Flail chest	Respiratory distress, paradoxical chest movement, crepitus	Early good analgesia, respiratory support, chest physio, humidified O_2. Chest drain likely
Cardiac tamponade	Becks triad—muffled heart sound, hypotension, and JVD	Thoracotomy (pericardiocentesis is not appropriate in the trauma setting)

JVD, jugular venous distension.

*Use clinical judgement—if the patient is stable and no skilled surgeon is present, then a watch-and-wait approach is appropriate. Use cell salvage (see below); bleeding often stops with lung re-expansion.

Sternal fracture

- Associated with cardiac contusions and arrhythmias.
- Use conservative management with good analgesia and monitor for arrhythmias and ischaemia.

Pain management and physiotherapy

- Fractured ribs are extremely painful and can hinder adequate ventilation and clearance of secretions making patients prone to pneumonia.
- Prescribe regular stepwise oral analgesia.
- Thoracic epidural is the gold standard, however, it is unlikely to be available.
- Intercostal nerve block can last between 4 and 24 h and can be repeated.
- Serratus anterior plane block works well (see 'Trunk Blocks' in Chapter 11, p. 254). If available a catheter may be left in place for further bolus dosing.
- Encourage lung expansion with exercises, e.g. using incentive spirometry. This can be homemade using a glove attached to a 20 ml syringe with the stopper removed.

Chest drain insertion and removal

Equipment

Intercostal drain (28G) (a Foley catheter may be used if no chest drain available), long-jawed clamp for blunt dissection, 2 or 3/0 silk on large handheld needle, 11 blade scalpel, 1% lidocaine, needle, syringe, connection tubing, sterile drapes, gauze, and skin prep.

Method

- If possible position the patient 45° head up with arm abducted.
- Safe triangle anatomy (Figure 9.1): fifth intercostal space, lateral edge of pectoralis major, and lateral edge of latissimus dorsi.
- Using sterile gloves +/− gown, prep and drape the area.
- Infiltrate the area with local anaesthetic down to the periosteum of the rib below the incision site.
- Make a 2–3 cm transverse incision in the intercostal space closer to the superior border of the lower rib (to avoid the neurovascular bundle).
- Blunt dissect until the pleura is breached (a pop may be felt as the tissue gives).
- Do a 360° finger sweep to ensure there are no adhesions.
- Pass the intercostal drain (without a trocar) into the pleural space ensuring all the holes are within the cavity. Guide the drain cephalad for a pneumothorax or caudad for a haemothorax.
- Connect the drain immediately using a Heimlich valve (may be improvised with an open glove finger) and collection bag or underwater seal system and secure the chest drain to the skin with sutures.
- Underwater seal:
  - Connection tubing volume = ½ patient's maximum inspiratory capacity (IC) (approx. 1 l).
  - Volume of water in bottle = ½ tidal volume (approx. 200 ml).

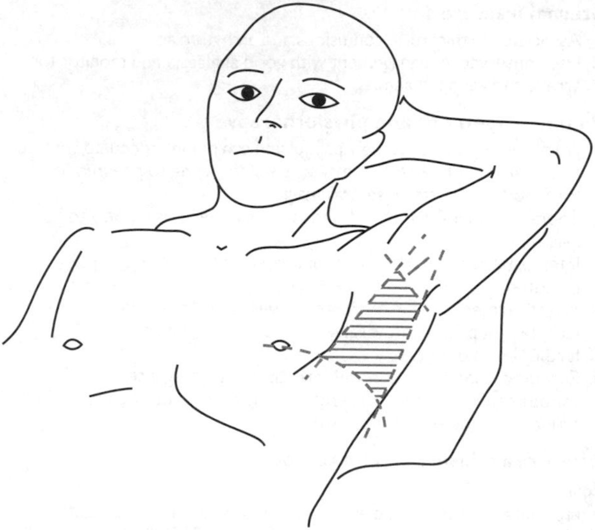

Figure 9.1 'Safe triangle' for chest drain insertion, bounded anteriorly by pectoralis major, posteriorly by latissimus dorsi, inferiorly by the fifth intercostal space, and superiorly by the axilla.

- The level of water/blood above the end of the tube should not exceed 4 cm, and may need to be adjusted as blood drains.
- The second vent tube should be open to the atmosphere.
- The drain should stay at least 45 cm below the patient.

- To remove the chest drain ask the patient to do a Valsalva manoeuvre as you remove the drain. Suture and cover the wound with a small dressing.

One lung ventilation (OLV)

There is rarely an absolute indication for OLV in trauma. Relative indications include:

- To enable optimal ventilation of uninjured lung in the presence of a massive air leak on the other side.
- To protect the lung from contamination from bleeding from the other side.
- To facilitate surgical access.

Methods of isolation

- Endobronchial intubation with a single lumen tube.
  - The easiest option in the absence of advanced equipment.
  - Use an uncut endotracheal tube (ETT) to ensure adequate length.
  - Avoid blocking the upper lobe with the ETT cuff (more common with right-sided placement).
  - To aid placement on the correct side: rotate bevel 90° to the required side, turn the head to face the opposite side; surgeons may help manipulate into place.
- Double lumen tube: rarely available.
- Bronchial blockers: very difficult to use in the absence of a fibreoptic scope.

Wound ballistics and blasts

Ballistics

From the anaesthesia perspective, it is important to understand the basic mechanisms of injury of a gunshot wound and the possible surgical implications.

Ammunition terms

A typical cartridge contains a case (with a primer and different amounts of gunpowder) and a bullet (the projectile). Most bullets used have a lead or steel core. This core is then either fully jacketed with a harder material like a copper alloy (full metal jacket (FMJ) bullets) or semi-jacketed (SJ) leaving the tip of the core exposed (soft point/hollow point bullets).

Energy transfer

- When gunpowder ignites, expanding gas is generated. The more gunpowder, the more gas is generated. Bigger cartridges like the ones used in assault rifles have much more gunpowder than smaller cartridges used in handguns.
- The extreme pressure generated by the expanding gas propels the bullet out of the case and through the weapon's barrel into the air. On impact, all the energy left in the bullet is transferred to the human body. The interaction of a bullet with the human body is called **wound ballistics**.
- The bullet of a typical 9-mm Luger cartridge used by many police forces has an average energy of 470 Joules (J). An AK47 Kalashnikov rifle's bullet has an average of 3,000 J.

Patterns of injury

- The pattern of injury is mainly determined by the type of bullet (FMJ vs SJ) and by the energy still left upon impact (handgun vs rifle).
- Rifle FMJ bullets penetrate deeper (Figure 9.2) before they start tumbling to create a temporary cavity—an area of deep tissue destruction.
- Handgun FMJ bullets do not create temporary cavities.
- SJ bullets deform or expand on impact, depositing most of the energy in the first centimetres after penetration. SJ bullets are used for hunting and by some police departments, but are prohibited for use in war.
- Bullets may ricochet around the body and cause injuries anatomically distant to the entry site.

Blast injuries

In today's conflicts and terror attacks, weapons containing explosives are causing a bigger share of the casualties, especially among civilian populations. It is important to understand how some of these weapons work, the similarities between them, and what are the main effects on the human body. These injuries should be excluded in any patient presenting from a blast.

Patterns of injury

- Pressure wave injuries:
  - The over-pressure wave generated by the detonation of a high explosive is a hypersonic wave that dissipates quickly as it travels. It has devastating effects on air/liquid interfaces.

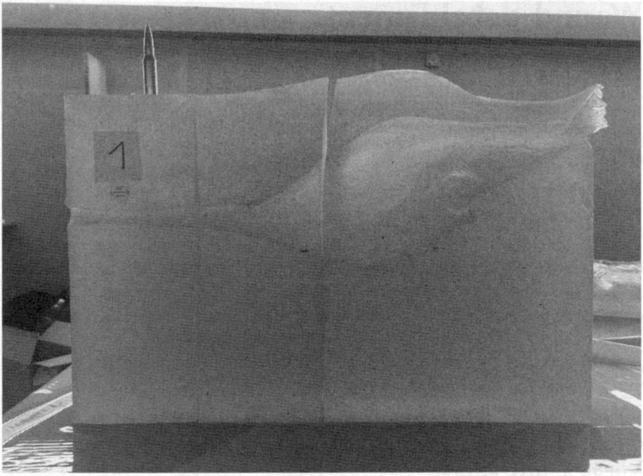

Figure 9.2 Full metal jacket rifle bullet, entering from left, showing deep cavity.

- Possible effects on the human body are mainly on **gas-filled structures**: blast lung (pulmonary barotrauma including pneumothorax and contusion); rupture of the tympanic membrane and middle ear damage; abdominal haemorrhage and perforation of hollow organs (sometimes delayed in time); rupture of the eye globe; and brain concussion without physical signs of head injury.
- **Externally there may be few physical signs**.

- Injuries by fragments:
  - The fragmented casing of the weapon and any additional material added (nails, bolts) are projected and can produce blunt or penetrating injuries in any body part.
- Blast wind injuries:
  - A subsonic wind is caused by the detonation.
  - If close to the detonation point this may be responsible for traumatic amputations.
  - If further away the wind may still be strong enough to throw a victim in the air and against solid objects.
- Thermal and chemical injuries:
  - The heat generated by the detonation may cause all types of burns depending on the victim's distance.
  - Inhalation injuries from toxic fumes, dust, or smoke must also be considered.
  - Chemical injuries depend on the type of chemical agent present in the weapon.
- Psychological injuries:
  - Short-term and long-term psychological injuries as acute stress reactions or post-traumatic stress disorder (PTSD) should not be disregarded.

Wound debridement

Debridement of penetrating wounds, open fractures, and burns is one of the commonest surgical procedures performed in low-resource settings and one of the most important in terms of limiting morbidity and mortality after trauma. Burns debridement will be considered separately in this chapter ('Burns', pp. 219–24).

Preoperative management

- All patients should be initially managed using the (c)ABCDE approach; consider blast injuries.
- High-energy projectile and blast injuries are highly contaminated.
  - Debride within 6 h of injury, if possible.
  - Give tetanus and antibiotic prophylaxis.
- Check Hb.
  - Blood loss should be anticipated in major debridements; check the availability of blood for transfusion.
  - Many patients return for multiple debridements, and slow blood loss is common: they may develop severe anaemia with few signs.

Surgical procedure

- A multi-stage approach should be taken with initial surgical debridement followed by a return to theatre for delayed primary closure.
- Primary closure at first visit is rarely appropriate.
- Gunshot wounds will require exploration of the whole tract to expose and debride the deep cavity if present.
- Small fragments that do not compromise vital organs can be left *in situ* with wound toilet.
- In many blast injuries, muscle and bowel viability cannot be fully assessed on the first procedure. Muscle may reveal itself to be necrotic on day 3 or 4 and delayed bowel perforation is not uncommon.

Intraoperative management

- Regional or general anaesthesia are both appropriate but in blast injuries, multiple sites for debridement often make regional alone impractical.
- If debridement is occurring as part of damage control surgery, only sufficient debridement for haemorrhage and sepsis control should be undertaken; further debridement can take place once stabilized—communicate with your surgeon.

Postoperative management

- Use analgesia and mobilization to preserve joint function.
- If ward dressing changes are planned, ensure adequate analgesia is prescribed.
- Ask about neuropathic pain symptoms and treat accordingly. See 'Pain Management' in Chapter 5 (p. 87).
- In patients with multiple debridements and wounds prescribe iron.
- Consider nutritional supplementation.

Open fractures

All open fractures are regarded as contaminated and at risk of infection, including osteomyelitis and tetanus. Surgical debridement should be performed within 6 h of injury if possible.

Preoperative management

- (c)ABCDE.
- Analgesia.
- Early reduction and stabilization of fracture to minimize blood loss.
- Intravenous prophylactic antibiotics and tetanus cover.

Surgical procedure

- Surgical debridement; wounds are left open.
- Postoperative surveillance of patients is often limited; if the patient is at risk of compartment syndrome, have a low threshold for fasciotomies.
- Carry out immobilization of the fracture with a plaster cast, traction, or external fixation as appropriate.
- Internal fixation is rarely appropriate due to:
    - mechanism of injury (war wounds can be very contaminated) or
    - context: insufficient sterility.
- The majority of patients will undergo further surgical procedures for delayed primary closure, muscle flap, or grafting of the wound.

Intraoperative management

- In major trauma, anaesthetic management will be dictated by the presence of other injuries, haemodynamic instability, or coagulopathy.
- Regional techniques, including spinal anaesthesia and peripheral nerve blocks provide excellent intraoperative and early postoperative analgesia and should be considered.
- The possibility of delay in the diagnosis of a compartment syndrome may dissuade anaesthetists from using regional techniques. There is no convincing evidence for this.

Postoperative management

- Intravenous antibiotic prophylaxis for 48–72 h.
- Regular simple analgesics with weak opioids.
- Early physiotherapy for affected joints and patient mobilization.
- Pressure area care for traction patients.
- Consider thromboprophylaxis for patients in traction and plaster casts.

Amputation

The decision to amputate a limb is difficult. Amputation is unacceptable to people from some cultures and religions, even for life-saving indications. Consent from wider family and community leaders may be required and a decision to decline amputation must be respected once full information including options for prostheses has been provided.

Indications for surgical amputation of a limb due to trauma

- Immediate:
  - Destruction of a limb or distal extremity at the scene of the injury, e.g. traumatic amputation.
  - Vascular injury to a limb in a patient with other life-threatening injuries, e.g. damage control procedure.
- Early:
  - Extensive tissue damage, nerve, or vascular injury, where an attempt at limb salvage is not considered appropriate.
- Late:
  - Failed attempt at limb salvage.
  - Severe infection.
  - Intractable pain.

Preoperative management

- (c)ABCDE.
- Check Hb and blood for transfusion.
- Documented consent—often there is a special form for amputation.

Surgical procedure

- Amputation with removal of all dead and infected tissue.
- The stump is usually left open with delayed primary closure or further debridement and stump revision at later procedures.

Intraoperative management

- In lower limb amputations, spinal anaesthesia with sedation is an excellent option if haemodynamic stability allows.
- General anaesthesia techniques with intraoperative opiate and ketamine for analgesia also work well.
- In both spinal and general anaesthetic techniques, regional blocks (brachial plexus or femoral/sciatic) should be considered for postoperative pain relief.
- A tourniquet should be used to minimize blood loss.
- Tranexamic acid 1 g (slow IV) also helps to reduce bleeding.

Postoperative management

- Patients require regular, stepwise analgesia, including morphine with early conversion to oral formulations.
- Postoperative use of ketamine may reduce opioid consumption.
- Phantom and neuropathic pain management. See 'Pain Management' in Chapter 5, Perioperative Care (p. 87).
- Mobilization to preserve joint function; referral for prosthesis.
- Psychological support.

Crush injuries, compartment syndrome, and reperfusion syndrome

These are easily missed, especially when working in a context where biochemical tests are not routinely available. A high index of suspicion based on the mechanism of injury is required.

Crush injuries

- Are time- and pressure-related; there is usually some history of entrapment.
- May not be associated with any fractures.
- Result in:
  - Direct muscle cell disruption.
  - Muscle cell death due to ischaemia from direct pressure.
  - Muscle cell death due to pressure on vascular structures.

Compartment syndrome

- Acute swelling of muscle in a fascial compartment.
- May be due to crush injury, haemorrhage into compartment, or ischaemia due to proximal vascular injury.
- Compartment pressure leads to muscle cell ischaemia and cell death.
- Is treated by fasciotomies, which should be performed prophylactically for high-risk injuries.

Reperfusion syndrome

This occurs when damaged muscle is re-perfused. The severity depends on the amount of muscle involved and ischaemic time. Clinical features and management include the following.

Shock

Due to acidosis and 'third space' fluid loss from leaky capillaries.

- Assessment: signs and symptoms of shock; cardiac arrest.
- Treatment: early aggressive fluid resuscitation, bicarbonate, inotropic support.

Hyperkalaemia

- Assessment: ECG changes, electrolytes, cardiac arrest.
- Treatment: insulin 10 units in 50 ml 50% glucose over 20 min; salbutamol nebulizer; calcium gluconate or chloride 10%, 10 ml IV over 2–5 min.

Myoglobinaemia

Leading to renal failure exacerbated by hypotension.

- Assessment: chocolate-coloured urine, urine dipstix.
- Treatment: urine alkalinization—add 20 ml 8.4% sodium bicarbonate to each litre of IV fluid; maintain a urine output of 2 ml/kg/h, which may need to be forced with furosemide or mannitol (after fluid resuscitation); short-term haemofiltration may be required.

Disseminated intravascular coagulation

- Assessment: excessive bleeding, clotting studies.
- Treatment: blood products if available.

Tetanus

An infection due to the bacillus *Clostridium tetani*, which produces a potent toxin blocking inhibitory central nervous system (CNS) neurotransmitters. Infection occurs via any break in skin or mucous membrane.

- High-risk wounds: umbilical cord in neonates, puncture wounds, burns, bites, avulsion, crush and blast injuries, any surgery in non-sterile conditions.
- Onset 3–21 days; shorter incubations result in more severe manifestation.

Diagnosis

Neonatal tetanus

- An illness occurring in an infant who has the normal ability to suck and cry in the first 2 days of life but loses this ability between days 3 and 28 of life and becomes rigid or has spasms.

Adult tetanus

At least one of:

- Trismus or risus sardonicus.
- Painful muscle spasms.
- Spatula test: reflex spasm of the jaw in response to touching the posterior wall of the pharynx with a soft instrument. Specificity 100% and sensitivity 94%.

Severe autonomic instability with arrhythmias may also be present.

Wound management

- Irrigate and debride except for umbilical cord infections.
- Antibiotics: metronidazole is preferred. Benzylpenicillin, tetracyclines, macrolides, clindamycin, cephalosporins, and chloramphenicol are also effective.
- Immunization (see Table 9.2).

Control of spasms

Diazepam

- Use 0.1–0.3 mg/kg slow IV bolus (3–5 min) every 1–4 h.
- If still symptomatic with hourly bolus start a continuous infusion at 0.1–0.8 mg/kg/h using a syringe driver if available.
- In neonates only use the emulsion preparation: the solution is unsuitable.
- Titrate to symptoms and respiratory rate:
  - ≥30 in children under 1 year
  - ≥25 in children 1–4 years old
  - ≥20 in children 5–12 years old
  - ≥14 in children over 12 years old
  - ≥12 in adults.
- Weaning:
  - Calculate the total 24 h IV dose and administer orally (PO) in four divided doses.

Table 9.2 Immunization management for tetanus.

Immunization status	All wounds	High-risk wound
	Vaccine	HTIG
Primary immunization complete, boosters up to date	No	Yes
Primary immunization incomplete or boosters not up to date	Booster dose and further doses to complete schedule	Yes
Not immunized or immunization status uncertain[2]	Immediate dose of vaccine followed by completion of full five-dose course	Yes

HTIG, human tetanus immune globulin.

Data from Medecins sans Frontieres clinical guidelines www.medicalguidelines.msf.org

- After the first oral dose decrease the rate of infusion by 50%; after the second oral dose stop the infusion.
- Once on an oral dose only wean by 10–20% every 24 h until a 6-hourly oral dose of 0.5 mg/kg is achieved.
- Then increase the time interval for oral dose to every 8 h for 24 h, then every 12 h, and then once a day before stopping.
- Wean more slowly if withdrawal signs appear.

Magnesium sulfate

- Use 5 g IV (or 75 mg/kg in children) given as a loading dose over 10–15 min followed by 1–3 g/h until the spasms are controlled.
- May be used as an alternative or as an adjunct to diazepam.
- Magnesium also treats autonomic dysfunction.
- Monitor toxicity using tendon reflexes (see also magnesium management in 'Pre-eclampsia and Eclampsia', Chapter 8, p. 187).

Respiratory support

- In severe cases intubation and ventilation may be required.
- Early tracheostomy may help for those with severe laryngeal spasm and to avoid mechanical ventilation.

Supportive management

- Close monitoring of respiratory rate (RR) and oxygen saturation (SpO_2) is essential; be alert for coughing, difficulty in breathing, or excess secretions.
- Nurse in a quiet, dark room to minimize stimulation. Use gentle suctioning of secretions. There should be minimal handling with adequate pain control and sedation.
- Nasogastric tube for hydration, nutrition, and oral medication. Neonates need expressed breastmilk/formula every 3 h and are at risk of hypoglycaemia.

Head injury

Diagnostic imaging and definitive neurosurgical treatment may not be available. Try and find out what the realistic options are before being faced with your first head-injured patient.

- What normally happens to these patients?
- Are there neurosurgeons or ventilatory support facilities?
- Is your hospital able to perform life-saving neurosurgical interventions (e.g. burr hole and elevation of a depressed skull fracture)?
- Is there an option for transfer to somewhere that can provide the above?

Prognostication in head injuries is difficult. There can be continued improvement over long periods. However, this needs to be taken in the context of resources available for long-term care and the impact on the patient's family.

Initial management

- Perform a (c)ABCDE assessment and treat other injuries as appropriate.
- Do not rush to intubate and ventilate the patient if they have a Glasgow coma score (GCS) <9. The purpose of intubation and ventilation in head injury is to minimize secondary brain injury by controlling CO_2, optimizing oxygenation and reducing cerebral metabolic requirement oxygen ($CMRO_2$) using appropriate sedation. If there are no ventilators, CO_2 monitoring, sedative infusions, or close BP monitoring then the risks are likely to outweigh the benefits. Fluctuations in ventilation, BP, and coughing on the tube will be detrimental.

Prevention of secondary brain injury

- This is achievable in low-resource settings and can significantly improve outcome.
- The aim is to maintain cerebral perfusion pressure (CPP) at 60–80 mmHg by controlling intracranial pressure (ICP) <20 mmHg and maintaining mean arterial pressure (MAP) >90 mmHg.

$$CPP = ICP - MAP$$

- Monitoring of these (other than MAP) is unlikely to be available.
- The patient should be in a critical care area with at least hourly observations including conscious level.

Maintain mean arterial pressure

- Appropriate fluid resuscitation and vasopressors.
- Treat other injuries causing bleeding.

Reduce intracranial pressure

- Nurse 30° head up and tape, rather than tie any ETT.
- Give O_2 to maintain SpO_2 at >95%.
- Maintain normocapnoea, ensure an unobstructed airway (Guedel or nasopharyngeal airway if required). If mechanical ventilation and capnography are available aim for CO_2 4–4.5 kPa, if there is no capnography ventilate at a tidal volume of 6 ml/kg RR 15.
- Reduce intra-abdominal pressure: urinary catheter; nasogastric tube; treat ileus.
- Reduce the brain's metabolic oxygen requirement ($CMRO_2$):
  - maintain normothermia (paracetamol and treat infections)

- adequate analgesia and sedation
- maintain normoglycaemia; insulin may be required
- control seizure activity/consider prophylaxis if GCS <10: load with phenytoin 20 mg/kg IV over 30 min (+ ECG and BP monitoring) or $MgSO_4$ 5 g over 10–15 min ($MgSO_4$ dose may be repeated). Treat further seizures with IV diazepam (1 mg/10 kg).

- Mannitol 20% (2 ml/kg) or hypertonic saline 5% (2 ml/kg) should be considered if signs of cerebral oedema (dilated pupil/Cushing's reflex) develop with lateralizing signs. This is a temporary measure only prior to definitive intervention, without which it is likely to cause intracranial hypertension over time and do more harm than good. Do not use if no further surgical intervention is planned.
- Steroids: there is no role for steroids in traumatic brain injury and the resultant hyperglycaemia is harmful. Do not use.

Prevent brain infections

- Use antibiotic prophylaxis in basal skull fractures and penetrating head injuries.

General supportive care to prevent complications

- Regular eye and mouth care.
- Regular suctioning of secretions.
- Regular turns with pressure area care.
- Ensure regular limb physio to prevent contractures.
- Prescribe stress ulcer prophylaxis.
- Commence enteral feeding via NG tube.

C spine immobilization in head injuries

C spine immobilization in this setting is not straightforward and the risks may well outweigh the benefits. Considerations include:

- How did the patient get to the hospital? (If carried for 3 h on the back of a motorbike etc. any damage is likely to have already happened.)
- Can the patient cooperate?
- Will you ever be able to clear the spine in the absence of a computerized tomography (CT) scan, C spine X-ray, and a reduced GCS?
- Is there a collar that will fit? Too small or too big may cause more harm than good for intracranial pressure (ICP) and pressure areas.
- Will putting on a collar and keeping the patient flat hamper pressure area care, increase aspiration risk, and/or raise ICP?

Burr holes

- Prompt removal of extradural and subdural haematomas will prevent the compression of the brain by the clot. This is a time-critical procedure and can be carried out safely by non-neurosurgeons.
- The outcome is usually favourable if done promptly compared with a high mortality and morbidity if delayed.
- Indication: GCS <8; imaging confirming diagnosis of extradural haematoma causing midline shifts and unequal pupils (strong clinical diagnosis with palpable fracture and ipsilateral dilated pupil is also acceptable); timely neurosurgical intervention not possible.

Anaesthesia for brain-injured patients

Patients with traumatic brain injury may present to theatre either for management of the primary brain injury or for other injuries.

Where possible the use of regional or local anaesthetic techniques is preferred; burr holes may be done under local anaesthetic. The general principle is to maintain secondary brain injury prevention measures during the anaesthetic.

Preoperative assessment

- Note GCS. For those with GCS ≤8 consider whether tracheostomy may be useful for postoperative management (see 'Tracheostomy Care' in Chapter 6, pp. 101–3).
- If it is not a damage control situation, ensure there is a full secondary survey so all injuries may be dealt with.

Induction

- Aspiration of NG tube if present.
- Position 30° head up.
- Prepare for possible difficult intubation—facial swelling, C spine control.
- Preoxygenation.
- Rapid sequence induction with ketamine (hypotension significantly increases mortality and morbidity in traumatic brain injury).
- Tape the ETT and position the head to minimize the obstruction to venous drainage.

Maintenance

- If possible maintain a head up tilt.
- The patient's head may be inaccessible—if so, ensure the tube is securely taped and unable to kink and that the patient's eyes are protected.
- Ventilate to normocapnoea or 6 ml/kg RR 15.
- Maintain BP, ketamine maintenance may help; vasopressor infusion may be required.
- Check temperature and blood glucose hourly and correct as required.
- Increasing hypertension, bradycardia, and an enlarging pupil require emergency management with hyperventilation and/or mannitol (see 'Head Injury' in this chapter, pp. 214–15).

Emergence

- Insert an NG tube (use caution in the case of basal skull fracture) and a urinary catheter if not already done.
- Extubation may be difficult in those with a low GCS (hence there should be consideration of a tracheostomy).
- Aim to extubate awake with minimal coughing and straining on the ETT.
- Discharge to a high care area for ongoing secondary brain injury prevention.

Spinal injury

Primary injury occurs due to cord compression, haemorrhage, or traction. There may then be secondary injury due to haemorrhage and oedema leading to ischaemia. Symptoms can deteriorate over the first 24 h.

Neurogenic shock

This is seen in injuries affecting the sympathetic supply (T2–T5) and causes bradycardia and hypotension with vasodilatation.

Spinal shock

This is loss of reflexes and flaccidity below the level of injury:

- Phase 1 (day 0–1) areflexic.
- Phase 2 (day 1–3) return of reflexes.
- Phase 3 (day 4–28) early hyperreflexia.
- Phase 4 (1–12 months) late hyperreflexia.

Autonomic hyperreflexia

- There is increased risk with higher injuries, reported from T10 and above.
- Causes acute life-threatening hypertension due to reflex sympathetic discharge.
- There is flushing and sweating above the level of injury, bradycardia, pupillary constriction, and nasal congestion (unopposed parasympathetic responses); and below the level of injury there is pale, cool skin and piloerection due to sympathetic tone and lack of the descending inhibitory parasympathetic modulation.
- It is generally triggered by pain/irritation below the level of the spinal lesion, e.g. bladder distension/surgery.
- Manage by: treating the trigger; sitting up and managing blood pressure—glyceryl trinitrate or nifedipine sublingual, hydralazine or $MgSO_4$ IV.
- General or spinal anaesthesia may be required for patients at risk needing surgery below the level of the lesion.

Management

Immobilization

Patients with suspected spinal injury should be immobilized to protect unstable fractures. This can be challenging in a limited-resources setting.

- No proper immobilization equipment.
- Limited imaging.
- Presentation can be delayed and the lack of pre-hospital care may mean that patients are not immobilized at the scene.
- The prolonged use of a spinal board must be avoided.
- Log-roll the patient and minimize the frequency of movement in unstable fractures but beware of pressure sores and thromboembolic risk.

There is ongoing debate about the use of C spine collars: see the 'Head Injury' section in this chapter (p. 215).

Airway assessment

- There is increased risk of aspiration (due to ileus/reduced sphincter tone).
- Intubation may be required due to apnoea or hypoventilation: rapid sequence induction with manual inline stabilization. Prepare for difficult intubation.
- Do not use suxamethonium from 72 h to 6 months after spinal injury (risk of hyperkalaemia).

Breathing

- Above C3—damage to the phrenic nerve. The patient will need long-term ventilation, which is unlikely to be appropriate in limited-resource contexts.
- C3–C5—partial damage to phrenic nerve, most patients will require ventilatory support.
- Above T8—loss of intercostals, may require some ventilatory support.
- Below T8—loss of abdominal component of ventilation.
- Spinal injury patients rely on diaphragmatic breathing so breathe better lying flat. Tilt the whole bed if required to reduce the risk of aspiration.

Circulation

- There is initial hyperreflexia due to catecholamine release.
- This is followed by neurogenic shock: hypotension/bradycardia plus warm and vasodilated peripheries (lesions above T5).
- Atropine/glycopyrronium may be needed for bradycardia.
- Cautious with fluid administration.
- Vasopressor support may be needed.

Disability and exposure

- Look carefully for associated injuries.
- Assess the neurological level and assess whether the injury is complete—look for sacral sparing and anal tone.

General care

- Meticulous nursing care with regular turns to prevent pressure sores.
- Bowel and catheter care regime.
- Pharmacological and mechanical thromboprophylaxis.
- Good nutrition.
- Physiotherapy and rehabilitation.

Considerations for anaesthesia in chronic spinal injury

- Increased risk of aspiration due to delayed gastric emptying.
- Spontaneously breathing general anaesthesia may lead to respiratory insufficiency dependent on injury level; spinal anaesthesia works well.
- Suxamethonium contraindicated between 3 days and 6 months.
- May require anaesthesia even for procedures below cord injury level if the patient is prone to autonomic hyperreflexia or reflex muscle spasms.
- Contractures may make positioning difficult.
- Vagal hypersensitivity may lead to bradyarrhythmias.
- Impaired thermoregulation.
- Increased thromboembolism risk.

Burns

Burns are frequent where open fires at home are common and the most vulnerable are young children, the disabled, and people with epilepsy.

Patients often present late as there are a number of local remedies that may be tried first. Acid burns are also common and have devastating consequences.

Treatment of burns requires access to extensive resources, fluids, blood, antibiotics, experienced personnel, theatre space and time, extra nutrition, dressings, and drugs for pain management. Patients who require grafting to >45% body surface area are highly unlikely to survive in the absence of high-resource intensive care management. It is essential to make an early decision whether or not to treat these patients and involve everyone (including relatives) so expectations are understood.

Principles of burns management are similar in adults and children except that children have a higher metabolic rate and are more susceptible to thermal loss, dehydration, and hypoglycaemia.

Assessment of burns

History

- Type of accident: check for other injuries.
- Type of burn: direct flame, hot water, etc. and length of exposure to the heat source.
- Length of time since burn and initial assessment.
- Being in a confined space increases the risk of inhalational injury.
- Potential toxic chemicals, e.g. cyanide.
- Treatment so far.
- Other injuries.

Initial assessment

- Check the airway and C spine.
- Treat life-threatening injuries first.
- Estimate the burn size and depth.
- If the patient is seen immediately, cool the burn site with water.
- Commence and monitor fluid resuscitation.
- Do a secondary survey.
- Commence burn wound management; remember analgesia and tetanus prophylaxis.

Burn assessment

- A major burn is defined as 15% body surface area (BSA) or 10% + inhalational injury.
- Burn size is measured as percentage of total body surface and is best assessed using a Lund and Browder chart (Figure 9.3).
- Full assessment often requires washing and dressing of burns under ketamine anaesthesia.
- Judging the depth of a burn by its appearance can often be remarkably difficult.
- The clinical assessment can be based on the presence or absence of blister formation and also on the colour of the wound, although these are not necessarily definitive.

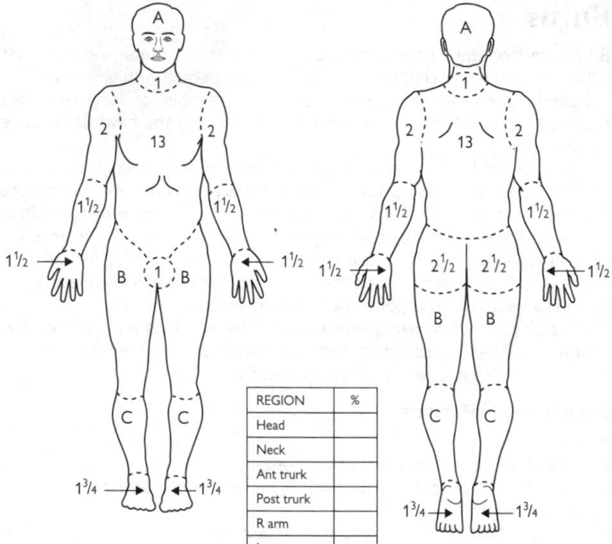

REGION	%
Head	
Neck	
Ant trurk	
Post trurk	
R arm	
L arm	
Buttocks	
Genitalia	
R leg	
L leg	
Total	

AREA	**0**	**1**	**5**	**10**	**15**	**Adult**
A = $\frac{1}{2}$ of head	$9\frac{1}{2}$	$8\frac{1}{3}$	$6\frac{1}{2}$	$5\frac{1}{2}$	$4\frac{1}{2}$	$3\frac{1}{2}$
B = $\frac{1}{2}$ of one thigh	$2\frac{3}{4}$	$3\frac{1}{4}$	4	$3\frac{1}{2}$	$3\frac{1}{2}$	$4\frac{3}{4}$
C = $\frac{1}{2}$ of one lower leg	$2\frac{1}{2}$	$2\frac{1}{2}$	$2\frac{3}{4}$	3	$3\frac{1}{4}$	$3\frac{1}{2}$

Figure 9.3 Lund and Browder chart for the assessment of burns.

The Lund Browder chart, in Lund CC, Browder NC. The estimation of areas of burns. *Surg Gynecol Obstet* 1944;79:352–358. Reprinted with permission from the *Journal of the American College of Surgeons*, formerly *Surgery Gynecology & Obstetrics*.

- The pinprick test is also very useful; light pressure with a sterile needle will establish the degree of sensitivity. Inability to perceive pain indicates a full thickness burn. Dullness to pain but awareness of touch is the most reliable objective test of a deep dermal injury. See Table 9.3.

Table 9.3 Clinical features for different burn depths.

Type of burn	Blistering	Appearance	Pin prick test
Superficial dermal	Present	Bright red/pink	Sensitive to pain
Deep dermal	Blisters are broken	Creamy coloured/ mottled	Dullness to pain, sensitive to touch
Full thickness	Absent	Grey/white or brown	No sensation

Initial fluid management

- IV access may be difficult: think of using a femoral, intraosseous, or even central line.
- Modified Parkland formula (2 ml/kg/%BSA) is recommended, using crystalloid for the first 24 h. Give half the required amount over the first 8 h from the time of burn and the rest over the subsequent 16 h.
- This formula is a guide; monitor fluid resuscitation closely as this will vary dependent on patient response.
    - If urine output is >2 ml/kg/h, reduce fluids; if urine output is <1 ml/kg/h, increase fluids.
    - If urine is positive for Hb maintain urine output at 2 ml/kg/h and, if required, promote diuresis with mannitol.
- Some patients may present very late, making these formulae redundant; in these cases base fluid resuscitation on urine output.

Management of inhalational injury

- Associated with high mortality >27%.
- Need high index of suspicion (prolonged exposure in confined space, headaches, seizures, low GCS, soot around nose, etc.).
- Upper airway injury:
    - Direct heat causes swelling of uvula, pharynx, epiglottis, larynx.
    - Leads to stridor, voice change, and obstructed breathing pattern.
    - Nurse head up.
    - Nebulized adrenaline may help.
    - Intubate early before airway management becomes a challenge and where ventilation on ICU is not safe, perform an early tracheostomy.
- Lower airway injury:
    - Toxic gases cause damage to epithelium, hypersecretion of mucus, and eventually airway obstruction.
    - May be exacerbated by fluid resuscitation.
    - Intubate and ventilate early if appropriate to context.
    - In the absence of an ICU these patients are very difficult to manage.

Anaesthesia for debridement and grafting

Surgery is an essential part of burn management and multiple painful interventions are often required. Good anaesthesia and multimodal analgesia in the beginning help with patient compliance and cooperation, especially with children, who can develop a phobia to the operating room. Blood loss can be extensive and blood products may be in short supply so use them judiciously and combine with haematinics.

Major considerations

- Heat conservation.
- Hypermetabolic state and continuous fluid loss.
- Cardiovascular instability due to systemic inflammatory response syndrome (SIRS) and intraoperative blood loss.
- Potential for massive blood loss (especially in paediatrics).
- Pharmacokinetic alterations:
  - Avoid suxamethonium between 24 h and 18 months post-burn injury (risk of hyperkalaemia).
  - Resistance to non-depolarizing muscle relaxants (may need to double dose if burns >20% BSA).
- Delayed gastric emptying.
- Difficult airway management.

Intraoperative management

- Keep the operating theatre as warm as possible. Avoid evaporative losses and use plastic bags to wrap the patient. Warm fluids (e.g. in buckets of warm water).
- Continue maintenance fluids.
- Replace blood loss (4 ml/kg of packed cells or 8 ml/kg of whole blood will increase Hb by 1 g/dl).
- Reduce blood loss:
  - Tourniquets.
  - Infiltration with adrenaline 1:100,000 and local anaesthetic solutions, especially to donor sites.
  - Tranexamic acid 10 mg/kg (up to 1g) slow IV and gauzes soaked in tranexamic acid/adrenaline applied locally.
- Use a combination of general anaesthesia or sedation and regional blocks to ensure good pain relief. Ketamine and halothane are used extensively in burns, and repeated halothane has been shown to be safe.
- Fascia iliaca block (see 'Lower Limb Blocks' in Chapter 11 pp. 251–2) is helpful for donor sites from anterior and lateral thigh. Donor sites are very painful: if unable to perform regional block use local infiltration of bupivacaine.

Postoperative care

Carrying out the basics well can improve the outcome of burns victims without complex equipment.

Sepsis

- Antibiotics are not required in the acute phase unless there is obvious infection.
- The burn area is susceptible to infection due to loss of natural barriers, so meticulous wound care is essential.
- Keep the patient separate from infected cases on the ward.
- Remember tetanus prophylaxis.

Pain management

- Pain is severe in superficial burns and from skin graft donor sites.
- Pain can become chronic if not managed appropriately.

- Early multimodal analgesia helps avoid development of complex pain.
- Regional analgesia is useful.
- Low-dose ketamine infusion is useful for postoperative pain relief especially in the first few days (see 'Ketamine', Chapter 4, p. 58).
- Amitriptyline, gabapentin, and carbamazepine are widely available and can be especially useful in adults (see 'Pain Management', Chapter 5, p. 87).
- Distraction with fun activities and the clinical psychologist can play a useful role.

Nutrition

- Burns patients have very high caloric requirements and nutrition must be started early to accelerate wound healing and reduce infection. This hypermetabolic state is worse with an inhalational injury.
- Maintain ambient temperature at 28°C so that heat loss and the need for thermogenesis to maintain body temperature are minimal.
- Enteral feeding is better than parenteral: it reduces the incidence of ileus, preserves gut integrity, and reduces the risk of stress ulceration.
- Add multivitamins, vitamin C, zinc, and ferrous sulphate syrup.
- Nutritional requirements: see Table 9.4.

Table 9.4 Nutritional requirements in burns.

	Minor burn	Major burn >15% TBSA
Protein	1.2 g/kg/day	1.5 2 g/kg/day
Carbohydrate	7 g/kg/day	8 g/kg/day
Fat	2 g/kg/day	2 g/kg/day
Water	1 ml per calorie	1.5–2 ml per calorie

TBSA, total body surface area.

In resource limited environments ready-made enteral feeds are often not available but the energy and protein requirements can be provided with local foodstuffs. See 'Nutrition' in Chapter 12 (pp. 264–5) for the recipe.

Ulcer prophylaxis

- Encourage oral or enteral feeding to reduce the risk of gastric ulcerations.
- Remember stress ulceration prophylaxis if unable to feed enterally.

Thromboembolism

- If the patient is immobile remember thromboprophylaxis.

Dressing changes

- Need to be done frequently and consume resources and theatre time.
- Dressing changes can be performed on the ward under oral sedation with appropriate resuscitation and monitoring equipment.
- An oral mixture of ketamine, diazepam, and paracetamol syrup works well if given 15–20 min prior to dressing change. Mix:
  - ketamine 15 ml (50 mg/ml) +
  - diazepam 10 ml (5 mg/ml) +

  - paracetamol 75 ml (24 mg/ml)
  - administer 0.5 ml/kg
  - there may be tachyphylaxis with repeated use.
- If burns are very extensive try soaking in a bath of water to allow dressings to fall off.

Anaesthesia for burn contractures or secondary reconstruction

Contractures around the mouth or neck may limit mouth opening or neck extension and make airway management hazardous.

- Maintain spontaneous respiration.
- If inhalational induction is chosen, parental presence may help relieve anxiety in a young child.
- Use ketamine either as an infusion or intermittent bolus for the entire procedure or just for surgical release of the neck contracture under local anaesthesia and then insert a laryngeal mask airway (LMA) or ETT if required. In paediatrics ketamine may cause secretions and an antisialogogue may be useful.
- In cooperative adults: anaesthetize the mouth, pharynx, and larynx with local anaesthetic, and then introduce an LMA. If there is a good seal induce the patient.
- Avoid excessive airway manipulations. Add dexamethasone 0.25 mg/kg IV to reduce airway oedema. Nebulized adrenaline (0.5–1 ml of 1:1000) in saline (4–5 mls) may also relieve laryngeal oedema.
- Avoid suxamethonium if the burn occurred within the preceding 18 months.
- Use combined regional and general anaesthesia for pain relief.
- Protect the eyes if ectropions are present.

Patient transfer

The most common reason for transfer is for more advanced care (e.g. ICU) or interventions (e.g. neurosurgery). The usual principles of patient stabilization and optimization pre-transfer should be applied.

Decision making for transfer

- Ask yourself, **can** the patient be transferred?
  - Is a higher care facility available?
  - Is the facility willing to accept the patient?
  - Is it within reasonable reach (distance and time)?
  - Who will pay?
  - Is there a means of transferring the patient?
  - Is it safe for the patient and personnel?
- And **should** they be transferred?
  - Will the patient benefit from the transfer?
  - Will the patient survive the transfer?
  - Do they (patient/relatives) agree to the transfer?
  - Are there adequate resources (equipment, drugs, and personnel) to allow the transfer without compromising other inpatient care needs?

Mode of transport

This will most likely be ground transport.

- Are there local ambulances and provider contact details (government vs private)? Who covers the cost?
- If utilizing air transport do not forget to organize ground transport and additional aviation paperwork.
- Don't forget to think about transport back to base and make prior arrangement for this.

Accepting hospital

- Contact details (with a named clinician) and location of the hospital. It is useful to have this written down and displayed prominently.
- If possible a planning visit to the facility will give invaluable information about the level of care available and build rapport. If not, talk to the local staff.
- Verbal contact with the accepting clinician prior to transfer including details of the destination (emergency department, theatres, or ICU) and the estimated time of arrival.
- It is important to discuss who will be covering the cost of transport and ongoing care.

Personnel

- There may be strict rules about staff movement imposed by your employer.
- Local staff may be inexperienced especially with critical care transfer. Organize a teaching session and have a means of communicating during transfer for advice.
- Road conditions may be poor and the journey long so think about personal comfort, safety provisions, and antiemetic.

- Don't forget the driver—they should also be trained, especially if driving at speed (blue light), be familiar with the vehicle and driving conditions, and briefed on the location and any safety issues (e.g. checkpoints).

Equipment

- The vehicle may vary from a fully equipped ambulance to a basic van/pick-up or four-wheel drive. Check what is available and make sure it is functioning.
- Having a transfer grab bag containing equipment and drugs needed can save time. The content will depend on availability but this may not be as comprehensive as what you are used to. A grab bag can also be used for stabilizing a sick patient within the hospital. Devise a sealing system to check visually that the bag is restocked after each use.
- Monitoring may be basic but ideally take at least an SpO_2 monitor. Auscultation can be difficult during transfer due to movement and a potentially noisy environment.
- A transfer ventilator is unlikely to be available so think about the feasibility of transferring a ventilator-dependent patient, especially over a huge distance.
- Anticipate and prepare for deterioration—bring emergency drugs and equipment (this must be balanced with the availability of spares and needs of other patients).
- Calculate requirements for O_2/drugs/fluid/battery-powered devices and have a plan for equipment failure/running out of things. A useful recipe for single-syringe transfer anaesthesia is provided in the 'Ketamine' section of Chapter 4 (p. 59). You may not have the luxury of unlimited supplies so be pragmatic.

Safety

- Road traffic accidents are common in LMICs and are a leading cause of morbidity and mortality.
- Roads may be poorly maintained or prone to weather-related hazards such as flooding and landslides. Local staff can provide useful information and the driver should be familiar with the roads.
- Vehicle maintenance should be up to date and spares available in case of breakdown.
- Seatbelts should be worn at all times and the trolley and equipment secured.
- Take into account the time of day. There are more road hazards in the night time with poorly lit roads and intoxicated drivers.
- If road blocks and checkpoints are present make sure you know the protocol for passing through.
- Maintain communication with base throughout (make sure there is phone reception throughout or radio contact).

Documentation and handover

- A referral letter should accompany the patient together with any results of investigations and details of interventions carried out in the referring hospital.

- Include contact details of the referring hospital.
- Use a chart to document patient's vital signs and any changes or interventions during transfer.
- Hand over patient to both the physician and nursing staff at the receiving hospital.

Top tips

- Pre-planning some of the logistical aspects of patient transfer and having a system in place is invaluable.
- Accept that transferring a patient is not always possible due to the challenges outlined. This can be difficult for the patient and family as well as the staff caring for the patient.
- Use a checklist to make sure nothing is forgotten. Ideally this should be customized to your environment but generic checklists can also be handy.

Further reading

Bonner S, Smith C (2013) Initial management of acute spinal cord injury. *CEACCP* 13 (6): 224–231.

International Committee of the Red Cross (2017) *Anaesthesia Handbook*. Geneva: ICRC.

International Committee of the Red Cross/World Health Organization (2016) *Management of Limb Injuries during Disaster and Conflict. Field Guide*. Geneva: ICRC/WHO.

Robinson J (2016) *Orthopaedic Trauma in the Austere Environment*. London: Springer International Publishing.

Rossaint R et al. (2016) The European guideline on management of major bleeding and coagulopathy following trauma, 4th edition. *Critical Care* 20: 100.

Skinner DV, Driscoll PA (2013) *ABC of Major Trauma*, 4th ed. Oxford: Wiley Blackwell.

Wilson MH et al. (2012) Emergency burr holes: 'How to do it'. *Scand J Trauma, Resusc Emerg Med* 20: 24.

World Health Organization (2010) *Current Recommendations for Treatment of Tetanus during Humanitarian Emergencies*. WHO Technical Note. Geneva: WHO.

Chapter 10

General and Urological Surgery

Lara Herbert and Ruth Tighe

For:
Liver abscess—see 'Tropical Abscess' in Chapter 7, p. 140.
Nephrectomy—see 'Wilms' Tumour' in Chapter 7, p. 144.

Laparotomy

General considerations

- Laparotomy is a common operation in low- and middle-income countries (LMICs) with high perioperative mortality due to late presentation and limited resources.
- The surgical diagnosis may not be clear preoperatively, so plan for all eventualities. Sepsis and obstructing cancers are common indications; less commonly, infectious diseases including typhoid, hydatid cyst, and Ascaris worm impaction may also necessitate laparotomy.
- Confirm the surgical plan preoperatively. Primary anastomosis after bowel resection is common, even if high-risk, to avoid stomas (which may be poorly accepted, hard to care for, and require a supply of bags), so anastomotic breakdown can occur postoperatively.

Preoperative

Assessment

History

- May be limited by the urgency of intervention, language.
- Establish comorbidities including recent fevers, previous surgery.
- The patient may have seen a traditional healer before coming to hospital, who may have marked or incised areas felt to be pathological, or administered various herbal remedies.

Examination

Follow a systematic approach: in the absence of extensive investigations, pay close attention to trends in clinical signs.

- Respiratory: an increase in respiratory rate may indicate pain, anaemia, and/or compensation for a metabolic acidosis. Measure oxygen saturation (SpO_2) if possible. Auscultate the chest.
- Circulatory: peripheral perfusion, capillary refill time (ideally central), pallor (conjunctivae, tongue, and gums), heart rate, pulse character, blood pressure (BP), and heart sounds (untreated structural cardiac disease may be present). Assess overall fluid status.
- Disability: assess conscious level and consider hypoglycaemia.
- General: assess nutritional status, examine the abdomen for distension, peritonism.

Investigations

- If available, consider a full blood count, urea and electrolytes, blood glucose, and testing for malaria and HIV.
- Send blood for grouping and/or cross-matching, as able (see 'Blood Transfusion' in Chapter 4, pp. 68–72).

Preoperative resuscitation

May occur on the ward or in theatre. Optimize:

- Respiratory function and oxygenation:
  - High-flow oxygen through a mask with a reservoir (if available).
  - Position semi-sitting as cardiovascularly tolerated.
  - Gastric decompression with a nasogastric (NG) tube.

- Volume status:
  - Ensure adequate IV access and administer warmed fluids. Fluid may be warmed in a bucket of warm water, a microwave (crystalloids only), or in the sun if there is no formal warmer.
  - Use fluid challenges and clinical signs to titrate volume replacement. In patients where fluid overload is a concern, haemodynamic response to a leg raise may indicate whether a fluid challenge is likely to be beneficial.
  - Fluid choices may be restricted: crystalloid is more commonly available than colloid.
- Monitoring: should commence as soon as possible and include pulse oximetry, BP, and three-lead electrocardiogram (ECG) monitoring, if available.
- Place a urinary catheter at this stage if not already present.
- Promote normothermia:
  - Cover patient with warming blanket if available.
  - Warmed bags of fluids should be placed around the patient.
  - Keep the patient covered as far as possible.
  - Switch the theatre air conditioning off.
- Give intravenous broad-spectrum antibiotics early to cover Gram positive, negative, and anaerobic organisms.
- Consider hyperkalaemia:
  - Acute kidney injury is not uncommon in late-presenting laparotomy patients; it is particularly relevant if suxamethonium (further potassium rise) and/or halothane (arrhythmia risk) are used.
  - In the absence of laboratory results, check urine output (if time allows) and the ECG for signs of hyperkalaemia (peaked T waves, widened QRS complexes).
  - If hyperkalaemia is suspected, consider: calcium gluconate 10 ml 10% intravenous (IV), inhaled salbutamol, an infusion (or slow injection by hand) of 50 ml 50% glucose with 15 international units of soluble insulin over 30 min, and/or 1 mg/kg IV lidocaine.
- Consider hypokalaemia:
  - More common in the patient with bowel obstruction or who has been vomiting for other reasons.
  - Can contribute to respiratory muscle weakness and insufficiency.
- Have a low threshold for NG tube insertion.

Perioperative

Preparation for induction

- Communicate with the surgical team: in particular, about the assistance that will be required at induction (e.g. cricoid pressure), the anaesthesia plan, and any specific concerns you have.
- Check the availability and location of emergency drugs, e.g. vasopressors. Do you need a vasopressor running prior to induction?
- Suction NG tube.
- Check oropharyngeal suction is available and working (if manual/pedal, assign someone to operate it).
- Ensure all your airway equipment (including emergency kit) is within reach and has been checked by you.

Induction

- Preoxygenate.
- Rapid sequence induction, e.g. with ketamine 1–2 mg/kg + suxamethonium 2 mg/kg IV. If suxamethonium is not available, see 'Absent Drugs and Work-arounds' in Chapter 4 (pp. 63–4) for alternatives.
  - Ketamine is a useful agent for the shocked patient; however, in extremis, even ketamine can cause cardiovascular collapse due to myocardial depression. Consider a reduced dose in this situation.
- Capnography may be available; if not, be meticulous about clinical tube position checking.

Maintenance

- May be dictated by availability. Halothane is widely used: limiting adrenaline infiltration by surgeons and tight CO_2 control will minimize arrhythmia risk.
- Muscle relaxation is advantageous but rarely absolutely essential: discuss with your surgeon. Consider what agent/s you have, the likely duration of surgery (it may be as short as 15 minutes with some expert operators), and the availability of neuromuscular monitoring, reversal agents, and recovery facilities.
- Ventilate according to the patient's preoperative respiratory rate, in the absence of capnography or blood gas measurements, to compensate for suspected metabolic acidosis.
- For the haemodynamically unstable patient:
  - Consider using a ketamine infusion rather than a volatile agent (see 'Ketamine', in Chapter 4, pp. 54–8).
  - IV hydrocortisone if adrenal insufficiency is suspected.
  - Run fluids and vasopressor on separate cannulae to allow independent control of each.
  - If possible, give blood only once bleeding has been controlled.

Analgesia

- Use opioids, paracetamol, and/or atypical analgesics such as gabapentin.
- Non-steroidal anti-inflammatory drugs (NSAIDs) are often available but should be used with caution/avoided in patients with possible kidney injury and/or delayed gut function.
- Regional techniques (transversus abdominis plane (TAP) or rectus sheath blocks) may be helpful.
- Seek local advice on the availability, risks, and use of postoperative opioid analgesia.

Postoperative

- Ideally admit to a high-dependency or intensive care unit (ICU) where the patient is most likely to receive regular observations, antibiotics, IV fluids, and analgesia. If not, regularly review the patient yourself.
- If agreed with the surgical team, encourage early mobilization and removal of lines; some centres still adhere to prolonged bedrest and fasting post-laparotomy, which may or may not be indicated.
- Encourage early enteral feeding, either by mouth or via NG tube.

- Utilize any allied healthcare provision within the hospital such as physiotherapists and dieticians.
- If the patient is on antiretrovirals, it is important that they continue to receive this treatment postoperatively.

Laparotomy under spinal anaesthesia

- It is possible to perform a laparotomy under spinal anaesthesia, e.g. with high-volume (3–4 ml) 0.5% heavy bupivacaine, +/− 100–200 μg intrathecal morphine.
- The technique may be useful in relatively stable patients where there is limited/no oxygen supply and/or critical care facility.
- Before opting for this, consider:
  - Haemodynamic and respiratory status of the patient and the likely impact on these of a spinal anaesthetic.
  - What vasopressors are available to you.
  - Whether you have access to preservative free opioid.
  - The potential for delayed respiratory depression after intrathecal opioid administration, and the likely level of nursing care postoperatively.
  - Discuss the duration of surgery with the surgeon: if the spinal wears off before the end, conversion to general anaesthesia or use of ketamine analgesia may be required.
- Note the following:
  - Rule out contraindications to spinal anaesthesia.
  - Better for lower abdominal surgery (below umbilicus), although surgical extent may not be known at the outset.
  - Ensure all monitoring is applied as available (SpO_2, BP, and ECG).
  - Ensure adequate IV access (ideally two cannulae, one for vasopressor and one for fast-flowing fluids) and preload.
  - A urinary catheter will be required.
  - Diaphragmatic pain may occur: encourage the surgeons to minimize handling close to the diaphragm. Low-dose supplemental ketamine at analgesic doses may be useful in this situation (e.g. 5 mg IV boluses titrated to response).

General anaesthesia and spinal

- In circumstances with limited/no opioid or muscle relaxant, and a relatively stable patient, a spinal followed by general anaesthesia provides good anaesthetic conditions for laparotomy, and with intrathecal opioid also confers postoperative analgesia.
- A lower local anaesthesia dose is needed than for sole anaesthesia (e.g. 1–1.5 ml 0.5% heavy bupivacaine with intrathecal morphine 100–200 μg).
- If intrathecal opiates are used, they must be preservative free, and there must be adequate postoperative monitoring to detect +/− treat delayed respiratory depression in a timely manner.

Anaesthesia for hernia repair

- Hernia may be incisional, umbilical, inguinal, or femoral.
- Affects all ages (for management in children, see 'Hernia repair' in Chapter 7, p. 132–3).
- May be elective, urgent (obstruction), or emergent (strangulation).

Preoperative

Assessment

- Look at the hernia: they are often massive due to late presentation.
- Is the hernia reducible? Is there evidence of bowel obstruction?
- Any other comorbidities?
- Is it amenable to spinal anaesthesia? This will depend on anatomical location of the hernia, likely duration of surgery, and likelihood of conversion to laparotomy (though see 'Laparotomy Under Spinal Anaesthesia').

Planning

- Spinal or general/local anaesthesia techniques may be used. If the hernia is massive (or if surgery may be prolonged), a general anaesthetic +/− rapid sequence induction +/− regional technique may be preferable.
- Unless truly emergent, ensure adequate fasting.
- Monitoring and IV access should be used as for any anaesthetic.
- Confirm side (if applicable) with the team.
- Give appropriate antibiotics (cover Gram positive, Gram negative, anaerobic organisms).

Perioperative

Spinal

- Exclude contraindications to spinal anaesthesia.
- A useful technique where recovery facilities are limited or likelihood of receiving postoperative analgesia is low.
- Local anaesthetic +/− opioid to achieve appropriate block height.
- In the author's experience (in Uganda), spinals were used with good effect in children down to roughly the age of 8, using doses of 0.3–0.5 mg/kg 0.5% bupivacaine.

General anaesthesia + local anaesthesia/ilioinguinal block for inguinal hernia repairs

- If you are concerned about bowel obstruction, consider rapid sequence induction.
- Ilioinguinal nerve block using a blind technique or ultrasound should be used if available.
- Alternatively, local anaesthesia infiltration of the inguinal canal should be carried out by the surgeon.

Postoperative

- Simple regular analgesia.
- Suggest a stool softener as locally available.
- Ensure early mobilization, eating and drinking, and removal of urinary catheter or NG tube if *in situ*.

Anaesthesia for open cholecystectomy

- More often listed as an elective case.
- If listed as 'exploration for obstructive jaundice', treat as emergency and use the laparotomy technique as on pp. 230–3.

Assessment

- Check for evidence of biliary tract obstruction and/or biliary sepsis.
- If the patient has evidence of biliary sepsis, consider postponing the surgery until the patient has been resuscitated and is stable (discuss with the surgical team).
- Liaise with surgeons regarding their approach and plan (most likely open right upper quadrant).
- Investigate as able (full blood count (FBC), urea and electrolytes (U&E), liver function tests (LFTs), clotting, group and save (G&S)).
- General anaesthesia. There is potential benefit from regional blocks (paravertebral/intrapleural/intercostal). Liaise with the local anaesthetists to find out what they normally do for analgesia for open cholecystectomy where no opioids are available.

Management

Preoperative management

- Ensure the patient is appropriately fasted, and that there is IV access and monitoring as available.
- Consider a ramped position for preoxygenation.

Intraoperative management

- Rapid sequence induction (if indicated) using an IV induction agent and suxamethonium.
- Give IV antibiotics according to local guidance.
- Maintain anaesthesia with a volatile agent.
- Paralysis will help the surgeon but is not mandated. If you are able to, ventilate with gentle positive end expiratory pressure (PEEP). Spontaneous ventilation is possible but is likely to reduce compensation for metabolic acidosis in the sicker patient (e.g. with biliary sepsis).
- Use a regional technique where possible, +/− simple and opioid analgesia.

Postoperative management

- Admission to a postoperative surgical ward is appropriate.
- If obstructive jaundice is present preoperatively, intrathecal opioids have been given, or there are intraoperative complications, then consider admission to a high-dependency unit (HDU) or ICU as available.
- Regular simple postoperative analgesia.
- The emphasis should be on deep breathing, early mobilization, eating and drinking early, and removal of the IV line and urinary catheter if *in situ*.
- If available, involve allied health professionals (such as physiotherapists and dieticians) in postoperative management.

Splenectomy

- May be required for:
  - trauma
  - portal hypertension (secondary to schistosomiasis)
  - hydatid cysts.
- Other causes of massive splenomegaly seldom require operative treatment but include malaria, lymphoma, and leukaemia.
- If possible, patients require:
  - Vaccination against *Streptococcus pneumoniae, Neisseria meningitidis, Haemophilus influenzae* type b, and influenza virus. Vaccinations may be given preoperatively (in elective cases) or postoperatively.
  - If 'high-risk' (e.g. <16 years, >50 years, no pneumococcal vaccination, underlying haematological malignancy): lifelong low-dose penicillin. The greatest risk is in the first 2 years after a splenectomy.
  - Advise the patient to present early if unwell. Malaria is particularly serious in the asplenic patient.

Trauma splenectomy

- Traumatic ruptured spleen management has altered in the resource-rich setting, with conservative management often favoured. This is in large part due to availability of imaging (sequential computerized tomography (CT) scans), plentiful blood transfusion resources, and reliable critical care.
- Splenectomy is often encompassed by 'trauma laparotomy in the unstable patient'. Please refer to 'Damage Control Laparotomy' in Chapter 9 (pp. 200–1). The diagnosis may not be clear preoperatively.

Non-trauma splenectomy

Schistosomiasis

- Causes portal hypertension and splenomegaly. Surgical treatment is the Sugiura procedure: all visible varices are tied off in an open operation and the spleen is removed.
- This is:
  - major, very high-risk surgery
  - a long operation (3–8 h)
  - not an emergency operation, thus there is time to optimize the patient, within available resources.
- Patients may present with variceal bleeding and tense ascites, but relatively normal liver function. There is a risk of losing the circulating volume from both a dilated portal system and a prolonged operation, therefore ensure blood is ready in theatre.
- A balance is struck between the extent of varices secured and the length of the procedure.
- Postoperative management is similar to that following laparotomy, with high-dependency care and opioid analgesia if possible.

Lymphoma

- Can be HIV-related (see 'HIV', Chapter 13, pp. 300–1).
- Chemotherapy may precipitate neutropaenic sepsis or worsen TB.
- Anti-retroviral therapy can worsen TB and disturb liver function.

Hydatid cyst excision

- Hydatid cysts secondary to *Echinococcus granulosus* occur most frequently in the liver, followed by the lungs and spleen. Clinical presentation may be related to cysts' mass effect or cyst rupture.
- Management may be conservative; alternatively cysts may be aspirated under radiological guidance or aspirated +/− excised in an open operation.
- Anaesthetic considerations depend on the location and size of cysts. Cyst rupture may cause local complications (such as aspiration in the case of pulmonary cysts) and systemic complications (fever, urticaria, and, rarely, anaphylaxis).

Appendicectomy

- This condition, common all over the world, has a relatively high mortality rate in low-income countries due to late presentation, peritonitis, and sepsis.
- Consider these patients at high risk for septic shock, especially those with known HIV. Young patients may compensate until relatively late.
- Patients presenting with longer than a 1-week history may have very difficult surgery due to friable tissues, multiple adhesions, and bowel inflammation. Where possible, consider treatment with antibiotics and delay surgery (>3 months) in these cases.

Assessment

- Warning signs:
  - raised respiratory rate (potential acidaemia)
  - prolonged capillary refill time
  - cool, clammy peripheries
  - tachycardia not resolving with analgesia
  - agitation/anxiety.
- Hypotension and oliguria are late signs of shock.

Management

- For generalized peritonitis—see the 'Laparotomy' section.
- For localized appendix—see the 'Hernia' section.

Bladder stone excision

- Large obstructing bladder stones are common, especially in the 'stone belt' across northern Africa, the Middle East, and the Far East.
- The operation is quick: suprapubic excision, extrusion of stone from bladder, and closure.
- Excision may be indicated for recurrent infection or for acute obstruction. There are therefore varying degrees of urgency.
- Stone recurrence is common due to urinary composition and predisposing factors remaining.

Assessment

- Assessment is as for any patient undergoing surgery, but in particular be alert for signs of systemic infection or acute/chronic renal failure (check haemoglobin (Hb) and U&E if possible).

Management

- Spinal: cover up to T10.
- Ketamine anaesthesia is very useful for this quick operation in patients who are potentially septic and have acute kidney injury.

Further reading

Datta PK, Lal P, De Bakshi S (2013) *Surgery in the Tropics* in Bailey & Love's Short Practice of Surgery, 26th edn. Williams N, Ronan O'Connell P. Boca Raton, FL: CRC Press. pp. 68–92.

Chapter 11

Regional Anaesthesia

Adrian Bosenberg and Jey Jeyanathen[1]

1 Dr Jey Jeyanathen is the chapter lead.

Consent and preparation

Regional techniques are particularly useful in low-resource settings. They allow the reduction or complete avoidance of general anaesthesia and therefore result in less postoperative sedation. This is an advantage where recovery room surveillance may be suboptimal and oxygen supplies erratic. They are especially useful for postoperative analgesia where ward opiates may be dangerous to administer and monitor. They may also have a role in the prevention of chronic pain.

Contraindications

These are largely relative and require review on a case-by-case basis.

- coagulopathy
- local infection at site of block
- local anaesthetic (LA) allergy
- patient refusal/unable to cooperate
- risk of masking the features of compartment syndrome (controversial).

Consent

Patient consent includes an explanation of the block process and ideally the relative risks vs benefits. Regional anaesthesia risks include:

- temporary or permanent nerve damage
- bleeding
- LA toxicity
- infection
- failure or patchy block.

Preparation

- Assemble:
  - assistance for positioning, block delivery, and aid in the event of an emergency
  - translator, if necessary
  - resuscitation equipment
  - LA with calculated maximum dose
  - monitoring of the patient to include blood pressure, pulse oximetry, and electrocardiogram (ECG) if available.
- Obtain IV access.
- Confirm correct side and site of block.
- Position the patient appropriately for the block.

Performance of block

- Aseptic technique.
- Always aspirate for blood before injecting.
- Never inject against high resistance (there is a risk of intraneuronal injection).
- Be vigilant for both cardiovascular system (CVS) and central nervous system (CNS) symptoms as indicators of LA toxicity during and after the block.
- Blocks in children are often performed under general anaesthesia or sedation.

Nerve localization

A variety of techniques can be used to localize nerves for regional block. The availability of equipment varies widely, so it is useful to be familiar with a range of techniques.

Landmark techniques

- Position of the nerve is assumed in relation to anatomical landmarks.
- Can be performed with only a normal (blunted) hypodermic needle.
- Paraesthesia may be sought in awake patients but can be uncomfortable.
- Failure rate is high in inexperienced hands.
- Relatively high volumes of LA are required to compensate for inaccurate needle position.

Needle nerve stimulator

- The *n*egative electrode should be connected to the *n*eedle and the *p*ositive electrode connected to the *p*atient using a standard ECG electrode. The stimulator should initially be set at 2 mA and 1–2 Hz.
- The needle should be advanced until the correct distal muscle contractions are elicited.
- The current should be decreased and the location of the needle adjusted until the maximum motor response is elicited with a low current of 0.3–0.5 mA.
- On injection of LA the muscle stimulation should immediately cease indicating a successful block is likely.
- The LA should not be injected if intense muscle contraction is elicited at <0.2 mA or if there is resistance to injection. Both suggest that the tip of the needle may be intraneural and that the nerve may be damaged by further injection.

Ultrasound

- Allows direct visualization of neurovascular structures and their relationship to the needle.
- Improves accuracy of needle positioning and therefore reduced LA volumes and potentially fewer complications.
- The ultrasound machine should be in the operator's line of sight so is often placed opposite to the operator and opposite to the side being blocked.
- Use a high frequency (6–13 MHz) linear probe. The depth should be adjusted so that target structures are in the centre of the screen. Optimize gain.
- Visualization of the needle along its course takes practice. Combined use with a nerve stimulator can be helpful.

Local anaesthetic drugs

The most commonly available agent is usually lidocaine but other agents such as bupivacaine may be available. Generally, these other longer-acting agents are in short supply so it is wise to reserve them for cases that really need them.

The maximum recommended doses for some of the more commonly found agents, their speed of onset, and their duration of action are given in Table 11.1.

Note:

- The duration of action of the block is dependent on the type of LA and the dose; lower doses are safer but the block is likely to be shorter.
- LA agents come in different concentrations, e.g. 1% = 10 mg/ml; 0.25% = 2.5 mg/ml. Make sure you know which concentration you have and calculate maximum doses accordingly.
- The volume of anaesthetic controls the spread of the block; where accuracy is likely to be poorer (e.g. landmark c.f. US guided techniques) a larger volume may be required. This may involve diluting the LA to stay below the maximum dose.
- The duration of action and maximum dose of some agents may be improved by the addition of 1:200,000 adrenaline (Table 11.1).
- Never use adrenaline around end arteries (fingers, penis).

Table 11.1 Commonly found local anaesthetic agents, their maximum allowable doses and properties.

Drug	Levobupivacaine (Chirocaine)	Bupivacaine	Lidocaine	Prilocaine	Ropivacaine
Onset	10–15 min	10–15 min	5–10 min	5–10 min	10–15 min
Max dose (without adrenaline)	2.5 mg/kg	2.5 mg/kg	3 mg/kg	6 mg/kg	2 mg/kg
Max. dose (with adrenaline)	2.5 mg/kg	2.5 mg/kg	7 mg/kg	8 mg/kg	2 mg/kg
Duration (without adrenaline)	3–12 h	3–12 h	1–2 h	1–2 h	3–12 h
Duration (with adrenaline)	4–12 h	4–12 h	2–4 h	2–4 h	4–12 h

Local anaesthetic toxicity

Systemic toxicity may occur either when a normal dose of LA has been inadvertently injected intravascularly or when a toxic dose of LA has been infiltrated leading to toxic serum levels. The risk can be reduced by always aspirating before and during LA injections and always calculating the maximum LA dose for the weight of the patient. LA toxicity may be fatal if not promptly recognized and treated. It is more difficult to treat and more severe when due to bupivacaine rather than lidocaine.

Clinical features

Central nervous system

- At low plasma levels of LA, initially excitatory symptoms, e.g. metallic taste, tingling around the mouth, tinnitus, agitation.
- These early signs and symptoms are not always apparent, and may be missed in the anxious or sedated patient.
- At higher plasma levels, seizures may be seen, and at very high levels massive cerebral depression occurs, leading to ventilatory compromise and coma.

Cardiovascular

- Depressed cardiac conduction manifests as cardiac dysrhythmias, including tachy/bradycardia or atrioventricular block.
- Hypotension.
- Cardiac arrest.

Management

- Is largely supportive and may have to be continued for a prolonged period of time.
- Stop LA injection.
- ABCDE approach to management and resuscitation.
- If available, administer IV lipid emulsion therapy (e.g. Intralipid).
  - Initial IV bolus of 20% Intralipid®: 1.5 ml/kg over 1 min.
  - Start IV infusion of 20% lipid emulsion at 15 ml/kg/h.
  - After 5 min give two further bolus doses if cardiovascular stability is not restored.
  - Double the infusion rate to 30 ml/kg/h if the patient is still unstable after 5 min. Continue infusion until the patient is cardiovascularly stable.
  - Do not exceed a maximum cumulative dose of 12 ml/kg.
- Intubate and ventilate if required—hypoxia and hypercarbia will exacerbate toxicity.
- Treat tachy- and bradyarrhythmias according to resuscitation guidelines (avoid lidocaine, calcium channel antagonists, and beta-blockers).
- If in cardiac arrest: start cardiopulmonary resuscitation and give adrenaline if required (lower doses may be appropriate).
- Control seizures with benzodiazipines, thiopental, or propofol.

Upper limb blocks

The motor and sensory innervation of the whole upper extremity is supplied by the brachial plexus with the exception of part of the shoulder (innervated by the cervical plexus); and the sensory innervation to the medial aspect of the upper arm (supplied by the intercostobrachial nerve, a branch of the second intercostal nerve).

The infraclavicular and the axillary approaches to the brachial plexus are considered the safest and easiest. Interscalene approach should be avoided in young children due to increased risk of intravascular injection, intrathecal injection, or temporary phrenic nerve palsy.

Axillary block

Indications

- Analgesia or surgical anaesthesia for elbow, forearm, and hand.
- The lateral aspect of forearm may require separate musculocutaneous nerve block as it lies outside the sheath at the level of the axilla.

Patient position

- Supine, head turned away from the side being blocked.
- Elbow flexed at 90°and arm abducted.

Suggested local anaesthetic volume and dose

- bupivacaine 0.25%, 0.2–0.3 ml/kg.

Ultrasound technique

- Place ultrasound probe transversely, where the pectoralis major insertion falls (see Figure 11.1).
- Identify the axillary artery.
- The nerves surround the axillary artery at the following clock face positions (Figure 11.2):
  - radial nerve (RN) 5–7 o'clock position
  - median nerve (MN) 9-12 o'clock position
  - ulnar nerve (UN) 12-3 o'clock position
- Deposit a quarter of the LA dose around each nerve (Figure 11.3).
- Use the remaining quarter dose for the musculocutaneous nerve, which should also be blocked at this time.

Nerve stimulator technique

- Palpate the axillary artery as high as possible in the axilla.
- Introduce an insulated needle:
  - immediately superior to the axillary arterial pulsation
  - at a 45–60° angle to the skin
  - directed parallel to the artery or towards the clavicle midpoint with the nerve stimulator set at 1–2 mA.
- On penetrating the sheath, distal muscle twitches are usually elicited in the median(finger flexion) or radial (wrist/finger extension) nerve distribution (rarely ulnar).
- Reduce the output of the nerve stimulator gradually to approximately 0.3–0.4 mA while the muscle twitch is maintained adjusting the position of the needle as needed.
- Inject LA.

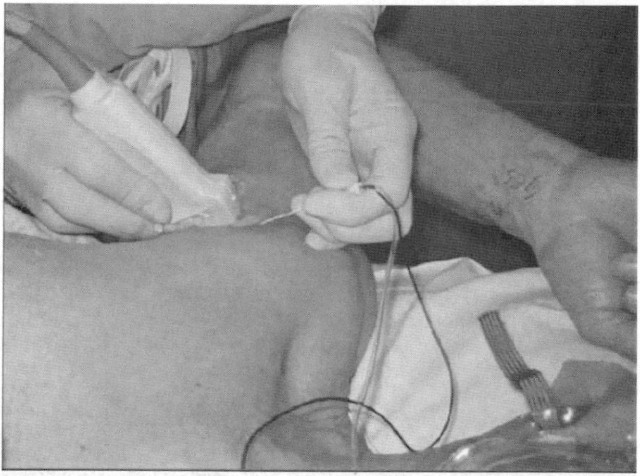

Figure 11.1 Position of patient and US probe for axillary block with the needle being placed for an in-plane view and technique.

With kind compliments from FUJIFILM SonoSite, Inc.

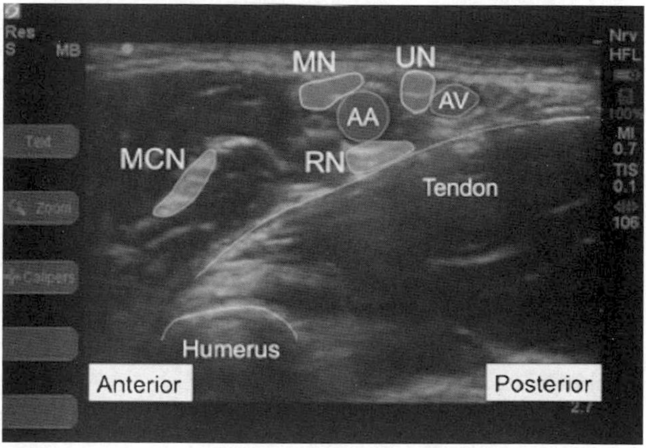

Figure 11.2 Ultrasound image with structures labelled including the axillary artery, axillary vein, musculocutaneous, radial, median, and ulnar nerves.

With kind compliments from FUJIFILM SonoSite, Inc.

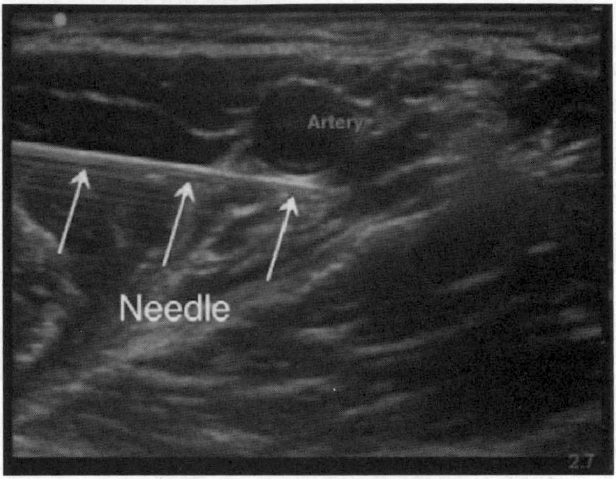

Figure 11.3 The axillary artery is demonstrated with the shaft of the echogenic needle seen slipping under the artery targeting the radial nerve.

With kind compliments from FUJIFILM SonoSite, Inc.

Note

- Multiple injection techniques have been described in both adults and children: there is little advantage in children because loose fascial attachments allow the even spread of a single injection to block the whole brachial plexus.
- Distal pressure may be applied during and immediately following injection while the arm is adducted: this decompresses the head of the humerus in its fossa, facilitating proximal spread of the solution and blockade of the musculocutaneous nerve.
- To block the musculocutaneous nerve separately (for procedures that involve the lateral forearm), advance a needle introduced perpendicular to the skin, just above the axillary pulsation, into the coracobrachialis muscle until forearm flexion is elicited using a nerve stimulator. Inject 0.5–1 ml LA just deep to the fascia.

Landmark technique

- Using either a nerve block needle or a well-blunted 22G hypodermic needle, introduce the needle as for the nerve stimulator technique.
- Feel for a definite pop as the sheath is entered. If using a hypodermic needle it should, if correctly positioned, be firmly gripped by the sheath when you let go of it and the hub should pulse strongly.
- Aspirate and then inject LA, which, if in sheath, should not cause the skin to bulge.
- It is not necessary to elicit paraesthesia.

- As above, distal pressure may encourage proximal spread.
- You are more likely to be successful with a larger volume of LA, e.g. 40 ml.
- If an artery is accidentally punctured, either remove the needle, press to stop bleeding, and start again, or advance through the artery until back bleeding stops. Aspirate very carefully and deposit LA deep to the artery.
- Note it is not uncommon to miss the musculocutaneous nerve with this technique.

Infraclavicular block

Indications

- Analgesia or surgical anaesthesia for elbow, forearm, and hand.
- Useful in those patients who find it too painful to move their arm for an axillary block.
- Most reliably performed using an ultrasound rather than nerve stimulator technique.

Patient position

- Supine, head turned away from the side being blocked.
- Arm by their side, forearm across the abdomen.

Suggested local anaesthetic volume and dose

- bupivacaine 0.25%, 0.2–0.3ml/kg.

Ultrasound technique

- Stand at the head of the patient, probe below the acromioclavicular joint (Figure 11.4)—at this point you are lateral to the apex of the lung so pneumothorax is unlikely.

Identify the subclavian artery (SA) and subclavian vein (SV) (Figure 11.5).

The brachial plexus at this level is divided into the lateral, medial, and posterior cords, surrounding the artery as hypoechoic (black) structures (Figure 11.6).

- Use an in-plane needle technique.
- Keeping the SA in clear view, direct the needle aiming to end with the needle tip at the 6 o'clock position just below the SA (Figure 11.6).
- Place sufficient LA to circumferentially surround the SA thus bathing the three cords of the plexus.

Nerve stimulator technique

- Insert the needle at the midpoint of the lower border of the clavicle at a 45–60° angle to the skin and directed towards the axilla.
- Aim to elicit pronation or flexion at the elbow.
- Once the nerve is located, reduce the voltage on the nerve stimulator to 0.2–0.3 mA.

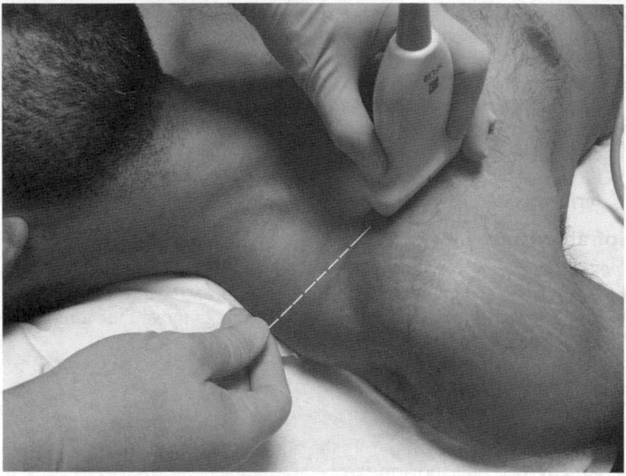

Figure 11.4 The US probe placement below the acromioclavicular joint, below the clavicle, with an in-plane needle approach.

With kind compliments from FUJIFILM SonoSite, Inc.

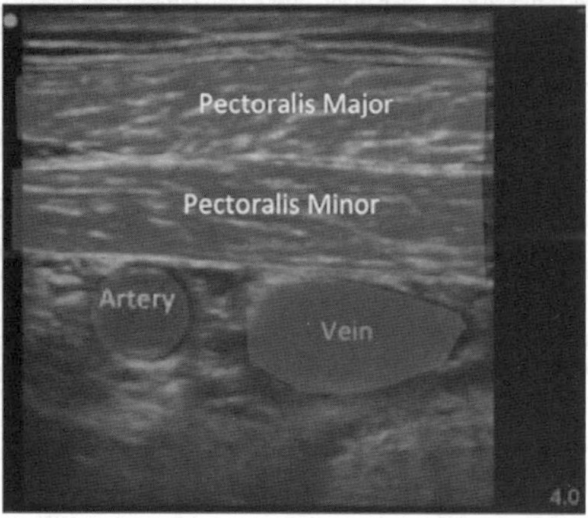

Figure 11.5 Ultrasound image with the pectoralis major and minor, alongside the cords surrounding the subclavian artery.

With kind compliments from FUJIFILM SonoSite, Inc.

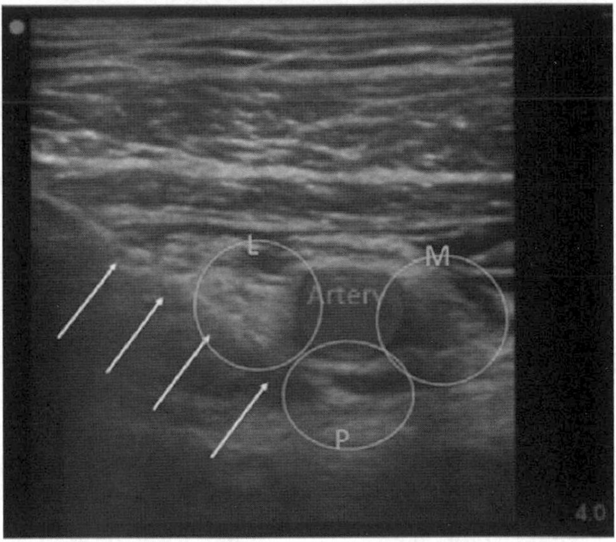

Figure 11.6 The subclavian artery surrounded by the lateral (L), posterior (P), and medial (M) cords, with the shaft of the needle seen approaching the desired 6 o'clock position.

With kind compliments from FUJIFILM SonoSite, Inc.

Interscalene block

Exercise caution in those with breathing difficulties as the phrenic nerve may become anaesthetized with subsequent compromised respiratory function.

Indications

- Analgesia or surgical anaesthesia for shoulder, clavicle, or upper arm.

Patient position

- Supine, head turned away from the side being blocked.

Suggested local anaesthetic volume and dose

- bupivacaine 0.25–0.5%, 0.2–0.3 ml/kg.

Ultrasound technique

- Place the probe over the neck in the oblique plane at the level of C6 (Figure 11.7).

The brachial plexus will be in a transverse view, with the plexus appearing as hypoechoic circles, in a 'traffic light' configuration. The plexus sits between the anterior scalene muscle (ASM) and the middle scalene muscle (MSM) (Figure 11.8).

The plexus is approached in or out of plane. For the in-plane approach, the needle enters from the lateral aspect of the probe traversing the MSM, before popping into the plexus sheath (Figure 11.9).

Careful hydrodissection observing for LA spread in around the brachial plexus will ensure the LA is deposited in the correct tissue plane. Dynamic scanning up and down the neck will demonstrate the spread of the LA.

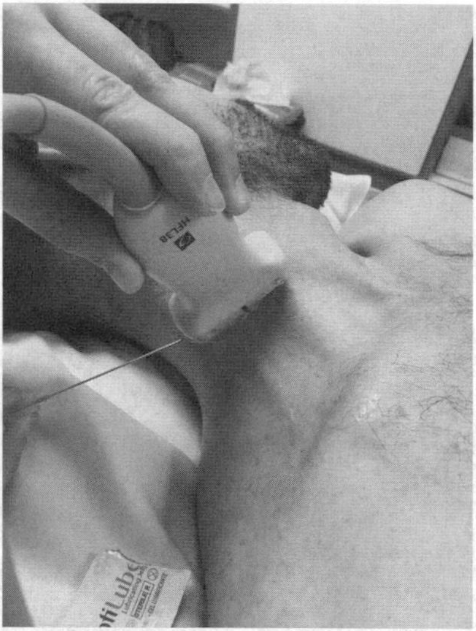

Figure 11.7 Ultrasound probe positioned in the oblique plane at the level of C6 for interscalene block.

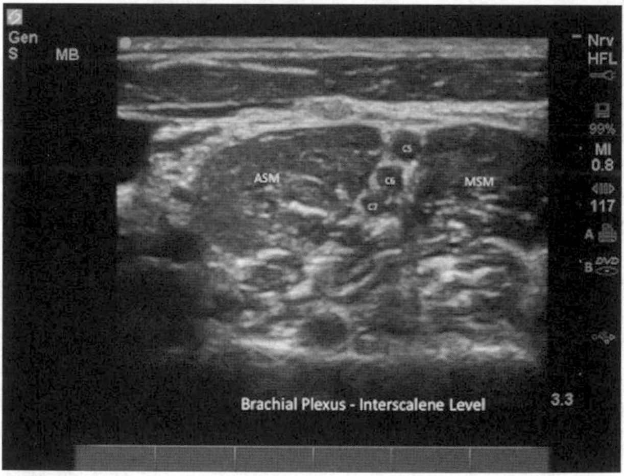

Figure 11.8 The brachial plexus at the level of C6, seen as hypoechoic circles in a 'traffic light' configuration, found between the anterior scalene muscle (ASM) and the middle scalene muscle (MSM), hence interscalene level.

With kind compliments from FUJIFILM SonoSite, Inc.

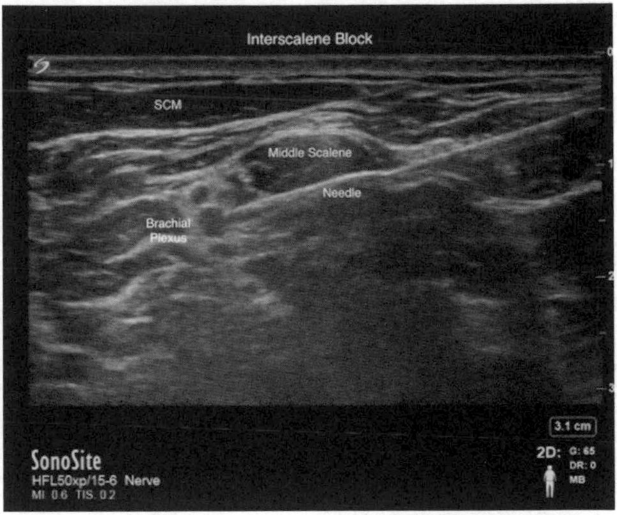

Figure 11.9 The interscalene brachial plexus, between the anterior scalene muscle (ASM) and the middle scalene muscle (MSM) with the needle at the plexus site.

With kind compliments from FUJIFILM SonoSite, Inc.

Lower limb blocks

Lower limb surgery is often most easily performed under spinal anaesthesia. Lower limb blocks can be used as sole anaesthesia but are also extremely useful in conjunction with either general or neuraxial anaesthesia for postoperative analgesia.

Femoral nerve block

Indications

- Analgesia or surgical anaesthesia for anterior thigh, shaft of femur, hip, or medial knee.
- Painless patient transfer, radiographic examination, and application of splints for femoral fracture.
- In combination with sciatic nerve for surgery on the knee and below.

Positioning

- Supine, with leg in the neutral position.

Suggested local anaesthetic volume and dose

- bupivacaine 0.25%, 0.2–0.3 ml/kg.

Ultrasound technique

- Place the ultrasound probe transversely, below the inguinal crease.
- Identify the femoral artery (FA) and the femoral vein (FV).
- The femoral nerve (FN) is deep to the fascia iliacus and above the iliacus muscle, and lies lateral to the FA (Figure 11.10).

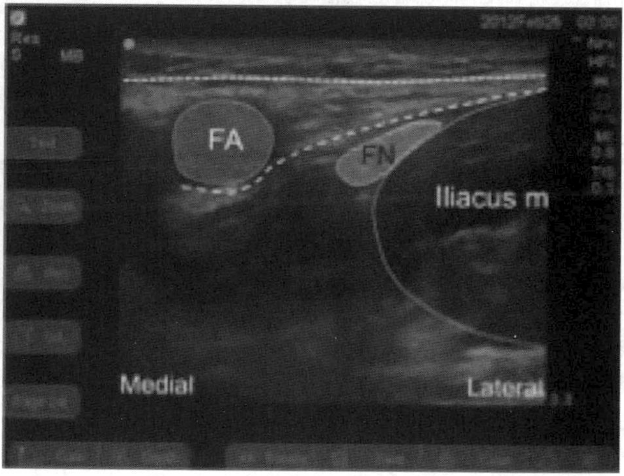

Figure 11.10 Ultrasound image with the femoral nerve and femoral artery.
With kind compliments from FUJIFILM SonoSite, Inc.

- Keeping the FA in clear sight, pass the needle lateral to medial, in-plane, aiming to place the needle tip under the fascial plane, where the FN sits.
- Place sufficient LA to surround the FN.

Nerve stimulator technique and landmark technique

- In children, the distance between the FA, inguinal ligament, and FN will vary according to the size of the child.
- Insert a short bevel insulated needle approximately 1 cm lateral to the femoral pulsation and 1 cm below the inguinal ligament (in adults).
- The nerve lies beneath the fascia lata and fascia iliaca and often two distinct 'pops' are felt as the needle traverses these layers.
- Seek contraction of the medial quadriceps. A 'patellar kick' confirms FN stimulation and should not be confused with direct stimulation of the sartorius muscle, which does not.
- Because of the close proximity of femoral vessels, intermittent aspiration for blood is obligatory prior to and during injection. Injection should feel easy.
- In the event of a femoral arterial puncture, apply pressure for at least 5 min to prevent haematoma formation.

Fascia iliaca block

Indications

- Any surgery above the knee.
- Particularly useful for the hip joint as more reliably blocks the lateral cutaneous nerve of thigh, femoral, and obturator nerves.
- Nerve stimulator cannot be used as there is no motor nerve in this area.

Position

- Supine, thigh slightly abducted and externally rotated.

Suggested local anaesthetic volume and dose

- bupivacaine 0.1–0.25%, up to 1 ml/kg (lower percentages produce less motor block)
- this block is most successful if a high volume is used.

Landmark technique

- Aim to deliver LA deep to the fascia iliaca and superficial to the iliacus muscle, where the three nerves of the lumbar plexus emerge from the psoas muscle.
- Draw/visualize a line from the pubic tubercle to the anterior superior iliac spine along the inguinal ligament.
- Insert a short bevelled needle perpendicular to the skin, 0.5–1 cm below the junction of the lateral and middle thirds of this line.
- Two 'pops' are felt as the needle pierces the fascia lata and then the fascia iliaca. A slight loss of resistance may be detected if light pressure is held upon the plunger of the syringe.
- After negative aspiration, inject LA.

Ultrasound technique

- As for femoral block but above inguinal ligament and more lateral. Identify both fascial planes and deposit LA under the fascia iliaca.

Sciatic nerve block

- Provides anaesthesia of the posterior aspect of the thigh and leg below the knee.
- Excludes the medial aspect of the lower half of the leg, the medial malleolus, and the medial aspect of the foot.
- Exact distribution depends on the level of block.

Indications

- Analgesia or surgical anaesthesia for ankle and foot.
- Combine with femoral block for total anaesthesia below knee.

Suggested local anaesthetic volume and dose

- bupivacaine 0.25%, 0.5ml/kg.

Ultrasound technique

- Position lateral with leg being blocked uppermost.
- Place ultrasound probe transversely, proximal to the popliteal fossa in between the hamstring muscle tendons (Figure 11.11).
- Identify the popliteal artery (PA). The compressible structure lying next to or beneath the artery is the popliteal vein (PV).
- Dynamic scanning from the popliteal fossa cranially, will show the sciatic nerve (SN) as one structure, which then divides into the common peroneal nerve and tibial nerve more distally.
- Identify the point where the SN begins to divide, giving the appearance of a dumbbell. This is an excellent point to block the nerves. This is often 2–5 cm above the popliteal fossa (Figure 11.12).

Using an in-plane technique, target the SN, with 1–2 ml hydrodissection to differentiate the tissue planes.

Inject LA to surround the nerve.

Nerve stimulator technique

- Position supine, hip and knee flexed to 90° (easier in children!).
- With exaggerated hip flexion, the glutei may be flattened and the SN becomes relatively superficial even in obese patients.
- Surface landmarks are the gluteal crease and the lateral border of the biceps femoris muscle.
- Insert an insulated needle at an angle of 70–80°, 1 cm distal to the gluteal crease along the lateral border of the biceps femoris muscle.
- Direct the needle cephalad.
- Confirm SN stimulation: plantar flexion, inversion, or dorsi-flexion at 0.3–0.4 mA.
- If bone contact is made before a motor response is elicited, withdraw and redirect the needle.
- The posterior cutaneous nerve of the thigh may be missed as it tends to separate more proximally in the thigh.

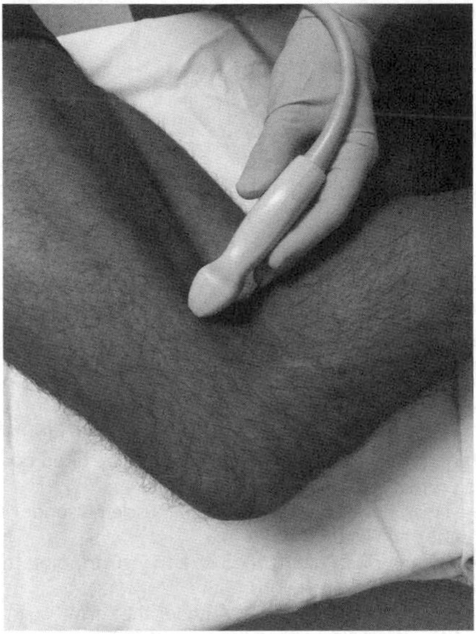

Figure 11.11 Patient positioned in the lateral position.
With kind compliments from FUJIFILM SonoSite, Inc.

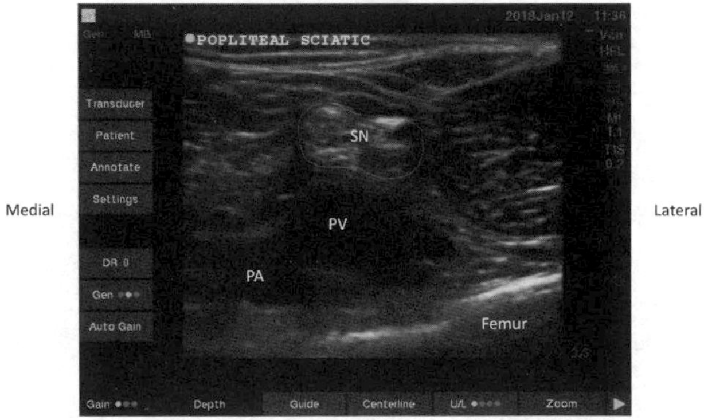

Figure 11.12 Ultrasound image demonstrating the sciatic nerve bifurcation into the common peroneal and tibial nerves.

Trunk blocks

Serratus anterior plane block

Indications

- Analgesia for multiple rib fractures.
- Analgesia for thoracic procedures.
- Analgesia for breast surgery (may need combination with pectoralis block).

Position

- Lateral with affected side up. Or
- Supine/sitting with arm raised to allow access to axilla.

Suggested local anaesthetic volume and dose

- bupivacaine 0.25%, 0.4 ml/kg.

Ultrasound technique

- Place the transducer coronally on the mid axillary line, at the level of the fourth rib or higher: the probe may need to be tilted posteriorly to obtain the correct view (Figure 11.13).
- Identify the latissimus dorsi (LD)—a thick muscle just under the skin.
- Identify the ribs and pleura.
- Follow the LD anteriorly until it reaches a triangular point; the serratus anterior will be lying over the ribs.
- Using an in-plane technique, place LA under the serratus anterior (Figure 11.14).

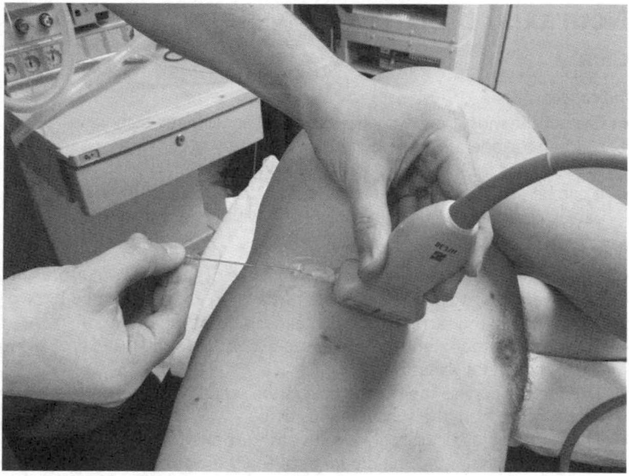

Figure 11.13 Coronal ultrasound probe position in the mid axillary line for serratus anterior plane block.

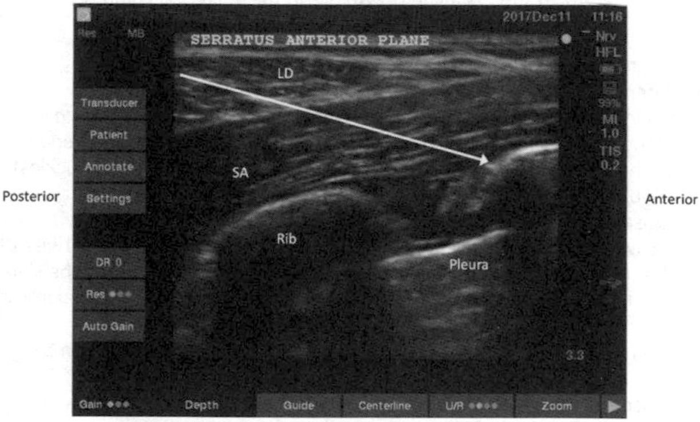

Figure 11.14 Ultrasound anatomy for the serratus anterior plane block. LD, latissimus dorsi; SA, serratus anterior, arrow, needle direction and placement for posterior approach.

Neuraxial Blocks

Caudal

Indications

- One of the most frequently used regional anaesthetic techniques in children for operations below the umbilicus.
- Widely used for initial postoperative pain relief.
- It can be used as the sole anaesthetic, particularly in ex-premature babies, but is usually used in conjunction with general anaesthesia.

Anatomy

- The sacral hiatus is formed as a consequence of failed fusion of the fifth sacral vertebral arch. The remnants of the arch are represented by two prominences, the sacral cornua, on either side of the hiatus.
- The sacral hiatus extends from the sacral cornua to the fused arch of the fourth sacral vertebra.
- The sacrococcygeal membrane covers the sacral hiatus separating the caudal space from the subcutaneous tissue.
- The sacral hiatus virtually always lies at the apex of an equilateral triangle, which has the line drawn between the posterior superior iliac spines as its base.
- A useful landmark for the sacral hiatus in chubby infants is where a line drawn from the patella through the greater trochanter with the hips flexed at 90° transects a line drawn down the vertebral column.

Technique

- Position: lateral decubitus, with both knees drawn up.
- Alternatively the prone knee–chest position may be useful when performing a caudal on the awake high-risk ex-premature neonate.
- Identify the sacral hiatus and cornua by palpation: they can be likened to the interspace between two metacarpal-phalangeal joints (knuckles) (Figure 11.15).
- Observe full asepsis.
- Introduce a short bevelled needle or 22G cannula held gently between the thumb and index finger, the needle at approximately 45° to the skin (i.e. the *bevel* parallel to the skin) at the sacral hiatus and advance until it pierces the sacrococcygeal ligament.
- A 'give' is felt as the needle tip enters the caudal space, which can be confirmed by loss of resistance.
- Once the needle position is confirmed and aspiration for blood and cerebrospinal fluid (CSF) is negative, inject the appropriate volume of LA. Note that aspiration should be gentle since strong negative pressure may cause the low-pressure epidural vessels to collapse before a positive aspiration test can be elicited.

Note

- Further needle advancement after entering the caudal space, as is described in adults, is unnecessary and increases the risk of dural puncture or bloody tap.

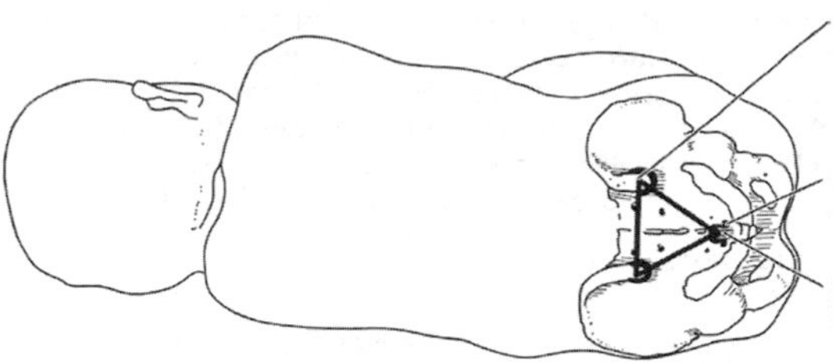

Figure 11.15 Anatomy for caudal puncture.

Reproduced from S. Berg and S. Campbell. Paediatric and Neonatal Anaesthesia. In: *Oxford Handbook of Anaesthesia*. K. Allman, et al. (Eds.). Oxford, UK: Oxford University Press. Copyright © 2015, OUP. Reproduced with permission of the Licensor through PLSclear. DOI: 10.1093/med/9780198719410.001.0001.

- Penetration of the sacrococcygeal membrane just above the sacral cornua carries a lower incidence of bloody tap.
- Failure to obtain loss of resistance after the sacrococcygeal ligament has been penetrated may indicate that the bevel is lying against the anterior wall of the caudal space. This can be overcome by simply rotating the needle through 180°.
- In the event of a 'bloody tap' the needle should be redirected or removed and carefully reinserted more cephalad. Injection of LA in these circumstances should proceed with caution in view of the greater risk of toxicity.

Dosage

- The most commonly used drugs for caudal block are bupivacaine and ropivacaine 0.25% or lidocaine 1%.
  - for sacro-lumbar dermatomes, 0.5 ml/kg
  - for lumbar thoracic dermatomes (subumbilical), 1.0 ml/kg
  - for mid-thoracic dermatomes (upper abdominal), 1.25 ml/kg.

At higher volumes use a lower concentration to stay below the toxic dose.

- Adding caudal clonidine 0.1–1 μg/kg improves the quality of block without increasing sedation and gives analgesia for up to 12 h.

Side effects and complications

- Failure.
- Apnoea in small neonates.
- Dural puncture and subsequent injection of LA may lead to a total spinal associated with cardiovascular collapse or respiratory arrest.
- Systemic toxicity may manifest as arrhythmia, cardiovascular collapse, or convulsions following accidental intravascular or sacral interosseous injections. The incidence of bloody tap varies with experience, the age of the patient, and the equipment used.

- Urinary retention and delayed micturition are related not only to the duration of preoperative starvation but also to the concentration of LA solution. The incidence is negligible when 0.25% bupivacaine is used.
- Motor blockade and inability to walk is also concentration dependent.
- Nerve injury and neurological defect have been reported but are extremely uncommon following caudal blockade and usually transient.

Spinal anaesthesia

Indications

- Suitable for surgery below the umbilicus, including lower limb surgery, lower segment Caesarean section (CS), gynaecological, and urological operations.
- May be used for upper abdominal surgery by extending the block with a slight head-down position. Small doses of IV ketamine, opiates, or benzodiazepines may be used to supplement.

Anatomy

- The spinal cord ends at L1 in adults and L1–L2 in children.
- To guide which interspace is being identified, a line joining the top of the iliac crests is at L3–L4.

Side effects and complications

- Hypotension: there must always be IV access with fluids attached and some means of supporting blood pressure, e.g. ephedrine, metaraminol, phenylephrine, or adrenaline.
- Failure or a patchy block may be treated with IV ketamine supplementation (titrate to effect, doses as low as 5 mg are often effective).
- A 'high' or total spinal leading to cardiovascular, respiratory, and neurological collapse.
- Post-dural puncture headache.

Technique

- Full aseptic technique.
- Infiltrate LA to the skin at the level of L3–L4 or L4–L5.
- Ideally use a pencil-point spinal needle (25–29G) with introducer.
- As the different tissue planes are passed the final give or pop felt will indicate breach of the dural plane.
- Remove the stylet: there should be free flow of clear CSF.

The patient should not feel or complain of sustained pain or discomfort, nor should there be free blood flowing. If either is encountered, stop the procedure and withdraw the spinal needle, before allowing to settle and then recommence.

For LA agents and adult doses see Table 8.4, p. 170.

Spinal drugs

- Bupivacaine—hyperbaric or 'heavy' 0.5% is often used, with a duration of 2 h. Isobaric or 'plain' 0.5% can also be used but can be associated with an unpredictable rise in the level of block.
- Spinal fentanyl 0.2 μg/kg can be used with caution where adequate postoperative monitoring is available. Take care that only preservative

free formulations are used. Spinal morphine is probably best avoided due to the risk of late respiratory depression.
- Spinal ketamine should not be used as the preparation contains a preservative that is neurotoxic.

Spinal anaesthesia in children

- See Table 11.2 for dosages.
- Usually performed under a small amount of sedation but in older children and infants the procedure is well tolerated.
- Useful technique in ex-premature infants and neonates at risk of apnoeas.
- Post-spinal cardiovascular instability is less common in infants and young children.
- Does not last as long as in adults, 1 h maximum in infants.
- Remember the spinal cord may terminate lower at L2 in children under 1 year.
- Approximate distance to the subarachnoid space:

$$\text{Distance skin to subarachnoid space (cm)} = 0.03 \times \text{height (cm)}$$

- In awake neonates and infants take care if positioning in the lateral position for spinal puncture that you do not inadvertently cause airway obstruction by flexing the neck.

Table 11.2 Spinal dosages in infants and children.

Weight	<5 kg	5-15 kg	>15 kg
Isobaric or heavy bupivacaine 0.5%	1 mg/kg (0.2 ml/kg)	0.4 mg/kg (0.08 ml/kg)	0.3 mg/kg (0.06 ml/kg)

Further reading

Warman P, Conn D, Nicholls B, Wilkinson D. (eds) (2014) *Oxford Specialist Handbook of Regional Anaesthesia, Stimulation and Ultrasound Techniques*. Oxford: Oxford University Press.
NYSORA.com, New York Society of Regional Anaesthesia.

Chapter 12

Critical Care

Polly Marshall-Brown, Francesca Mazzola, Bruce McCormick, and Kate Stephens[1]

(For:
Head injuries
Burns
Thoracic trauma
Spinal injury
Tetanus
see Chapter 9, p. 197)

1 Dr Bruce McCormick and Dr Kate Stephens are the chapter leads.

Limits and challenges

Effective critical care is achieved by simple interventions such as:

- a high ratio of nurses to patients
- good basic nursing care
- regular frequent monitoring of the patient
- regular frequent medical review.

Critical care units in low- and middle-income countries (LMICs) may range from high-dependency units (HDUs) (single organ support) to, more rarely, a full intensive care unit (ICU) (ventilation and/or multi-organ support). When working in critical care in a low-resource setting, consider the following when making patient care decisions:

Human resources and equipment

- See also: 'Critical Care' in Chapter 2, pp. 32–4.
- Nursing staff may have had no specific critical care training.
- There may be no resident medical staff.
- You may be the only critical care trained doctor.
- Equipment such as ventilators and pumps if available may:
  - have had no servicing
  - not be fully functional
  - not have working alarms
  - not have any staff trained to use them.
- Oxygen and electricity supplies may be erratic.

Admission criteria

Capacity is always limited. A critical care facility should have local admission and discharge criteria, appropriate for the context and regularly reviewed by audit of admissions and outcomes. Of note:

- In some contexts even the requirement for intravenous (IV) or intramuscular (IM) opiates, or oxygen therapy, may be enough to warrant admission.
- Training for ward staff in the identification and prompt management of the sick and deteriorating patient should be provided.
- Patients admitted to critical care should have a reversible pathology and sufficient physiological reserve to allow a reasonable chance of good recovery.
- Thought should be given to local customs and policy regarding withdrawal of active treatment. Prolonged, futile treatment may bankrupt the family.

Disease profile

- Patients often present late and so can be profoundly ill.
- General health may be compromised by poor living conditions, poor nutrition, and infectious diseases such as HIV and TB.
- Surgical emergencies, obstetric complications, and trauma are all common. Tropical illnesses, such as tetanus, malaria, typhoid, etc. may be present (see Chapter 13, p. 293).

General care

The combination of good nursing care, regular observations, and timely treatment can result in excellent outcomes.

Nursing care

- A nurse or attendant should be present at the bedside at all times; patients with organ failure may die quickly if organ support is interrupted, e.g. blocked/displaced endotracheal tube, failure of oxygen supply.
- Observations should be recorded at least every 1 or 2 h.
- Give medications as prescribed.
- The patient should be turned every 4 h and padding should be used to prevent pressure sores.
- Mouth and eye care are important.
- Regular suctioning of secretions/aspiration of nasogastric (NG) tubes should be carried out if required.
- A physiotherapist should assess the patients daily.

Medical care

- Initial management of a critically ill patient is with an 'ABCDE' approach and any urgent interventions should be performed immediately and the response assessed. Then a thorough system-based approach can be continued.
- Patients should be reviewed twice daily with:
  - a head to toe physical examination
  - a review of observations, fluid balance, medication chart, and lab results
  - documentation of findings and treatment plan.
- The FASTHUG mnemonic is useful for remembering important daily considerations (Box 12.1).

Box 12.1 FASTHUG mnemonic.

F **Feeding.** Ensure that the patient is taking an adequate oral diet. If not consider starting nasogastric (NG) feeds.

A **Analgesia.** Adequate analgesia should be given to all patients. Use pain scoring.

S **Sedation.** Avoid over- or under-sedation of patients. Perform a daily sedation hold.

T **Thromboprophylaxis** (pharmacological and mechanical) should be given as all critical care patients are at increased risk of deep vein thrombosis.

H **Head up.** Patients should be nursed at 30° head up as this helps to prevent ventilator-associated pneumonia.

U **Ulcer prophylaxis** should be prescribed when patients are ventilated or not on established enteral feeds.

G **Glucose control.** Regular blood sugar measurements should be taken and you should aim for levels between 6 and 10 mmol/l.

Reproduced with permission from Vincent JL. Give your patient a fast hug (at least) once a day. *Crit Care Med.*, 33(6):1225–1229. Copyright © 2005 by the Society of Critical Care Medicine and Lippincott Williams. doi: 10.1097/01.CCM.0000165962.16682.46.

Nutrition

Patients should receive oral nutrition as soon as they are able to eat. Early enteral feeding reduces stress ulceration, preserves gut integrity, and reduces ileus. If they are unable to tolerate oral intake within 24–48 h, start feeding via an NG or nasojejunal feeding tube.

- Insert the NG tube and confirm position (chest X-ray or pH paper (pH ≤5.5)).
- Aspirate every 4 h (accept gastric aspirates of <250 ml).
- Gastric stasis is common—promotility agents such as metoclopramide 10 mg IV every 8 h may help.
- Nurse head up 30°.
- Continuous feeding is preferable to bolus feeds, however either is far better than none at all.

Feeds and feeding regimens

Specially designed enteral feeds may not be available. Alternatives include:

- Therapeutic milks, feeds, or dietary supplements.
- Liquidized meals, soup.
- Milk and eggs.
- Oral rehydration solution can be a useful source of electrolytes.
- An enteral feed can be made by mixing local food stuffs according to the quantities in Table 12.1, with boiled water to a volume of 1,000 ml. Each 100 ml of feed provides 129 kcal and 4 g protein.

Normal adult daily requirements are:

- Calories 25–35 kcal/kg/day.
- Protein 0.8–1.5 g protein /kg/day.
- Fluid 30–35 ml/kg/day plus replacement of losses.

Calorie requirements may be increased by 50% in critical illness—a catabolic state—and in burns patients even higher, with protein requirements reaching 2 g/kg/day (see 'Burns' in Chapter 9, p. 223).

Initiate feeds at 10–20 ml/h increasing to the target rate over 6–8 h. NG tube position should be confirmed prior to each bolus feed by aspiration and ideally pH testing.

Table 12.1 Quantities and nutritional values for locally sourced enteral feed components, to be made up to 1,000 ml of feed with boiled water.

	Energy (kcal)	Protein (g)	Carbohydrate (g)	Fat (g)
150 g whole milk powder	726	39	56	42
30 g sunflower oil	270	-	-	30
75 g sugar	295	-	79	-
Total	1,291	39	135	72
% Energy Contribution		12%	37%	50%

Refeeding syndrome

This is metabolic derangement seen after feeding severely malnourished patients, consisting of:

- Hypoglyacemia.
- Low phosphate, potassium, and magnesium leading to arrhythmias, heart failure, seizures, and coma.

Risk factors

- One of the following:
  - Body mass index (BMI) <16.
  - Unintentional weight loss of >15% in the past 3–6 months.
  - Little/no oral intake for >10 days.
  - Already low plasma levels of potassium, magnesium, or phosphate.
- Or two or more of the following:
  - BMI <18.5.
  - Unintentional weight loss of >10% in the past 3–6 months.
  - Little or no intake for >5 days.
  - History of alcohol abuse, or drug use including insulin, chemotherapy, or diuretics.

Prevention

- High-risk patients: feed with 10 kcal/kg/day and then gradually increase to full calorific intake over 4–7 days.
- In extreme cases (BMI <14 or no oral intake for >15 days) restrict the initial intake to 5 kcal/kg/day and increase gradually.
- Continuous cardiac monitoring is advised if possible.

Additional considerations

- Give thiamine 200–300 mg, Vitamin B compound one or two tablets three times a day (t.d.s.) and multivitamins for 10 days.
- Likely daily needs of electrolytes are potassium 2–4 mmol/kg/day, phosphate 0.3–0.6 mmol/kg/day, and magnesium 0.2 mmol/kg/day IV or 0.4 mmol/kg/day orally.
- Ideally daily bloods for phosphate, potassium, calcium, and magnesium should be taken and corrected as necessary.
- Fluid balance needs to be carefully managed to prevent fluid overload, oedema, and heart failure.
- Use an input/output chart and perform regular clinical assessment.

Respiratory support

Options for respiratory support may be limited and come with increased risks. Prevent respiratory complications in postoperative patients by:

- Using lung protective ventilation during surgery.
- Good analgesia.
- Chest physiotherapy.
- Early mobilization.

Options for respiratory support include the following.

Physiotherapy techniques

- Oro-nasal suctioning.
- Deep breathing exercises.
- Saline nebulizers.
- Mobilization.
- Incentive spirometry—inflating gloves/balloons.

Oxygen therapy

- Supplied by oxygen cylinder or oxygen concentrator (if possible ensure cylinder back-up for power failure).
- Aim for oxygen saturation (SpO_2) of 92–95% (or lower in chronic type 2 respiratory failure).
- Humidify if possible or use intermittent nebulized saline.

Mask continuous positive airway pressure (CPAP)

- Improves oxygenation but will not improve CO_2 clearance.
- Effective in cardiac failure, pulmonary contusion, and atelectasis post abdominal surgery. May help in acute respiratory distress syndrome (ARDS).
- CPAP circuits can be improvised using a Klausen harness and facemask attached to a Waters type circuit with an adjustable pressure limiting (APL) valve (Figure 12.1). Ideally the APL valve is left open with a positive end expiratory pressure (PEEP) valve attached to its expiratory port. Improvised circuits need high-flow oxygen (10–15 l/min minimum), which can be provided using two oxygen concentrators with their oxygen tubing joined by a Y-connector. They have several downsides:
  - Exact oxygen concentration cannot be controlled and some concentrators can only deliver 95% oxygen.
  - At lower flow rates CO_2 may be rebreathed.
  - If used just with the APL valve the amount of CPAP is uncertain.
- CPAP machines for use in LMICs that can run off room air with supplemental oxygen from a concentrator exist and may be available.
- Potential problems/contraindications include:
  - Lack of patient cooperation.
  - Pressure injury from mask.
  - Retained secretions due to dry gases (use a heat moisture exchanger (HME) filter).

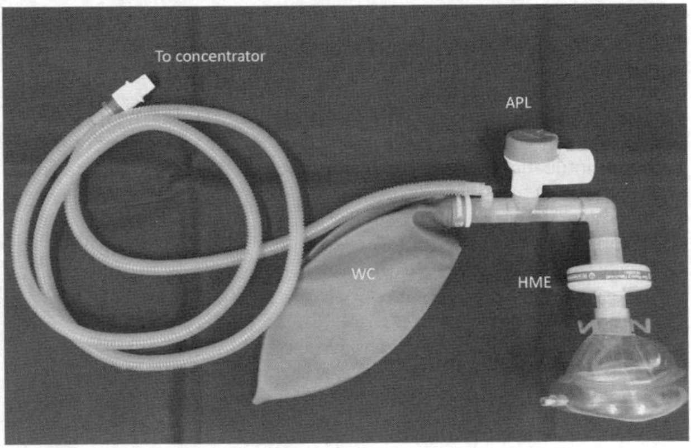

Figure 12.1 Improvised facemask continuous positive airway pressure circuit. WC, waters circuit; APL, adjustable pressure limiting valve; HME, heat and moisture exchange filter.

- Gastric distension requiring NG tube; avoid after gastric and oesophageal surgery.
- Use only with caution in patients at risk of pneumothorax who do not have functioning chest drains.

Non-invasive ventilation (NIV)

- Improves oxygenation and CO_2 clearance.
- Effective for conditions that benefit from CPAP and also in hypoxia with raised CO_2.
- Can be delivered either by an ICU ventilator in NIV mode (requires pressurized oxygen) or by commercially available home bilevel positive airway pressure (BiPAP) machines, which will run using an oxygen concentrator.
- Provides most of the benefits of invasive ventilation but no airway protection. Depending on the context it may still be a safer option than intubation in patients with a reduced conscious level.
- Problems and contraindications: as for CPAP.

Tracheal intubation and ventilation

Mechanical ventilators may not be available but, if they are, the potential risks and benefits must be considered:

- Poorly maintained and functioning equipment.
- Lack of trained staff to recognize and manage blocked or displaced tracheal tubes.
- Inadequate access to sedation to facilitate ventilation.
- Intermittent electricity.

- Unreliable oxygen supplies.
- Once patients are intubated and ventilated it may be culturally unacceptable to withdraw treatment. There should be agreed indications for intubation.
- Patients with a reduced conscious level may be safer nursed on their side, with an NG tube to reduce aspiration risk, than exposed to the risks of intubation, ventilation, and sedation without adequate staffing or monitoring.
- Dependent on the context, consider invasive ventilation for:
  - apnoea
  - respiratory failure
  - Glasgow coma score (GCS) <9: airway protection and neuroprotection
  - upper airway obstruction (consider early tracheostomy)
  - inability to clear secretions
  - need for sedation, e.g. tetanus or head injury management.

Lung protective ventilation

- Tidal volumes of 6 ml/kg ideal body weight.
- Plateau pressures <30 mmHg
- You may need to tolerate a higher CO_2 to achieve this (if no raised intracranial pressure); exercise caution if using halothane.
- Apply appropriate PEEP to improve oxygenation (raise PEEP if the fractional inspired oxygen concentration (FiO_2) is high.
- Titrate FiO_2 to achieve SpO_2 92–95%.

Weaning ventilation

- If possible use a ventilation mode synchronized to respiratory effort.
- Pressure support and PEEP is better tolerated on minimal sedation.
- Trial spontaneous breathing with a T-piece.
- For some patients requiring longer-term ventilation a tracheostomy may help ventilatory weaning and clearing of secretions, see "Tracheostomy Care" in Chapter 6, pp. 101–3.

Physiotherapy in ventilated patients

- Manual and ventilator hyperinflation (delivery of larger tidal volume breaths to a peak pressure of 40 cm H_2O).
- Percussions and vibrations.
- Variable positioning: 30° head up and alternating sides.
- Suctioning.
- Saline nebulizers or instillation.
- Mobilization.

Cardiovascular support

Important questions that need to be considered before commencing inotropes include:

- What would the local staff usually do in this situation?
- What level of observation and care will the patient receive when you are no longer at the bedside?
- How are we to establish safe and secure intravenous access?
- Do we have enough medication supply to last?
- How likely is it that there could be drug calculation errors?
- How are we to safely control the infusion rate?
- How will we monitor blood pressure regularly?
- Would the team be able to recognize and deal with the common and rare complications associated with the use of these agents with their extremely narrow therapeutic window?

Venous access

Central venous access may not be possible and peripheral administration may need to be considered. Regarding peripheral administration of vasopressors and inotropes:

- Vasoactive drugs can cause severe tissue necrosis if they extravasate.
- Be aware that phentolamine and other dilators may not be available to reduce the sequelae of extravasation.
- Plastic surgery reconstruction may be unavailable.

If peripheral administration of these agents is considered appropriate:

- A dedicated cannula should be used.
- Use dilute solutions as described below.
- The line should have no injection ports.
- The cannula site should not be obscured by excessive bandaging.
- The cannula site should avoid the hand, wrist, cubital fossa, and dominant arm if possible. The forearm is best.
- Close supervision of the cannula site for signs of extravasation is mandatory.

Infusions

A syringe driver or IV fluid pump is ideal. If unavailable then consider using a drip set, but this needs **constant supervision**. Small changes in the drip rate could be fatal. If you decide that you must run vasoactive medication (or other infusion) using an intravenous drip set, below is an example of an adrenaline infusion set up based on Médecins Sans Frontières (MSF) clinical guidelines. See also Table 12.2.

Adrenaline/epinephrine

- Adults
  - Dilute 10 ampoules of 1 mg in 1 ml (1:1,000) adrenaline in 1 l of 5% glucose or 0.9% sodium chloride to obtain a solution containing 10 μg/ml.
  - Check on your infusion set packaging that 1 ml = 20 drops.
  - Infusion rate should be between 0.05 and 0.5 μg/kg/min. For example, for a 50 kg adult, the drip rate will be between 5 and 50 drops/min (15–150 ml/h).

    - For lower infusion rates and greater safety, a paediatric burette (1 ml = 60 drops) may be filled with only 1 h's worth of infusion.
- Children
    - Dilute 1 ampoule of 1 mg in 1 ml (1:1,000) adrenaline in 100 ml of 5% glucose or 0.9% sodium chloride to obtain a solution containing 10 μg/ml.
    - Check your infusion set is **paediatric**; that 1 ml = 60 drops.
    - Infusion rate should be between 0.05 μg/kg/min and 0.5 μg/kg/min. For example, for a 10 kg child, the drip rate will be between 3 and 30 drops/min (3–30 ml/h).

Table 12.2 Drug infusions.

Drug	Preparation	Infusion (50 kg adult), adult set, 20 drops/ml
Noradrenaline	8 mg in 1,000 ml of 5% glucose = 8 μg/ml	0.05–0.5 μg/kg/min = 6–60 drops/min
Dopamine	200 mg in 500 ml 5% glucose = 400 μg/ml	Low dose: <10 μg/kg/min High dose: >10 μg/kg/min 10 μg/kg/min = 25 drops/min
Isoprenaline	5 mg in 1,000 ml 5% glucose = 5 μg/ml	0.02–0.2 μg/kg/min = 4–40 drops/min

Vasopressors

- Phenylephrine and metaraminol are safe to give through a peripheral cannula.
- A phenylephrine infusion can be made up containing 100mcg/ml.
- Infusion rate should be between 0.5 and 5 mcg/kg/min. For example for a 50kg adult the drip rate will be between 5 and 50 drops/min (15–150ml/h).

Management of extravasation

- Stop infusion.
- If the patient is inotrope-dependent move infusion to another limb.
- Do not flush the cannula.
- Do not remove the cannula initially.
- Attempt to aspirate the cannula.
- Consider injecting phentolamine 5–10 mg (adult dose) through the cannula if available.
- Aspirate as you remove the cannula.
- Measure and mark the extravasated area.
- Assess distal circulation.
- Immobilize and elevate the limb.
- Obtain early plastic surgery input if available.
- Local necrosis may heal with conservative management.
- Surgical debridement and reconstruction may be necessary for full thickness skin necrosis.

Acute kidney injury (AKI)

AKI is a reduction in kidney function within 48 h. This can be defined as:

- Absolute increase in serum creatinine of >0.3 mg/dl (>26.5 μmol/l) from baseline.
- Increase in serum creatinine to 1.5× baseline.
- Reduction in urine output (<0.5 ml/kg/h for >6 h).

Rapid corrective action is required; progression to renal failure is often a death sentence due to lack of renal replacement options.

Initial management of acute kidney injury

1. Identify and treat the underlying cause.
   - Pre-renal: reduced renal blood flow due to shock from any cause and some drugs, e.g. non-steroidal anti-inflammatory drugs (NSAIDs).
   - Renal: acute tubular necrosis (ATN) due to shock (especially shock caused by sepsis); acute interstitial nephritis (AIN) due to drugs especially penicillins; myoglobinuric renal failure.
   - Post-renal: kidney damage due to urinary obstruction.
2. Stop nephrotoxic drugs.
3. Ensure the patient is euvolaemic.
   - Carry out clinical evaluation for signs of dehydration.
   - Administer a fluid bolus of 10–20 ml/kg crystalloid or colloid over 30 min (caution in malnourished or septic children (see 'Resuscitation of the Sick Child' in Chapter 7, pp. 152–3)).
   - If there are symptoms or signs of fluid overload give furosemide; high doses may be required.
   - Low-dose dopamine does not improve outcomes.
4. Maintain adequate mean arterial pressure (MAP).
5. Manage hyperkalaemia:
   - Start continuous electrocardiogram (ECG) monitoring if possible.
   - ECG signs suggesting potassium (K^+) >6.5 mEq/l include peaked T waves, loss of P waves, widening of QRS complexes, PR prolongation, asystole.
   - Provide membrane stabilization urgently:

- Calcium gluconate 10%, 10 ml IV. May be repeated three times; effect lasts for approx. 30 min (or calcium chloride 10%, 10 ml IV, more slowly, once only).
   - Drive K^+ into cells:
- Ten units of fast-acting insulin in 250 ml 10% glucose over 1 h (or 10 units in 50 ml 50% glucose over 30 min if available) should reduce K^+ by 1 mEq/l.
- Give salbutamol 10 mg by nebulizer.
- If acidotic, sodium bicarbonate may be helpful.
   - Reduce total body potassium:
- Loop diuretic, e.g. furosemide 20 mg IV initially.
- Calcium polystyrene sulfonate 15 g per os (PO) t.d.s.

Renal replacement therapy (RRT)

RRT in LMICs is not widely available, even for short-term replacement. Prevention of AKI is vital and there should be a high index of suspicion for conditions that may cause AKI, e.g. crush syndrome, reperfusion injuries. Establish on arrival at your hospital what possibilities, if any, there are for referral for RRT.

Indications for RRT

AKI with:

- Fluid overload (unresponsive to diuretics).
- Hyperkalaemia (K^+ >6.5).
- Severe metabolic acidosis (pH <7.1).
- Rapidly climbing urea/creatinine (or urea >30 mmol/l).
- Symptomatic uraemia: encephalopathy, pericarditis, bleeding, nausea, pruritis.
- Oliguria/anuria.

Types of RRT

- Peritoneal dialysis.
- Intermittent haemodialysis.
- Continuous renal replacement therapies (CRRT).
    - This can be haemodialysis, haemofiltration, or haemodiafiltration.

Postoperative patients

Avoidable postoperative mortality is often high and tends to occur during the first 24 h post-surgery. Postoperative care may be suboptimal because of shortages of staff, oxygen, and monitoring, leading to undetected hypoxia, hypotension, or haemorrhage. High-risk patients should preferably be admitted to a ward with the best possibilities for regular observations. In some contexts this may include anyone requiring IV or IM opiates or oxygen therapy. Attention to detail and basic interventions in this period can have a huge impact.

Airway and respiratory management

- If a patient is hypothermic, and cardiovascularly unstable, extubation may be delayed if there are critical care facilities.
- Encourage basic chest physio, early sitting out, and mobilization.
- Oxygen if required—should be humidified if possible.

Cardiovascular management

- Monitor closely for signs of any ongoing bleeding—observations, drains, and dressings.
- Check haemoglobin (Hb).
  - If further bleeding is expected or if the patient is critically ill transfuse if Hb <7 g/dl ('Blood Transfusion', Chapter 4, pp. 68–72).
  - In healthy patients with chronic anaemia use a threshold of 5 g/dl.
- Aim for MAP of >60 mmHg for a fit patient; higher in hypertensive patients or patients with abdominal compartment syndrome.
- Consider thromboprophylaxis.

Fluid management

- In patients with hypotension, low urine output, or cold peripheries, give a fluid bolus (preferably Ringer's lactate or equivalent) of 250–500 ml then reassess—repeat the bolus if the patient improves.
- Maintenance fluids: 25–30 ml/kg/day of balanced salt solution and 50–100 g/day glucose.
- Replace drain/NG outputs with 0.9% NaCl or balanced salt solutions.
- Aim for a urine output of 0.5 ml/kg/h (chart hourly input/output).
- Monitor electrolytes if possible and replace as needed.
- Encourage oral fluids and stop IV fluids when no longer needed. NG fluids or enteral feed is preferable to IV fluids. Oral rehydration solution is a useful source of electrolytes.
- Oral intake or enteral feed can be commenced in the absence of bowel sounds. After elective laparotomy this can be started the day of surgery.
- Monitor blood glucose, aiming for 6–10 mmol/l.

Pain management

- Use local and regional anaesthesia where possible.
- Low-dose ketamine may be a useful adjunct especially if no opiates are available.
- See 'Pain Management' in Chapter 5, pp. 68–72.

Sepsis

Sepsis has a high mortality rate. Whilst many of the pathogens are familiar, other causes of sepsis may not be. Consider: malaria, TB, HIV, tetanus, measles, seasonal viral (e.g. Dengue, Zika), and epidemic viral (e.g. Ebola) diseases (see Chapter 13, p. 293).

Definitions

Sepsis

A life-threatening organ dysfunction caused by a dysregulated host response to infection: diagnosed by two or more of:

- Hypotension: systolic blood pressure (BP) ≤100 mmHg.
- Altered mental status (GCS <15) including anxiety and agitation.
- Tachypnoea: RR ≥22.

Septic shock

A subset of sepsis with profound circulatory, cellular, and metabolic abnormalities, this is associated with a higher mortality and characterized by:

- Hypotension requiring use of vasopressors to maintain MAP ≥65 mmHg (i.e. not responding to fluids). **And**
- Arterial lactate >2 mmol/l persisting despite adequate fluid resuscitation.

Awareness, early detection, and treatment of sepsis are vital. Any patient with suspected infection who is causing concern should be managed as below—do not wait until definitions are met.

Clinical assessment

- History, focusing on risk factors and likely source of infection.
- Examination to identify source.
- Regular repeated vital signs including RR.

Investigations

Often very limited availability, but if possible:

- Blood tests—full blood count (FBC) (white cell count (WCC), haemoglobin (Hb), platelets, haematocrit), urea and electrolytes (U&E), liver function tests (LFTs), clotting, glucose, lactate.
- Urine dip.
- Imaging.
- Cultures as appropriate—blood, urine, sputum, pus, wounds, catheters, cerebrospinal fluid (CSF).

Treatment

Prompt recognition, resuscitation, and treatment is vital. If the patient is not responding to initial treatment and has sepsis/septic shock, then consider critical care admission.

Airway and breathing

- Give oxygen to maintain SpO_2 >92%.
- NIV or intubation may be required if appropriate in the context.
- If the decision is made for intubation, be prepared for rapid desaturation and hypotension on induction; use lung protective

ventilation strategies (see 'Respiratory Support' in this chapter, p. 268–70).

Circulation

- Large-bore IV or intraosseous access, take blood for investigations.
- Fluid resuscitation for hypotension up to 30 ml/kg in first hour.
- Exercise caution in children and the malnourished as rapid fluid resuscitation may lead to pulmonary oedema.
- Aim for MAP >65 mmHg.
- Further fluid may be given if the patient is responsive.
- If the patient is not responsive to fluid, consider vasopressors but be aware of potential pitfalls (see 'Cardiovascular Support', in this chapter, pp. 271–2).
- If there are signs of reduced oxygen delivery despite fluid resuscitation and adequate BP (e.g. rising lactate, reduced GCS), consider blood transfusion to Hb 7–9 g/dl (to increase O_2 carrying capacity).

Other priorities

- Antibiotics, antimalarials, and surgical source control:
  - Antibiotics should be given within the first hour (Table 12.3).
  - Removal of source of infection, i.e. laparotomy, debridement.
- Glycaemic control and FASTHUG (see 'General Care', p. 265).

Table 12.3 Possible first-line antibiotic choices (consult local guidelines).

Origin	Antibiotic	Alternative
Cutaneous: *Staphylococcus* or *Streptococcus*	Cloxacillin + gentamicin	
Pulmonary: *Pneumococci, Haemophilus influenzae*	Ampicillin or ceftriaxone +/− gentamicin; clarithromycin for atypical cover	Co-amoxiclav or ceftriaxone + ciprofloxacin
Intestinal or biliary: enterobacteria, anaerobes, enterococci	Co-amoxiclav + gentamicin	Ceftriaxone + gentamicin + metronidazole
Gynaecological: *Streptococcus*, gonococci, anaerobes, *Escherichia coli*	Co-amoxiclav + gentamicin	Ceftriaxone + gentamicin + metronidazole
Urinary: enterobacteria, enterococci	Ampicillin + gentamicin	Ceftriaxone + ciprofloxacin
Other or undetermined	Ampicillin + gentamicin	Ceftriaxone + ciprofloxacin
Critical care acquired: Gram negative aerobic bacilli; *Staphylococcus*; *Candida*	Meropenem or piperacillin/tazobactam; vancomycin; fluconazole	

Arrhythmias

Tachyarrhythmia

Causes

Ischaemia, sepsis, hypoxia, hypovolaemia, pain, anaemia, thyrotoxicosis, electrolyte abnormalities, and halothane.

Assessment

- Assess patient's airway, breathing, and circulation.
- Administer oxygen.
- Attach to monitoring, including 12-lead ECG.
- Obtain IV access and check Hb and electrolytes.
- Seek and treat reversible cause/s.

Adverse signs present—unstable patients

- Shock: systolic BP <90 mmHg, pallor, sweating, cold, impaired conscious level.
- Syncope.
- Myocardial ischaemia: chest pain, ECG changes.
- Heart failure: pulmonary oedema.

Treatment for unstable patients

- Synchronized direct current (DC) cardioversion—up to three attempts.
  - Sedation will be required for cardioversion in conscious patients, e.g. ketamine 0.25–0.5 mg/kg IV.
  - Broad complex and atrial fibrillation (AF): 120–150 J in increasing increments.
  - Regular narrow complex: 70–120 J in increasing increments.
- If synchronized cardioversion fails, or is not available or safe:
  - Amiodarone 300 mg IV over 15 min followed by 900 mg IV over 24 h.
  - Administer centrally or through a large and well-flushed peripheral vein.

Cardioversion for AF may not be successful whilst the underlying cause is still present, e.g. sepsis. Risk/benefit analysis may favour trying amiodarone/digoxin as a first-line treatment even if adverse features are present.

Treatment for stable patients

Narrow complex tachycardia (QRS <0.12 s or three small squares)

- Regular rhythm:
  - Vagal manoeuvres.
  - Adenosine 6 mg by rapid IV injection, followed by a further two 12 mg boluses if no effect.
  - Verapamil 2.5–5 mg IV over 2 min can be used if adenosine is not available; do not give with beta-blockers.
  - If sinus rhythm is restored, then diagnosis is likely to be paroxysmal supraventricular tachycardia (SVT).
  - If sinus rhythm is not restored, atrial flutter may be the diagnosis: consider rate control with beta-blocker, e.g. propranolol 10–30 mg PO every 4 or 6 h, or 1 mg by slow IV injection, repeated up to 5 mg.

- Irregular rhythm:
  - Likely to be AF.
  - First choice = beta-blocker.
  - Amiodarone or digoxin may also be used.
  - Digoxin regime: loading dose 8–12 μg/kg IV or 10–15 μg/kg PO. Give half of the loading dose initially, then quarter every 8 h for two further doses. Maintenance = 3 μg/kg IV or 4–5 μg/kg PO once a day.

Broad complex tachycardia (>0.12 s or three small squares)

- Regular rhythm:
  - If VT (or uncertain): amiodarone 300 mg IV over 15 min followed by 900 mg IV over 24 h.
  - If known SVT with bundle branch block (BBB) treat as for regular narrow complex tachycardia.
- Irregular rhythm:
  - If possibly AF with BBB: treat as narrow complex tachycardia.
  - If pre-excited AF: treat with amiodarone.

Bradyarrhythmia

Causes

- Physiological: sleep, athlete.
- Cardiac: atrioventricular (AV) node block.
- Non-cardiac: increased vagal stimulation, hypothermia, hypothyroid, raised intracranial pressure (ICP), hyperkalaemia, typhoid fever.
- Drug-related: beta-blockers, digoxin, organophosphates.

Assessment

- As for tachyarrhythmia.

Adverse signs present (as for tachyarrhythmia)

Treatment:

- Atropine IV, 500 μg. Assess response. Can be repeated up to 3 mg.
- Adrenaline, 2–10 μg bolus IV.
- Transcutaneous pacing.
- Low-dose adrenaline or isoprenaline infusions can be considered (see Table 12.2, 'Cardiovascular Support', p. 277).

No adverse features

- If there is a risk of asystole (recent asystole/Mobitz II AV block/complete heart block/ventricular pause >3 s): treat as per adverse features. The patient may require transvenous pacing if it is available.
- Otherwise observe.

Myocardial ischaemia

Pathophysiology

Myocardial ischaemia or acute coronary syndrome (ACS) can be split into unstable angina (UA), non-ST elevation myocardial infarction (NSTEMI), and ST elevation myocardial infarction (STEMI).

Signs and symptoms

- Chest pain—typically tight, heavy, pressure feeling in the chest that may radiate up into the neck or down the arm.
- Palpitations.
- Breathlessness.
- Nausea/vomiting.
- Hyper/hypotension.
- Cardiovascular collapse.

Diagnosis

- Twelve-lead ECG is the most important diagnostic test. STEMI will have ST-segment elevation on the ECG. NSTEMI and UA may show permanent or transient ST changes on ECG, e.g. ST depression.
- Blood tests for cardiac enzymes (troponin/creatine kinase).
- Chest X-ray—cardiomegaly, pulmonary oedema.
- Echocardiogram.

Treatment

- Assess ABC.
- Administer oxygen.
- Establish IV access and take bloods (FBC, electrolytes, glucose, cardiac enzymes).
- Analgesia: morphine (2–10 mg IV).
- Coronary artery dilation: nitrates, glyceryl trinitrate (GTN) (two puffs unless hypotensive).
- Antiplatelet therapy: aspirin 300 mg and clopidogrel 300 mg.
- Beta-blocker if no contraindication, e.g. metoprolol 2.5 mg every 5 min up to 15 mg.
- NSTEMI or UA: anticoagulant therapy—enoxaparin 1 mg/kg subcutaneous (SC) every 12 h, continued for 1 week or until stabilized. Unfractionated heparin may be used but monitoring of activated partial thromboplastin time (APTT) is rarely available.
- STEMI: thrombolytic therapy or percutaneous coronary intervention (PCI) or, if neither available, enoxaparin 30 mg IV + 1 mg/kg SC followed by 1 mg/kg SC every 12 h continued for 2 weeks.

If all the above drugs are not available even giving just aspirin, analgesia, and a beta-blocker will significantly reduce mortality.

Complications

- Ventricular fibrillation /pulseless ventricular tachycardia—requires prompt cardiopulmonary resuscitation (CPR) and cardioversion.
- Arrhythmias (see 'Arrhythmias', pp. 278–9).
- Pericarditis—management of pain.
- Heart failure (see 'Heart Failure', p. 281).
- Pericardial tamponade.

Heart failure

Common causes

- Myocardial infarction/ischaemia.
- Atherosclerosis.
- Hypertension.
- Infection (rheumatic heart disease/Chagas/HIV cardiomyopathy).
- Valvular disease.
- Peripartum cardiomyopathy.
- Thiamine deficiency.
- Anaemia.
- Alcoholic cardiomyopathy.

Clinical features

- Pulmonary oedema with acute breathlessness and pink, frothy sputum.
- Increasing dyspnoea and peripheral oedema.
- Chest pain/palpitations.
- Cardiogenic shock: hypotension and poor peripheral perfusion.

Investigations

- ECG—looking for signs of ischaemia.
- Chest X-ray—pulmonary oedema, cardiomegaly.
- Echocardiogram—assess contractility of the heart and valve competence.

Treatment

Acute heart failure

- Assess ABC, give high-flow oxygen and obtain IV access.
- Sit patient upright.
- Give morphine (2–5 mg IV or 5–10 mg SC) and furosemide (40–80 mg IV).
- Give GTN spray or sublingual tablet if not hypotensive.
- The patient may benefit from CPAP or NIV.
- Cardiogenic shock may require inotropic support—consider whether the pathology is reversible and whether aggressive treatment is appropriate in the context.
- Selected patients with hypotension due to isolated right heart failure may benefit from a fluid bolus (e.g. right ventricular infarction).
- Treat the specific cause, e.g. acute rheumatic fever, thiamine deficiency, anaemia.
- Longer-term treatment includes diuretics, angiotensin-converting enzyme (ACE) inhibitors, and bisoprolol introduced gradually.

Diabetes

Management of hyperglycaemic emergencies is extremely difficult in the absence of electrolyte monitoring.

Check whether your glucometer/sticks measure in mmol/l or mg/dl (to convert mg/dl to mmol/l, divide by 18).

Hyperglycaemia

Hyperglycaemia in hospitalized patients is associated with adverse outcomes. However, in low-resource settings with limited glucose monitoring, hypoglycaemia poses the greater risk and moderate hyperglycaemia may be tolerated.

Causes

- Stress response to illness—commonly seen on HDU.
- Poor compliance with medication/inadequate medication.

Features

- May be symptomless and found on glucose testing.
- Polyuria, polydipsia.

Management

- Target blood glucose is 6–10 mmol/l: accept levels of 4–12 mmol/l.
- Follow the flow diagram in Figure 12.2.

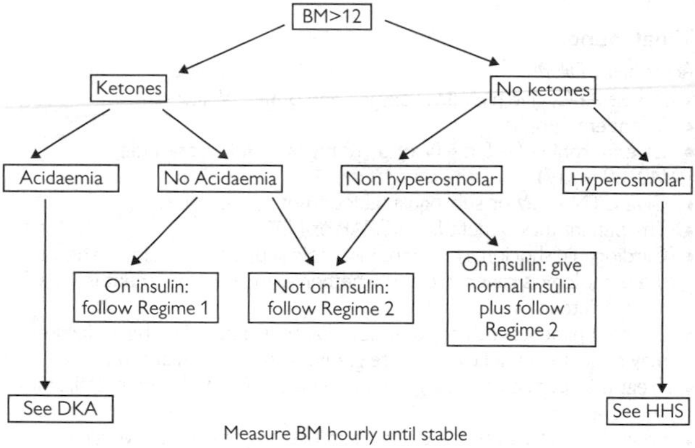

Figure 12.2 Management of hyperglycaemia. Regime 1: Calculate total daily dose of insulin. Give 20% extra as fast-acting subcutaneous insulin in three divided doses. Regime 2: Assume 1 unit of fast-acting insulin lowers the blood sugar by 3 mmol/l and give an appropriate single subcutaneous dose.

Data from *British National Formulary*

Variable rate insulin infusions (VRIIs)

If control is not gained using regime 1 or 2 above then a VRII may be indicated (see Table 12.4).

- Continue long-acting insulin (stop fast-acting doses).

Table 12.4 Variable rate intravenous insulin sliding scale (can also be given as subcutaneous bolus).

Blood glucose		Insulin rates (ml/h) (units/h)		
mmol/l	mg/dl	Insulin sensitive (<24 units/day)	Standard rate	Insulin resistant (>100 units/day)
<4	<72	Treat for hypoglycaemia		
4.1–8	73–144	0.5	1	2
8.1–12	145–216	1	2	4
12.1–16	217–288	2	4	6
16.1–20	289–360	3	5	7
20.1–24	361–432	4	6	8
>24	>433	6	8	10

- Mix 50 units of fast-acting insulin with 49.5 ml 0.9% saline to make 50 ml (1 unit/ml)
- Must run with glucose substrate.
  - First choice = 0.45% NaCl + 5% glucose + 0.3% K^+ (40 mmol/l) at 125 ml/h.
  - You may also use 0.9% NaCl + 5% glucose, particularly if the patient is hyponatraemic.
  - Or 5% glucose + 0.3% K^+ (40 mmol/l) at 125 ml/h. (This may cause hyponatraemia. Ringer's lactate or 0.9% NaCl can be given in addition but beware of fluid overload).
  - If K^+ >5.5 mmol/l do not add K^+.
- Hourly blood glucose measurement aiming for 6–10 mmol/l.
- If blood glucose levels are persistently above 12 mmol/l and not falling, move up to the insulin-resistant rate.
- If blood glucose level <4 mmol/l stop the infusion and treat for hypoglycaemia.

Aim to convert back to their usual medications when the patient is improving and eating and drinking.

Diabetic ketoacidosis (DKA)

DKA is characterized by hyperglycaemia, acidosis, and ketonaemia.

Clinical features

- Hypovolaemia from osmotic diuresis causing polyuria.
- Nausea/vomiting.
- Abdominal pain.
- Hyperventilation/Kussmal breathing to compensate for metabolic acidosis.
- Ketotic breath.
- Reduced conscious level.

Investigations

- Blood glucose is usually very elevated.
- Urine analysis or blood test for ketones (capillary ketones >3 mmol/l or urinary ketones >2+).
- Bicarbonate <15 mmol/l and/or pH <7.3).
- Laboratory blood tests—FBC, electrolytes.
- ECG and ideally cardiac monitoring.
- Investigations for suspected source of infection (blood cultures, chest X-ray).

Management

Use an ABC approach.

Fluid resuscitation in adults

- Restore circulating volume. If systolic BP <90 mmHg give 500 ml 0.9% saline over 15 min. Recheck BP; if still low, repeat.
- When systolic BP is >90 mmHg give the doses in Table 12.5.
- Start 10% glucose IV when blood glucose <14 mmol/l and run at 125 ml/h alongside the 0.9% saline, until the patient is eating and drinking adequately.
- Exercise caution in elderly or pregnant patients and those with cardiac or renal failure.

Table 12.5 Adult fluid resuscitation in diabetic ketoacidosis.

Infusion fluid	Infusion duration
1,000 ml 0.9% saline	Over 1 h
1,000 ml 0.9% saline + KCl 40 mmol	Over 2 h
1,000 ml 0.9% saline + KCl 40 mmol	Over 2 h
1,000 ml 0.9% saline + KCl 40 mmol	Over 4 h
1,000 ml 0.9% saline + KCl 40 mmol	Over 4 h
1,000 ml 0.9% saline + KCl 40 mmol	Over 6 h

Fluid resuscitation in children and young people

The risk of cerebral oedema is greater in children and young adults. Use a slower rate of fluid replacement in people under 25 years and use the following guidelines:

- Children who are alert, not clinically dehydrated, and not vomiting usually tolerate oral rehydration and subcutaneous insulin.
- Give a fluid bolus only if shocked and start with 10 ml/kg.
- Assume a 5% fluid deficit in children with pH >7.1, and 10% if pH <7.1. Replace over 48 h.
- In addition, give a reduced volume of maintenance fluid:
  - Weight <10 kg give 2 ml/kg/h.
  - Weight 10–40 kg give 1 ml/kg/h.
  - Weight >40 kg fixed rate 40 ml/h.

- Use 0.9% saline with 40 mmol KCl/l. Once the blood glucose is <14 mmol/l, add glucose (0.9% NaCl with 5% glucose and KCl 40 mmol/l, which can be made by adding 50 ml 50% glucose to a 500 ml bag of NaCl with 40 mmol/l KCl).

Potassium replacement

Initially potassium is high but falls rapidly with treatment.

- K^+ >5.5 mmol/l requires no replacement.
- K^+ 3.5–5.5 mmol/l add 40 mmol K^+ per litre.
- K^+ <3.5 mmol/l will require higher concentrations of K^+.
- If K^+ cannot easily be measured, add 40 mmol K^+ to the second/third litre of 0.9% saline (adults), if the patient has adequate urine output.

Insulin therapy

Start a **fixed**-rate insulin infusion **after** fluid therapy has commenced.

- In a syringe driver mix 50 units of short-acting insulin with 49.5 ml 0.9% saline. Start a fixed-rate IV insulin infusion at 0.1 units/kg (e.g. for a 70 kg person start at 7 ml/h).
- Insulin may be infused in the same line as the IV fluid but a one-way valve **must** be used to prevent insulin collecting in the IV fluid tubing.
- A bolus dose of IM insulin 0.1 units/kg may be given if there will be a delay setting up an infusion.
- If no syringe driver is available, appropriately calculated amounts of insulin may have to be added to the IV fluid with very careful rate monitoring—use of a paediatric burette can be helpful.
- Long-acting insulin, if normally taken, should be given as usual.

Antibiotics

- Appropriate broad-spectrum antibiotics should be started if there is evidence of infection.

Targets

- A reduction in ketones by 0.5 mmol/l/h.
- A reduction in blood glucose by 3 mmol/l/h.
- An increase in bicarbonate by 3 mmol/l/h.
- If any of these three targets are not achieved, then increase the insulin infusion rate by 1 unit/h.
- Maintain K^+ between 4 and 5 mmol/l.
- Convert back to a subcutaneous regime when ketones <0.3 mmol/l, pH >7.3, and bicarbonate >18 mmol/l.

Complications

- Cerebral oedema:
  - A significant cause of mortality particularly in children and adolescents.
  - Initial signs are headache, irritability, and confusion leading to decreased conscious level and seizures.
  - Exclude hypoglycaemia.
  - Administer 5 ml/kg 20% mannitol.
  - Restrict fluids to two thirds of maintenance, replaced over 72 h.
  - Consider intubation and ventilation.
  - Computerized tomography (CT) scan if available.

- Aspiration pneumonia: insert an NG tube if the patient conscious level is reduced.
- Hypokalaemia.
- Pulmonary oedema:
  - Rarely seen in DKA.
  - Elderly patients and those with cardiac history are most at risk.
- Thrombosis—give thromboprophylaxis to prevent deep vein thrombosis (DVT).

Hyperosmolar diabetic emergencies (HHS)

More commonly seen than DKA in LMICs. It has a slower onset than DKA so dehydration and metabolic disturbances can be more severe. Mortality is higher than DKA and can be complicated by myocardial infarction (MI), stroke, and thrombosis.

Diagnosis

- Hypovolaemia.
- Hyperglycaemia (blood glucose >30 mmol/l) without significant ketones or acidaemia.
- Osmolality >320 mosmol/kg (2 × (Na + glucose + urea)).

Treatment

- Estimate the fluid deficit (usually in the range of 100–220 ml/kg).
- Calculate osmolality regularly to assess the response to treatment.
- Give 0.9% saline to correct dehydration. A fall in Na^+ should not exceed 10 mmol/l in 24 h.
- Aim to replace 50% of the calculated fluid loss in the first 12 h and the remaining replacement fluid over the next 12 h.
- A total of 40 mmol/l of K^+ should be added to each bag of fluid if the patient's K^+ is between 3.5 and 5.5 mmol/l.
- Regularly assess for signs of fluid overload.
- Any fall in blood glucose level should be no more than 5 mmol/l/h.
- Low-dose IV insulin (0.5 units/kg/h) should only be commenced if blood glucose level is not falling with fluid correction or if there are ketones present.

Thyroid emergencies

Thyroid crisis (thyroid storm)

Thyroid crisis is a life-threatening form of extreme thyrotoxicosis with a high mortality rate. It is most commonly associated with Graves' disease and can be seen during thyroidectomy in patients with inadequate antithyroid therapy. It usually has a precipitant such as infection, surgery, MI, pregnancy, or abrupt cessation of medication (e.g. carbimazole).

Clinical signs

- Pyrexia.
- Tachycardia.
- Agitation/confusion.
- Heart failure.

Management

- In a suspected thyroid storm initiate treatment before waiting for blood results.
- Actively cool the patient (tepid sponging/exposure/cool fluids). Antipyretics can be given but avoid salicylates (aspirin), which can displace thyroid hormone from thyroid-binding globulin.
- Tachyarrhythmias should be treated (see 'Arrhythmias', p. 278–9).
- Beta-blockers, propranolol (1-5 mg IV then 20-80mg PO every 6 hours) should be given to control the effects of catecholamines.
- Carbimazole (20–30 mg every 4–6 h) or propylthiouracil (loading dose 600 mg followed by 200 mg every 4–6 h) should be given to prevent further formation of thyroid hormone.
- One hour later give potassium iodide to block thyroxine synthesis, (400mg IV over 2hours then 2g/day PO).
- Dexamethasone 2 mg IV every 6 h helps to prevent T4 to T3 conversion.
- Requires careful management of fluids and electrolytes.
- Treat precipitating illness.

Myxoedema coma

Patients present with extreme features of hypothyroidism. Myxoedema often has a precipitant such as infection, hypothermia, or surgery.

Clinical signs

- Patients usually have classic signs of hypothyroidism (weight gain, lethargy, cold intolerance, constipation, eyelid oedema, ptosis, hair loss especially the outer third of the eyebrow, delayed deep tendon reflexes).
- Bradycardia.
- Hypotension.
- Hypothermia.
- Reduced conscious level.

Management

- Investigations include bloods (FBC, thyroid function test (TFT), electrolytes, blood glucose level, arterial blood gas (ABG)), ECG, chest X-ray, infection screen.
- Intubation and ventilation may be indicated if the patient has reduced conscious level or is hypoxic/hypercarbic.
- IV fluids for hypovolaemia and correction of electrolytes.
- Correct hypoglycaemia.
- Gradual rewarming.
- ECG monitoring. Treat arrhythmias.
- Levothyroxine 300 μg IV loading followed by 100 μg daily.
- NG thyroxine may be tried if an IV preparation is not available but absorption is likely to be very delayed.
- Hydrocortisone 100 mg every 6 h to treat adrenal insufficiency.

Organophosphate poisoning

Organophosphates are used as pesticides, nerve agents (chemical warfare), and as an antihelminth. Ingestion is sometimes intentional. In LMICs, predominately in rural areas, they cause a significant clinical burden, with an estimated 200,000 fatalities annually. They can be absorbed through the skin, inhaled, or ingested.

Clinical features

Organophosphates block acetylcholinesterase, therefore increasing the amount of acetylcholine at muscarinic and nicotinic receptors:

- **Central nervous system**—agitation, confusion, drowsiness, seizures, coma.
- **Neuromuscular junction**—muscle weakness, fasciculation.
- **Muscarinic (parasympathetic) stimulation**—miosis, bronchospasm/bronchorrhoea, salivation, lacrimation, bradycardia, vomiting, diarrhoea, urinary incontinence.

Treatment

- Avoid self-contamination, wear full personal protective equipment.
- Remove any clothing that may be contaminated and wash the patient with soap and water to prevent further absorption.
- Support the patient's airway and breathing if compromised. Intubation may be necessary. Note that suxamethonium is likely to have a prolonged effect due to inhibition of plasma cholinesterase.
- Give atropine for bradycardia (1–3 mg, 0.02 mg/kg in children) and monitor effect.
- If there is little effect after 5 min, be prepared to give further doses of atropine until you see an improvement in symptoms (heart rate >80 beats/min, systolic BP >80 mmHg, clear chest).
- When an improvement of symptoms is seen, an atropine infusion can be started at 0.02–0.8 mg/kg/h titrated to effect (too little and cholinergic symptoms will reappear, too much and the patient may become agitated, pyrexial, have absent bowel sounds, and develop urinary retention). Very large doses of atropine may be required.
- Pralidoxime reactivates phosphorylated anticholinesterase before it is deactivated and is used to reverse effects at the neuromuscular junctions at a dose of 30 mg/kg followed by an infusion of 8 mg/kg/h.
- Atropine requirement is maximal on day 1 and should be decreased over the next few days. Pralidoxime infusion can be stopped when atropine has not been needed for 12–24 h and the patient is extubated.
- Benzodiazepines should be given for agitation and seizures.
- Rebound toxicity can occur after days/weeks with some organophosphates as they are lipid soluble.

Other compounds

Organochlorines, e.g. endosulfan

- Antagonize gamma-aminobutyric acid (GABA) and glycine causing neuronal hyperexcitability and toxicity.
- High morbidity and mortality.
- Presents with prolonged treatment-resistant seizures.
- Other features include vomiting, paraesthesia, hypertonia, coma, respiratory failure, congestive cardiac failure, hyperpyrexia, metabolic acidosis, and renal failure.
- Management is supportive, with treatment of status epilepticus and arrhythmias.

Paraquat

- Buccal and oesophageal burns, renal and hepatic damage, pneumonitis, and pulmonary fibrosis, which may be exacerbated by oxygen and is usually fatal.
- Ingestion of more than 15 ml causes shock, pulmonary oedema, metabolic acidosis, arrhythmias, coma, convulsions, and death usually within 24–48 h.

Snake envenomation

Agricultural workers are at high risk of bites, with males bitten twice as often as females. Death has been attributed to:

- antivenom (inadequate dose or use of monospecific/inappropriate specificity preparation)
- delay in seeking hospital treatment
- inadequate artificial ventilation or failure to ventilate
- failure to treat hypovolaemia in shock
- airway obstruction
- complicating infections.

Clinical features

- Localized:
  - Fang marks, pain, bleeding, bruising, lymphangitis, blistering, necrosis.
- Systemic:
  - General: nausea, vomiting, weakness, abdominal pain, drowsiness.
  - Cardiovascular: dizziness, collapse, shock, hypotension, arrhythmias, pulmonary oedema.
- Cytotoxic:
  - Progressive pain and swelling.
- Neurotoxic:
  - Progressive weakness, paraesthesia, disturbance to taste/smell, ptosis, paralysis of facial muscles, difficulty swallowing secretions, respiratory depression.
- Haemotoxic:
  - Local bleeding, epistaxis, intracranial haemorrhage, haemoptysis, malaena, haematuria, disseminated intravascular coagulopathy.
- Skeletal muscle breakdown:
  - Pain, stiffness, myoglobinuria, hyperkalaemia, acute renal failure, oliguria/anuria, uraemia.

Examination

- For the features above. **And**
- Assess ABC, give oxygen and IV fluids.
- Monitoring including oxygen saturations and ECG.
- Monitor the circumference of the bitten extremity.
- Identification of the snake is useful but do not attempt to catch it!

Investigations

- If available send blood for tests: FBC, U&E, clotting, glucose, creatine kinase.
- These may show anaemia, leucocytosis, low platelet count, deranged clotting, AKI.
- An ABG may show hypoxaemia or hyperkalaemia with respiratory acidosis.
- Urine examination for haematuria, proteinuria, myoglobinuria, and haemoglobinuria.
- A 20-min whole-blood clotting test can be performed:
  - Put 2 ml of venous blood in a clean, dry glass vial.

- Leave for 20 min undisturbed.
- Tip the vessel: if it is liquid/unclotted this suggests coagulopathy.
- NB: this test has low sensitivity and should not delay antivenom administration.

Treatment

First aid/prehospital

- Give reassurance (death rate is <10% in untreated patients).
- Immobilize the limb and preferably the whole patient to delay spread.
- Transfer promptly to hospital.
- Tourniquets are not recommended but a pressure pad over the bite site is.
- Incision and suction is ineffective.

Antivenom

- May be monovalent (specific to one species) or polyvalent (active against several species).
- Used only for life- or limb-threatening bites (most can be managed without).
- Can cause anaphylaxis so have adrenaline ready.
- Repeat doses may be required.

Anticholinesterase drugs

- Bites with neurotoxic features caused by blockade of D-tubocurarine receptors have similar pathophysiology to myasthenia gravis.
- Neostigmine may be given 0.02 mg/kg in adults and 0.04 mg/kg in children IM.
- If improvement in neuromuscular transmission (loss of ptosis, increased peak flow) is seen over 30–60 min, then regular treatment should be initiated.
- Glycopyrronium/atropine may be required with the neostigmine.

Surgical treatment

- Compartment syndrome is uncommon but may require fasciotomy (relatively contraindicated in coagulopathy).
- Debridement may be needed for necrotic tissue (best left for 5–7 days so tissue is clearly demarcated).

Supportive measures

- HDU care will be required for severe envenomation.
- Ventilatory support may be needed.
- Treatment of hypotension and shock may require inotropes.
- Blood transfusion for haemolysis/bleeding.
- Correct coagulopathy with fresh frozen plasma and platelets if possible, tranexamic acid may be of benefit. **Fresh whole blood is ideal.**
- Some patients may require dialysis for renal complications.
- Analgesia should be given.
- Treat hyperkalaemia.
- Prophylactic antibiotics are not indicated.

End-of-life care

The World Health Organization (WHO) defines palliative care as 'an approach that improves the quality of life of patients and their families facing the problems associated with life-threatening illness, through the prevention and relief of suffering by means of early identification and impeccable assessment and treatment of pain and other associated problems, physical, psychosocial, and spiritual' (http://www.who.int/cancer/palliative/definition/en).

Death is common in critical care so it is an important aspect of care. It is a sensitive subject to approach with patients and their families at any time but when ethnic, cultural, religious, and spiritual differences are encountered it becomes an even more challenging topic. Local staff are a valuable source of information.

Cultural issues

- In some cultures, death is a taboo subject. It may be believed that it is disrespectful to discuss and it may cause bad luck or bring about death sooner.
- Family may try to protect the patient from a terminal diagnosis and believe that it should not be discussed with them as it may cause them to give up hope.
- Extended family may be involved in collective decision making.
- Removing a patient from life support may be seen as killing them.
- Patients may be used to a doctor-centred approach and are not used to being asked to make decisions.
- Pain may be seen as a positive sign that the body is fighting the illness or it may be seen as a weakness to take pain killers; therefore, patients may not ask for pain relief.

Religious issues

- There may be a strong belief in prayer and the power of God to heal the patient.
- It may be considered appropriate for a religious leader to be involved in delivering the diagnosis.
- Different religions will have different approaches to end-of-life care. There may be specific customs or rituals that it is important to know about and try to accommodate:
  - Muslims may wish for the dying patient to face towards Mecca.
  - Pacific islanders may leave a window open so that the soul can escape.
  - Hindus may wish to wash the deceased's body themselves.

These are just a few considerations to think about but you must gain cultural awareness of where you are working and understand the patient's beliefs and expectations. Asking specific questions may help guide your management:

- Do they wish to receive the diagnosis of their illness?
- Would they prefer treatment decisions to be made by their family?
- Who do they wish to be present?
- What are their religious beliefs?

Practical aspects

Overall the comfort of the patient is your main consideration. Making a decision to move to end-of-life care is a difficult one but ultimately the patient should not be distressed or discomfort prolonged:

- Unnecessary treatments should be stopped, including ventilatory support, cardiovascular support, and antibiotics. Lines should be removed.
- Analgesia: patients should be kept comfortable. Paracetamol, ibuprofen, and regular opioid analgesia is often required.
- Other symptom control options include:
  - Morphine for dyspnoea.
  - Hyoscine for secretions.
  - Benzodiazepines for anxiety.
  - Antiemetics for nausea and vomiting.

Decisions should be made by the team caring for the patient. It is often easier for families to accept that a transition to focus on comfort care rather than prolonging life is a medical decision made in consultation with them, and not a choice they are being asked to make. Guidance from local staff about how to address any issues appropriately and sensitively is key.

Further reading

Biccard B, Mabadagan H, Kluyts HL et al. (2018) Perioperative patient outcomes in the African Surgical Outcomes Study: a seven day prospective observational outcome study. *Lancet* 391: 1589–1598.

Dunser MW, Festic E, Dondorp A et al. (2012) Global intensive care working group of European Society of Intensive Care Medicine. Recommendations for sepsis management in resource limited settings. *Intensive Care Med* 38: 557–574.

Watters DAK, Wilson IH, Leaver RJ, Bagshawe A (1991) *Care of the Critically ill Patient in the Tropics and Subtropics*. London: Macmillan Education.

Further reading

Chapter 13

Tropical Medicine for Anaesthetists

Victoria Howell

Introduction

Many tropical diseases have implications for the anaesthetist: some may require surgery as part of the treatment for the condition or its complications, some may need high-dependency or intensive care, and the treatment of others may interact with anaesthetic drugs. With increasing global travel, these diseases may be seen outside the tropics. However, it is within tropical countries that these conditions are most problematic, given the limited resources in many low- and lower-middle-income countries (LMICs).

The tropical diseases outlined in this chapter frequently overlap with conditions of poverty, such as anaemia or malnutrition, often prevalent in these areas, and which also have implications for anaesthesia.

Sources of information on tropical diseases

- The Centers for Disease Control and Prevention website provides good information about a range of tropical diseases https://www.cdc.gov/globalhealth/index.html
- The World Health Organization website has a wealth of information and guidelines. It also has factsheets on various tropical diseases http://www.who.int/topics/tropical_diseases/factsheets/en
- NaTHNaC (National Travel Health Network and Centre) is a UK government organization providing travel health guidance for healthcare professionals http://nathnac.net
- The 'Yellow Book' (CDC Health Information for International Travel) contains vital information for anyone considering travelling or working abroad https://wwwnc.cdc.gov/travel/page/yellowbook-home

Malaria

Malaria is one of the most common infectious diseases worldwide. It is endemic in 106 countries, with an estimated 212 million malaria cases in 2015, and over 425,000 malaria deaths. Young children and pregnant women are particularly at risk of developing severe disease, with 70% of deaths occurring in children under 5 years.

Aetiology

- Caused by the parasite *Plasmodium*, of which five species are known to cause disease in humans.
- *Plasmodium falciparum* is found throughout the tropics and causes the greatest number of deaths. *Plasmodium vivax* is mainly found on the Indian subcontinent, Mexico, Central America, and China. *Plasmodium ovale* is found in West Africa. *Plasmodium malariae* has a varied distribution throughout the tropics and temperate climates. *Plasmodium knowlesi* was previously thought to only affect monkeys in South East Asia, but is now known to also cause human disease.
- Transmitted by the bite of an infected female *Anopheles* mosquito, the parasite is found in the saliva of the mosquito, and travels through the blood to the liver, where it matures and is subsequently released, infecting red blood cells.
- Malaria is also transmittable through maternal–foetal placental transfer, blood transfusions, and organ donations.

Pathophysiology

- The multisystem manifestations of malaria are due to changes in parasitized erythrocytes.
- Infection leads to reduced membrane deformability with increased fragility of red blood cells, accelerated haemolysis causing anaemia, and bone marrow suppression.
- Increased adherence to other erythrocytes and the vascular endothelium causes sequestration of red cells and microvascular capillary obstruction of splenic, renal, hepatic, cardiac, and cerebral circulations.
- Released pro-inflammatory cytokines, interleukin-1 (IL1), and tumour necrosis factor (TNF) cause a systemic inflammatory response.

Clinical features

Clinical features include intermittent fever, malaise, headache, myalgia, and minor gastrointestinal symptoms. Anaemia and splenomegaly may be seen on examination. See Box 13.1 for the clinical features of severe malaria.

Diagnosis

- Examination of peripheral blood slide for parasites:
  - Thick film for determining presence of malaria.
  - Thin film for determining species of malaria and degree of parasitaemia.
  - Microscopy is the most sensitive method of diagnosis, but requires training and equipment.

Box 13.1 Severe malaria.

Severe malaria is usually caused by *P. falciparum* and occurs in 1–2% of malarial infections. Defined as one or more of the following:

- **Prostration**—unable to sit or stand without assistance.
- **Impaired consciousness**—Glasgow coma score (GSC) <11, or Blantyre Score <3 in children.
- **Multiple convulsions**—more than two episodes in 24 h.
- **Pulmonary oedema**—seen on chest X-ray, or saturations <92% in room air, respiratory rate >30, or respiratory distress with crepitations heard on auscultation.
- **Significant bleeding**—recurrent or prolonged bleeding from nose, gums, or venepuncture sites; haematemesis or melaena.
- **Shock**—may be compensated shock with prolonged capillary refill time (>3 s) or limb temperature gradient but no hypotension. Or decompensated shock, with a systolic blood pressure <70 mmHg in children or <80 mmHg in adults, with evidence of impaired perfusion.
- **Hyperparasitaemia**—>10% parasitized red blood cells.
- **Severe malarial anaemia**—Hb <50 g/l in children or <70 g/l in adults.
- **Hypoglycaemia**—blood or plasma glucose <2.2 mmol/l or <40 mg/dl.
- **Acidosis**—base deficit >8 mEq/l, plasma bicarbonate <15 mmol/l or venous plasma lactate ≥5 mmol/l. Clinical signs of acidosis may be seen as respiratory distress with rapid, deep, laboured breathing.
- **Renal impairment**—plasma or serum creatinine >265 μmol/l or >3 mg/dl or blood urea >20 mmol/l.
- **Jaundice**—plasma or serum bilirubin >50 μmol/l or >3 mg/dl.

Severe malaria is a medical emergency with a mortality rate of 10–20% and death may occur rapidly within hours of admission.

Treat severe malaria with IV or intramuscular (IM) artesunate for at least 24 h (2.4 mg/kg b.d. in adults, 3 mg/kg b.d. in children <20 kg). Once tolerating oral medication, complete a 3-day course of ACT. If artesunate is not available, use IM artemether (3.2 mg/kg first dose then 1.6 mg/kg once daily) in preference to quinine.

Patients with severe malaria may require high-dependency or intensive care. Patients should be closely monitored for vital signs, urine output, and coma score. Blood glucose measurements should be done every 4 h. Supportive treatment may be required for any of the complications of severe malaria listed above.

Blood transfusion may be required if Hb <50 g/l in a high transmission area or <70 g/l in a low transmission area (consider higher thresholds if undergoing surgery). Antibiotics should be given to children with malaria as bacterial co-infection is common.

- Rapid diagnostic tests (RDTs) detect the presence of parasitic antigens in a drop of blood.
  - Can detect all *Plasmodium* species, or antigens specific to one species.
  - Detection of *P. falciparum* is important as this has the potential to cause severe disease.
  - Asymptomatic infection is common in high transmission areas.
  - Low levels of parasitaemia, not detected by RDT, may cause significant illness in non-immune individuals.

Management

Treat uncomplicated malaria with oral artemisinin-based combination therapy (ACT) for 3 days. See Box 13.1 for treatment of severe malaria.

Anaesthetic implications

Elective surgery should be postponed until an acute episode of malaria has been treated. Routine testing of patients preoperatively may be advocated. Surgical stress may cause reactivation of dormant *P. vivax* or *P. ovale* from the liver.

- Central nervous system (CNS)—cerebral malaria may cause impaired consciousness, raised intracranial pressure (ICP), and seizures. An anaesthetic that minimizes rises in ICP and maintains cerebral perfusion is ideal.
- Pulmonary—a dry cough is common in malaria. Severe malaria may lead to acute lung injury from cardiogenic or non-cardiogenic pulmonary oedema. Intraoperative ventilation may be challenging in these patients, and postoperative intensive care is required.
- Cardiovascular—usually only problematic in severe malaria. Congestive cardiac failure may result from profound anaemia and ischaemic cardiomyopathy from coronary microvascular obstruction.
- Haematological—anaemia, thrombocytopenia, and coagulopathy may all complicate malaria. Caution should therefore be exercised when considering neuraxial anaesthesia in these patients. Transfusion may be required if haemoglobin (Hb) <50 g/l in high transmission areas and 70 g/l in low transmission areas, although consider higher thresholds for surgery with anticipated blood loss.
- Renal—acute kidney injury may result from severe malaria, caused by a combination of hyperparasitaemia, hypovolaemia, sepsis, haemolysis, and rhabdomyolysis. Children with *P. malariae* infection may develop malarial nephrotic syndrome. Blackwater fever is due to quinine-induced lysis of red blood cells.

Tuberculosis (TB)

Caused by *Mycobacterium tuberculosis*, TB is endemic in most tropical countries, with one third of the world's population thought to harbour the bacilli.

Pathophysiology

- *Mycobacterium tuberculosis* is spread by inhalation of infected droplets. Usually close and prolonged contact is required, but only a few bacteria are necessary to acquire infection.
- The usual site of infection is the upper lobe of the lung—a 'Ghon focus'.
- Bacteria replicate within macrophages, followed by a T-cell-mediated response, which forms a granuloma.
- These bacteria within the granuloma may become dormant, resulting in the latent phase, when the patient is asymptomatic.
- Only 5–10% of those infected develop active TB: those at risk include children under 5 years, people in the first year of infection, and immunocompromised individuals.
- Co-infection with HIV increases the risk of acquiring new infection and developing active disease.

Clinical features

These include persistent cough, usually productive of sputum, haemoptysis, fever, night sweats, malaise, and weight loss or failure to thrive. Extrapulmonary TB can present in any other organ. Typical sites are the bones, lymph nodes, abdomen, meninges, pericardium, and pleura.

Diagnosis

- Isolation of *M. tuberculosis* from a sample takes 2–12 weeks to culture.
- Microscopy of sputum with a Ziehl–Neelsen stain may show acid-fast bacilli.
- Automated nucleic acid amplification tests (NAATs) are now used for near-patient testing, for example Xpert MTB/RIF (*Mycobacterium tuberculosis* and resistance to rifampicin), which has good sensitivity and specificity, and can detect rifampicin resistance as a surrogate for multidrug resistance.
- Tuberculin skin tests may be used, but false positives occur in those who have been vaccinated and false negatives in immunocompromised individuals.
- Chest X-rays may not show the typical apical cavitating lesion.

Management

- Six months of combination therapy is required and direct observation of therapy (DOT) used to ensure patient compliance.
- Drug regimens are complex, depend on HIV co-infection, drug sensitivity testing, and the likelihood of multidrug resistance.
- Rifampicin, isoniazid, ethambutol, and pyrazinamide are all first line.
- Multidrug resistant (MDR) TB is defined as resistance to isoniazid and rifampicin.
- Extensively drug-resistant TB (XDR TB) is a rare type of multidrug-resistant tuberculosis that is resistant to isoniazid and rifampin, plus any fluoroquinolone and at least one of three injectable second-line drugs (i.e. amikacin, kanamycin, or capreomycin).

Anaesthetic considerations

All elective surgery should be postponed until the patient is no longer infectious. Anaesthesia may be required for diagnostic procedures, such as lymph node biopsy or bronchoscopy, or to treat complications of TB, such as splenic abscess, intestinal obstruction, or hydrocephalus.

- Patients may be cachectic and anaemic, or have pancytopenia or deranged liver function tests from disseminated TB.
- Mediastinal lymphadenopathy may cause bronchial compression.
- Pleural effusions, consolidation, and cavitations may compromise respiratory function, with longstanding TB causing bronchiectasis and/or pulmonary fibrosis.
- Drug interactions may occur (see Box 13.2).
- The anaesthetist is at risk of contracting TB from infectious patients, particularly during laryngoscopy, tracheal intubation, and suctioning.
- Gloves, eye protection, and a filtering face piece (FFP3) mask should be used if available.
- Prevent contamination of anaesthetic equipment and use filters on breathing circuits.
- If significant exposure to TB occurs, a tuberculin skin test may be required, and 6–9 months of chemoprophylaxis with isoniazid may be required if positive, to prevent progression to active disease.

Box 13.2 Anaesthetic implications of drugs used to treat TB.

Drug interactions

- **Rifampicin** is a potent inducer of CYP3A4, the cytochrome P450 enzyme responsible for the metabolism of midazolam, fentanyl, alfentanil, and lidocaine. This may result in reduced therapeutic effects, or increased generation of potentially toxic metabolites.
- **Isoniazid** inhibits CYP3A4, but does not predictably cancel out the effects of rifampicin. There is an increased risk of halothane hepatitis as isoniazid induces CYP2E1, which is responsible for halothane metabolism.
- **Streptomycin** can potentiate non-depolarizing muscle relaxants. However, enzyme induction may also increase metabolism of rocuronium and vecuronium.

Side effects

Known side effects of anti-tuberculous therapy may impact upon anaesthesia. Drug-induced hepatitis may occur with isoniazid, rifampicin, or pyrazinamide. It usually occurs within first 2 months of therapy with symptomatic hepatitis having a mortality of around 5%. Rifampcin may cause thrombocytopenia, causing spontaneous bleeding, so may be a contraindication to neuraxial anaesthesia. Isoniazid may also cause thrombocytopenia, but more commonly anaemia or agranulocytosis. Hypersensitivity reactions may also occur, leading to disseminated intravascular coagulation.

Human immunodeficiency virus (HIV)

HIV is a global disease, though it is of particular significance in LMICs, where more than 95% of those with HIV live. In 2018 it is estimated there were 37.9 million people living with the condition, and it is the sixth biggest cause of death globally.

Pathophysiology

- It is caused by two distinct viruses, HIV-1 and HIV-2.
- It is transmitted in body fluids and spread through sexual intercourse, vertical transmission from mother to child, blood transfusions, and shared intravenous needles.
- HIV enters helper T-cells and macrophages, which have CD4 surface antigens, where the viral RNA is transcribed to DNA and is combined into host DNA.
- This allows billions of new HIV particles to be produced every day, to which the immune system response is to destroy infected cells.
- In time, the capacity of the host to replace T-cells is exceeded.
- Reducing numbers of CD4 cells results in reduced cell-mediated and humoral immunity, and an increase in opportunistic infections.
- The opportunistic infections that occur depend on geographically endemic diseases and the degree of immunosuppression.

Clinical features

Acute seroconversion illness occurs in around 50% of patients 2–5 weeks after infection with variable non-specific features of fever, sore throat, malaise, myalgia, arthralgia, headache, generalized lymphadenopathy, and a maculo-papular rash. This is usually followed by an asymptomatic stage, and symptoms tend not to occur until the immune system is significantly compromised. Persistent generalized lymphadenopathy may develop. Weakness, weight loss, reduced functional capacity, diarrhoea, and peripheral neuropathy may all occur as the CD4 count declines, together with the onset of opportunistic infections.

Diagnosis

- RDTs are commonly used to detect anti-HIV IgG and IgM in samples of oral fluid, whole blood, plasma, or serum.
- Serial testing is recommended to confirm a positive test.
- During seroconversion, antibody tests may be negative, weakly positive, or discordant (one test positive, another negative).
- Fourth-generation immunoassays are used when laboratory facilities are available, with greater sensitivity and specificity.

Management

- Current WHO guidance is that antiretroviral treatment should be started for everyone with HIV regardless of CD4 cell count. Interactions with anaesthetic drugs may occur (see Box 13.3).
- Three main classes of antiretrovirals are used:
  - nucleoside analogue reverse transcriptase inhibitors (NRTIs)
  - non-nucleoside analogue reverse transcriptase inhibitors (NNRTIs)
  - protease inhibitors (PIs).

Box 13.3 Anti-retroviral drug interactions.

Protease inhibitors inhibit the cytochrome P450 enzyme CYP3A4, which also metabolizes fentanyl, pethidine, alfentanil, and midazolam. Dexamethasone and thiopental can reduce protease inhibitor concentration.

Nevirapine, an NNRTI, induces cytochrome P450 enzymes. Patients on combination therapy may be taking drugs that both inhibit and induce hepatic enzymes, leading to an unpredictable response to co-administered anaesthetic agents.

Tenofovir, an NRTI, is associated with a small but significant risk of kidney injury, and therefore nephrotoxic drugs such as gentamicin or non-steroidal anti-inflammatory drugs should be avoided perioperatively.

- First-line therapy for adults is currently tenofovir, lamivudine, and dolutegravir, although many alternative regimens exist and the latest guidelines should be consulted.
- TB prophylaxis with 6 months of isoniazid should be given to those without clinical evidence of active TB.
- Co-trimoxazole prophylaxis is recommended for adults with severe or advanced HIV clinical disease and/or CD4 counts ≤350 cells/mm^3. This helps to prevent many bacterial infections including *Pneumocystis jirovecii* and *Toxoplasma gondii*.

Anaesthetic implications

HIV infection alone is not associated with an increased postoperative risk of death, however those with advanced disease may have comorbidities and infections that may impact upon anaesthesia.

- Respiratory—acute respiratory infections are common, with bacterial pneumonia being the usual cause, but TB should always be excluded. Empyemas should be looked for and drained if appropriate. Pulmonary Kaposi's sarcoma or lymphoma may also have an impact on respiratory function.
- Cardiac—myocarditis progressing to a dilated cardiomyopathy is common and usually precipitated by an infectious cause. Bacterial infections may result in endocarditis and congestive cardiac failure.
- Gastrointestinal—chronic diarrhoea and weight loss are common and may result in fluid and electrolyte imbalance.
- CNS—neurological complications are common, ranging from peripheral neuropathy to meningitis and encephalitis.
- Anaemia, thrombocytopenia, and leucopenia are common.
- Universal precautions should be used for all patients with or without HIV; this is especially important in areas of high prevalence.
- Post-exposure prophylaxis (PEP) for health professionals should be started as soon as possible after exposure to high-risk body fluids, which may occur following a needle-stick injury. Current recommendations for PEP are for tenofovir with emtricitabine plus lopinavir with ritonavir for 28 days.

Dengue

A mosquito-borne viral infection, clinically separated into dengue fever with or without warning signs (see Box 13.4), and severe dengue, previously known as dengue haemorrhagic fever. It is endemic in more than 120 countries in the tropics, and 3.2 million cases were reported in 2015.

Aetiology

- Dengue is mainly transmitted by the female *Aedes aegypti* mosquito.
- These day-biting mosquitoes breed in collections of water around the house and bite multiple hosts during feeding, increasing their role as vectors.
- Dengue is a flavivirus and has four serotypes that affect humans.
- Infection by one serotype confers immunity to it, but cross-immunity to other serotypes is only partial and transient. Severe dengue may develop from subsequent infection with other serotypes.

Pathophysiology

- The pathology of dengue haemorrhagic fever occurs due to the host's immune response.
- Previous dengue infection causes antibody-dependent enhancement, which increases entry of a second dengue virus into macrophages, leading to increased severity of infection.
- A massive increase in vascular permeability leads to plasma leakage from capillaries.
- Abnormal haemostasis occurs with thrombocytopenia and activation of clotting and fibrinolytic pathways, which may lead to disseminated intravascular coagulation.

Clinical features

Dengue fever may cause severe flu-like symptoms with a high fever, headache, retro-orbital pain, nausea and vomiting, lymphadenopathy, myalgia, arthralgia, and rash. Symptoms usually last 2–7 days.

Criteria for severe dengue include severe plasma leakage leading to shock or fluid accumulation with respiratory distress. Severe haemorrhage may be a feature. Severe organ impairment may be characterized by liver transaminase >1,000 iu/l, impaired consciousness, or severe involvement of the heart or other organs.

Diagnosis

- Dengue virus may be detected by polymerase chain reaction in acute infection, or by IgG and IgM antibodies in later illness.

Management

- Most cases of dengue fever are self-limiting and can be managed with oral fluids and paracetamol.
- Dengue haemorrhagic fever may require fluid resuscitation, blood transfusion, and invasive monitoring.
- A vaccine to dengue fever has been developed but is recommended only in areas with a high burden of disease.

Box 13.4 Warning signs of severe dengue.

Usually occur 3–7 days after first symptoms, and are associated with a reducing temperature. They include:

- Abdominal pain or tenderness.
- Persistent vomiting.
- Haematemesis.
- Respiratory distress.
- Mucosal haemorrhage.
- Fatigue or restlessness.
- Increase in haematocrit, with rapid decrease in platelet count.

Zika virus

Zika virus is also a flavivirus and is transmitted by *Aedes* mosquitoes. Two strains of the virus have been identified—Asian and African. Over recent years, an increased number of outbreaks have been occurring, associated with Guillain–Barré syndrome (GBS). It has been associated with microcephaly in foetuses due to placental transmission.

Clinical features

The majority of people are asymptomatic, with about one fifth experiencing non-specific illness of fever, maculopapular rash, arthralgia, headache, and conjunctivitis.

Diagnosis

- Blood tests can detect Zika RNA, or the antibody response to it with IgG and IgM levels.
- Cross-reactivity may occur with dengue and other flaviviruses.

Treatment

- There is no specific treatment for Zika virus; treatment is supportive.
- Pregnant women need particular support during pregnancy if they contract Zika virus.

Anaesthetic considerations

- Thrombocytopenia may occur especially if there is co-infection with dengue or chikungunya.
- Neuraxial anaesthesia may be relatively contraindicated during active viral infection.
- The risks of anaesthesia may be increased in those with GBS as patients may have profound weakness requiring ventilatory support.
- Suxamethonium is contraindicated in GBS as it can precipitate hyperkalaemia due to the upregulation of acetylcholine receptors.
- Anaesthetists may theoretically be at risk of contracting Zika virus, although there has been no reported transmission in a healthcare setting.

Schistosomiasis

Schistosomiasis, or bilharzia, affects around 200 million people worldwide, the majority of whom live in Africa. Found in freshwater lakes, the parasite typically affects children aged between 10 and 15 years old, who have greatest exposure, but also those who work in the water.

Pathophysiology

- Caused by the blood fluke *Schistosoma*, three types affect humans.
- *Schistosoma haematobium* causes urogenital schistosomiasis, whereas *Schistosoma mansoni* and *Schistosoma japonicum* cause liver and bowel disease.
- The parasites replicate in an aquatic snail before being released into the water to find a human host, where they penetrate the skin and enter the circulation, travelling through the lungs to reach the liver.
- They mature in the liver and migrate to their destination in the mesenteric veins or vesical plexus where they deposit eggs.

Clinical features

Acute schistosomiasis, or Katayama fever, causes a mild illness, with fever, skin rashes, urticaria, dry cough and wheeze, malaise, myalgia, nausea, and vomiting or diarrhoea. More severe disease occurs in later life and is due to eggs leaving the body or causing tissue reactions.

- Urinary schistosomiasis typically causes terminal haematuria, but may also cause perforations in the bladder wall leading to microalbuminaemia.
- Bladder calcification and fibrotic changes lead to bladder contraction and ureteric strictures causing hydronephrosis. Chronic schistosomiasis is associated with squamous cell bladder cancer.
- Around 1% of those with chronic schistosomiasis may develop pulmonary hypertension if the eggs escape the portal system and end up in the lungs. Similarly, portal hypertension may develop from a periportal granulomatous response to eggs in the liver. This may lead to oesophageal varices, with associated bleeding, and massive splenomegaly, which may require splenectomy for symptom control or due to spontaneous rupture.

Diagnosis

- Direct diagnosis is by observing viable eggs.
- Eggs from the bladder are typically voided around midday and can be detected by sedimentation or filtration.
- Stool sample or rectal biopsy is required for eggs in the gut.
- Immunodiagnosis detects circulating antibody, but cannot distinguish between past and active infection, cannot distinguish between species, and does not become positive until 3 months after infection.

Management

- A single oral dose of praziquantel effectively treats the parasite.
- Praziquantel may be used for mass chemotherapy in endemic areas.

Filariasis

Lymphatic filariasis is endemic in more than 80 countries throughout the tropics, and affects around 120 million people.

Pathophysiology

- The majority of cases of lymphatic filariasis are caused by *Wurchereria bancrofti*, which is transmitted by mosquitoes.
- These thread-like worms are between 4 and 10 cm long and can live for more than 10 years.
- Infection usually occurs in childhood, but the chronic manifestations of the disease develop months or years after acute symptoms.

Clinical features

A wide range of clinical effects from the infection may be seen, ranging from asymptomatic, to filarial fever, acute filarial lymphangitis, or tropical pulmonary eosinophilia.

- Chronic lymphatic filariasis is caused by obstructed lymphatics leading to lymphoedema of the extremity and elephantiasis. Chyluria, chylous diarrhoea, and chylous ascites may occur if the dilated lymphatics rupture. Acute epididymitis or more commonly a unilateral hydrocele may develop, requiring surgery.

Diagnosis

- A finger-prick immunochromatographic card test can rapidly detect both adult worms and microfilariae, with high sensitivity and specificity.
- Identification of filarial parasites in blood or hydrocele fluid confirms the diagnosis, but patients may be amicrofilaric.
- In endemic areas, the WHO recommends that all hydrocele are presumed to be caused by filariasis unless proved otherwise.

Management

- Antihelminthic treatments with albendazole, ivermectin, or diethylcarbamazine have traditionally been used, but do not kill the adult worms and are associated with adverse effects.
- Doxycycline may be used to kill the parasites by targeting *Wolbachia*—symbiotic bacteria living within the worms.
- A 6-week course has been shown to eliminate worm nests from the scrotum of men with filarial hydroceles.
- Hydrocelectomy may be required for those unresponsive to drug therapy. Local anaesthesia with a spermatic cord block and local infiltration has been shown to be effective.
- The WHO has a global programme to eliminate lymphatic filariasis. It advocates annual mass drug administration in endemic areas, continued for 4–6 years to interrupt transmission of the disease. It also focuses on morbidity management and disability prevention, which includes the surgical treatment of hydroceles.

African trypanosomiasis

African trypanosomiasis, or sleeping sickness, is caused by *Trypanosoma brucei*, of which there are two species that affect humans and cause differing symptoms. Transmission occurs through the bite of the tsetse fly, which is only found in sub-Saharan Africa.

Clinical features

A trypanosomal chancre may occur 3 days after the bite, with local lymphadenopathy. An acute severe illness may develop with fever, headache, arthralgia, lymphadenopathy, and eventually CNS involvement with behavioural and psychiatric manifestations, and disordered sleep patterns.

Diagnosis

- Blood films or lymph node aspirates will show parasites.

Management

- Suramin or pentamidine may be used for early disease.
- Melarsoprol, an arsenic compound, is used for later disease as it will penetrate the CNS, but is associated with significant toxicity.

South American trypanosomiasis

Also known as Chagas' disease, caused by *Trypanosoma cruzi*, and transmitted by reduviid or kissing bugs. Transmission may also occur through maternal–foetal infection, blood transfusion, or organ donation.

Clinical features

Acute infection usually occurs in children, although about one third are asymptomatic. Swelling at the entry site of the infection—a chagoma—lymphadenopathy and hepatosplenomegaly may be seen.

- Chronic Chagas' disease can occur after 10–20 years. A dilated cardiomyopathy with conduction system scarring may lead to heart block or arrhythmias. Mortality may be due to sudden cardiac death, from ventricular tachycardia or fibrillation, or less commonly from refractory heart failure or thromboembolism.
- Dilatation of the gastrointestinal tract from destruction of the autonomic ganglia can result in megacolon or megaoesophagus, which may require surgery with an increased risk of aspiration.

Diagnosis

- Microscopy in the acute phase will demonstrate the parasites.
- Serological tests may be used in chronic disease.

Management

- Nifurtimox or benznidazole will eliminate the parasites in the acute phase and help to prevent chronic disease.

Typhoid

Typhoid, or enteric fever, is caused by *Salmonella enterica* serovar Typhi. There are approximately 21 million cases per year, with a mortality rate of about 1%. It is most common in children and young adults.

Pathophysiology

- The Gram negative bacilli are usually transmitted in contaminated water and food.
- The duration of incubation and severity of illness are related to the bacterial load ingested.
- Asymptomatic carriers are important reservoirs of infection.
- The ingested organisms penetrate intestinal mucosa before being transported to lymph nodes from where they enter the bloodstream.
- The bacilli multiply within macrophages in the bone marrow, liver, spleen, and gallbladder. Release of infected bile leads to secondary invasion of the bowel.
- Typhoid nodules can occur in various organs, and more diffuse organ involvement may also occur.

Clinical features

It commonly presents with non-specific symptoms of fever, a non-productive cough, myalgia, headache, anorexia and abdominal pain, with diarrhoea or constipation. Rarely, meningitis may be the only manifestation of typhoid.

- Complications occur in 10–15% of patients. Intestinal perforation is the most serious and the commonest cause of death from typhoid.
- Necrosis of Peyer's patches occurs throughout the ileum, leading to multiple perforations. Mortality may be up to 30% despite surgery, where segmental resection is preferable to simple suturing due to friable tissue. Patients may be critically ill, requiring aggressive fluid resuscitation and postoperative high-dependency care. Gastrointestinal haemorrhage may occur, but it is usually self-limiting. Typhoid abscess is a late complication and can occur at various locations.

Diagnosis

- Usually the diagnosis is made clinically.
- Bacteria may be cultured from blood, bone marrow, or bile.
- The Widal agglutination test, widely used to diagnose typhoid fever, is unreliable due to low sensitivity and specificity.
- RDTs have been developed, but have similar issues with sensitivity and specificity.

Management

- Ciprofloxacin for 5–7 days is usually very effective.
- Drug resistance is emerging but third-generation cephalosporins are useful, although the response may be slower.
- Typhoid vaccines are available for those in endemic areas and for use during outbreaks.

Diarrhoea

Infective diarrhoea is the third highest cause of death from infections in the world, with approximately 80% of these deaths occurring in children under 2 years. Diarrhoea is very common in tropical countries, where high rates of malnutrition and HIV infection compound the problem.

Acute diarrhoeal disease can be subdivided into whether there is the presence of blood (dysentery, Box 13.5) or not (enteritis).

Shigellosis

- Shigellae are Gram negative bacteria, of which four species are described with various subtypes. Some are more common in the tropics, and some more prone to cause epidemics.
- Transmission is faecal–oral, via water, food, flies, and person-to-person contact.
- There are an estimated 165 million infections per year, causing 1.1 million deaths.
- Around 70% of cases occur in children under 5 years, resulting in 60% of deaths.

Clinical features

- Mild illness may cause watery diarrhoea without blood or mucus.
- Severe disease causes fever, tenesmus, cramps, and frequent bloody mucoid stools, often described as redcurrant jelly.
- Dehydration, hypoglycaemia, and hyponatraemia may occur.
- Complications include toxic megacolon, perforation, protein-losing enteropathy, post-dysenteric colitis, and rectal prolapse in children.
- Shiga toxin, an extotoxin produced by *Shigella dysteneriae* type 1, is a neurotoxin producing CNS effects, such as confusion, meningism, and convulsions in children, and haemolytic uraemic syndrome (HUS), which usually occurs 1–5 days after the onset of dysentery.

Management

- Bedside dipstick testing of faeces can detect *Sh. dysteneriae* type 1.
- The WHO recommend all cases of dysentery to be treated with antibiotic therapy, although multidrug resistance is common.
- Ciprofloxacin is usually recommended.
- Oral rehydration solution for mild cases or IV fluids for more severe cases, and blood transfusions may be required.

Box 13.5 Causes of dysentery.

Usually a sign of ulceration of the large bowel, causes include:

- *Shigella* (bacillary dysentery)
- *Campylobacter*
- *Entamoeba histolytica* (amoebic dysentery)
- enterohaemorrhagic *E. coli*
- *Salmonella* enterocolitis
- *Yersinia* enterocolitis
- *Balantidium coli* enterocolitis
- *Trichuris* infection
- *Schistosomiasis mansoni* or *Schistosomiasis japonicum* infection.

Amoebiasis

- *Entamoeba histolytica* is an intestinal protozoa that affects around 48 million people worldwide, although only 10% are symptomatic.
- Symptoms may develop years after initial infection.
- Transmission is faecal–oral, usually contaminated food and drink, although sexual transmission is also possible.

Clinical features

- Dysentery (bloody diarrhoea) with crampy abdominal pain.
- Complications include abscess formation, colonic strictures, haemorrhage, post-dysenteric colitis, toxic megacolon, peritonitis, and amoeboma formation—a chronic inflammatory mass that may lead to intestinal obstruction or intussusception.
- Amoebic liver abscesses may occur when the parasites destroy hepatocytes causing multiple small abscesses that coalesce. Right upper quadrant pain, fever, and cough may be features. Rupture occurs in about 20% of patients, and may cause an empyema, peritonitis, hepatobronchial fistula, or rarely cardiac tamponade.

Management

- A 5–10-day course of metronidazole is usually effective.
- A luminal amoebicide is recommended for eradication of cysts, e.g. diloxanide or paromomycin.
- Surgery may be required for management of the complications or for aspiration and drainage of liver abscesses.
- Aggressive resection of bowel in severe colitis has a high mortality.

Trichuriasis (whipworm)

- *Trichuris trichiura* are small worms 3–4 cm long that inhabit the colon and rectum after ingestion of faecally contaminated soil.
- Affects approximately 25% of the world's population.

Clinical features

- Mild infections may be asymptomatic.
- Co-infection with hookworms, *Ascaris lumbricoides*, may cause abdominal distension, flatulence, vomiting, and weight loss.
- Heavy infection causes haemorrhage, mucopurulent stool, dysentery, and rectal prolapse.
- Severe anaemia and protein-losing enteropathy can occur.

Management

- One dose of albendazole or mebendazole is usually effective.
- Heavy infection may require a 3-day course.

Tapeworms

- Tapeworms can measure from 10 mm to 2 m in length.
- Infection occurs from eating cysts in undercooked meat, usually beef (*Taenia saginata*) or pork (*Taenia solium*).
- Infection may also arise from ingestion of eggs of *T. solium*, which leads to cysticercosis, which causes the development of tissue cysts.

Clinical features

- Intestinal infections are usually asymptomatic, but worms may appear in the faeces or occasionally in vomit.
- Complications may occur when the worm migrates to the pancreatic or bile ducts, or to the appendix.
- Cysticercosis may cause pain and swelling with eosinophilia, as cysts develop in the tissues.
- Brain cysts may be intraparenchymal and cause diffuse cerebral oedema called cysticerci encephalitis.
- Extraparenchymal cysts, causing obstructive hydrocephalus or arachnoiditis, are rarer in children and have a poorer prognosis.

Management

- A single dose of praziquantel is recommended for those with a single brain lesion and positive serology.
- Active parenchymal neurocysticercosis can be treated with albendazole for 8–15 days.
- Dexamethasone helps to reduce the effect of inflammation around damaged cysts; seizures can be treated with anticonvulsants.
- Surgical intervention may be required for obstructive hydrocephalus or intracranial hypertension.

Ascariasis (roundworms)

- *Ascaris lumbricoides* affects over 800 million people worldwide, most commonly children aged between 3 and 8 years old.
- The eggs of these helminths contaminate vegetables and are ingested, releasing larvae that pass through intestinal mucosa.
- These enter the bloodstream and lymphatics and reach the lungs around 4–16 days after initial infection.
- The larvae eventually migrate to the small intestine where adult worms develop, growing to 15–40 cm in length.

Clinical features

- Ascaris pneumonitis causes cough, dyspnoea, wheeze, fever, and urticaria, which usually resolves within 10 days.
- Chest pain, cyanosis, and haemoptysis may indicate severe infection.
- Intestinal worms are rarely noticed, but heavy infections may cause intestinal obstruction, volvulus, perforation, and peritonitis.
- Obstruction of biliary ducts by the worms is more common in adults leading to biliary colic, cholangitis, pancreatitis, or liver abscesses.
- Occasionally wandering worms may block endotracheal tubes or cause airway obstruction.

Management

- A single dose of albendazole or a 3-day course of mebendazole is usually effective, though heavy infections may need a prolonged course.
- Ascaris pneumonitis may be treated symptomatically with bronchodilators and steroids.
- Intestinal obstruction is usually managed conservatively, but surgery may occasionally be required.

Cholera

Vibrio cholerae is a Gram negative bacteria causing a severe watery diarrhoea that may be rapidly fatal. It is estimated there are between 1.3 and 4 million cases of cholera a year, with up to 140,000 deaths.

Classification of cholera subtypes is important to determine the global epidemiology of outbreaks. There are two biotypes of Serogroup 01—classical and El Tor—each can be divided into Ogawa, Inaba, or Hikojima serotypes. *Vibrio cholerae* 0139 is a newer serogroup seen only in Asia.

Pathophysiology

- Spread occurs directly via the faecal–oral route, or indirectly through infected food and water.
- Cholera toxin released by the bacteria, once in the gut, binds to epithelial cells and allows entry of the toxin into the cells.
- The toxin activates cyclic AMP resulting in efflux of water, chloride, and bicarbonate, leading to dehydration and electrolyte imbalance.

Clinical features

Clinical features range from asymptomatic infection or mild self-limiting diarrhoea to profuse, watery 'rice water' diarrhoea of up to 30 l a day. The diarrhoea may lead to a metabolic acidosis, electrolyte imbalances, and profound dehydration that may lead to death within hours. Vomiting follows onset of the diarrhoea, and shock follows around 12 h later, with hypovolaemia and hypoglycaemia contributing to reduced consciousness. Complications include ileus, renal failure, and cardiac arrhythmias prior to death.

Diagnosis

- In epidemics, the diagnosis is made clinically.
- Culture of a stool specimen remains the gold standard.
- Laboratory diagnosis can determine the serogroup and serotype.
- Immuno-diagnostic dipsticks (Crystal VC®) can be used in the field, but have suboptimal sensitivity and specificity.

Management

- Rehydration is essential, and this may be orally with oral rehydration solution (ORS), or with IV fluids in cases of hypovolaemic shock.
- Large volumes of either fluid may be required, and Ringer's lactate (Hartmann's solution) is ideal if IV resuscitation is necessary.
- Azithromycin as a single dose helps to reduce the volume and duration of the diarrhoea in severe illness.
- Doxycycline is an alternative, or erythromycin in children.
- Oral cholera vaccines are available. Dukoral® is suited to travellers and provides 65% protection for 2 years. Two other vaccines are more suited to outbreak control in emergencies and have been stockpiled by the WHO for this purpose.

Further reading

Beeching N, Gill G. (2014) *Tropical Medicine: Lecture Notes*, 7th edn. Chichester: Wiley.
Davidson R, Brent A, Seale A (2014) *Oxford Handbook of Tropical Medicine*, 4th edn. Oxford: Oxford University Press.
Mabey D et al. (2013) *Principles of Medicine in Africa*, 4th edn. Cambridge: Cambridge University Press.
World Health Organization (2015) *Guidelines for the Treatment of Malaria*, 3rd edn. Geneva: WHO.
World Health Organization (2017) *Guidelines for Treatment of Drug-susceptible Tuberculosis and Patient Care*. Geneva: WHO.

Appendices

Vaporizer recognition

The vaporizers shown in Figures A.1 to A.5 are all suitable for draw-over.

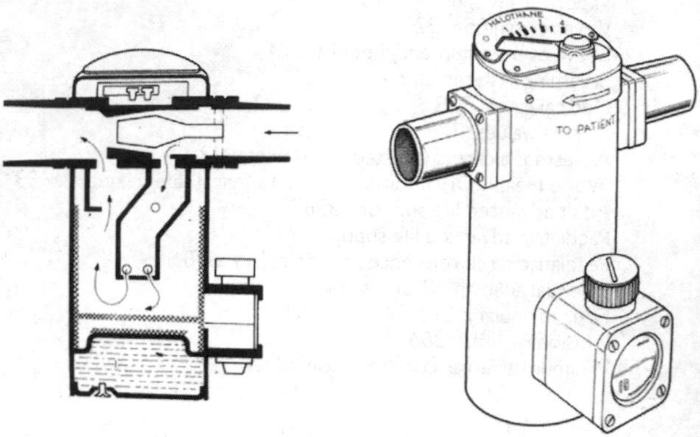

Figure A.1 OMV (Oxford miniature vaporizer).

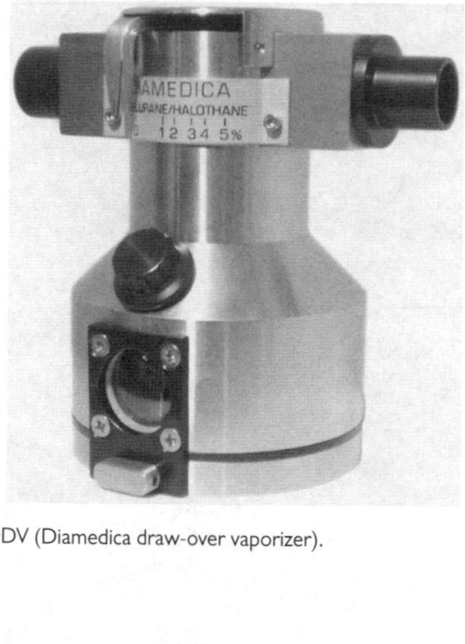

Figure A.2 DDV (Diamedica draw-over vaporizer).

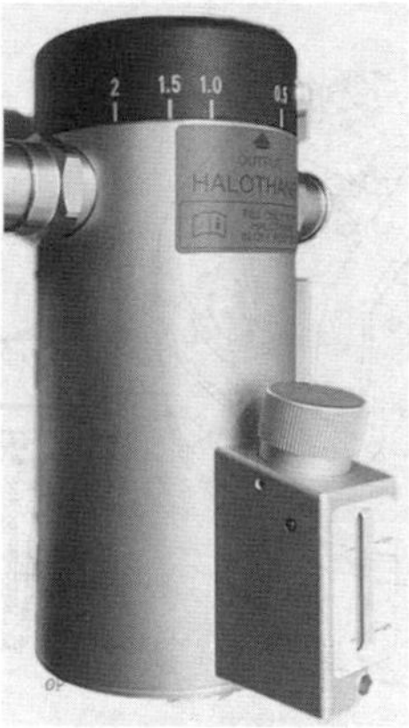

Figure A.3 UAM/OES (universal anaesthesia machine vaporizer).

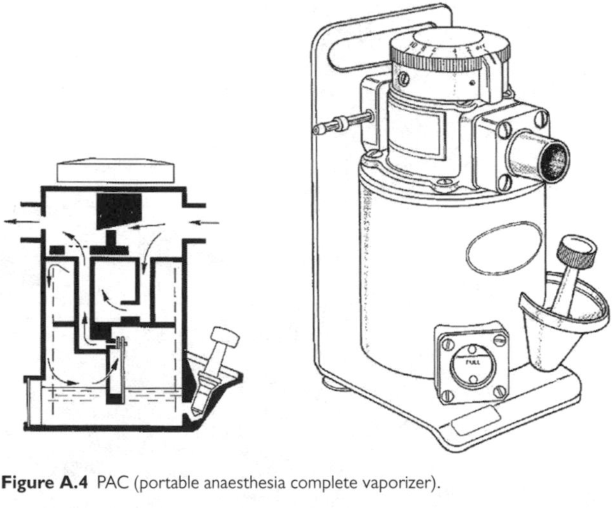

Figure A.4 PAC (portable anaesthesia complete vaporizer).

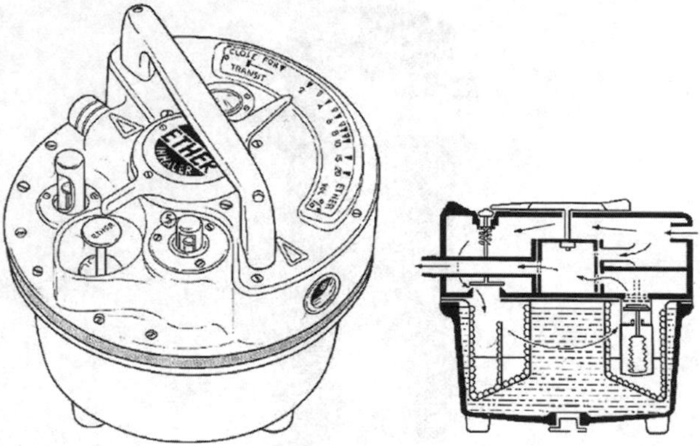

Figure A.5 EMO (Epstein Macintosh Oxford) ether vaporizer.

Valve recognition

- The valves in Figures A.6 to A.8 are all suitable for draw-over with both spontaneous and controlled ventilation.
- There are many other valves, most unsatisfactory and some (copies of the ones illustrated here) that are dangerous if mistaken for the valves shown.

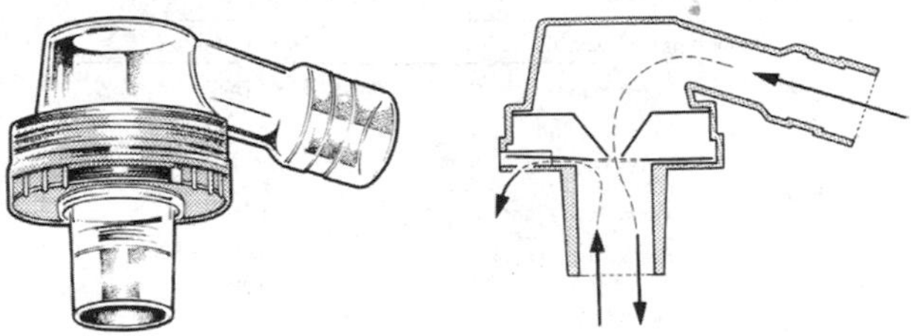

Figure A.6 Laerdal valve.

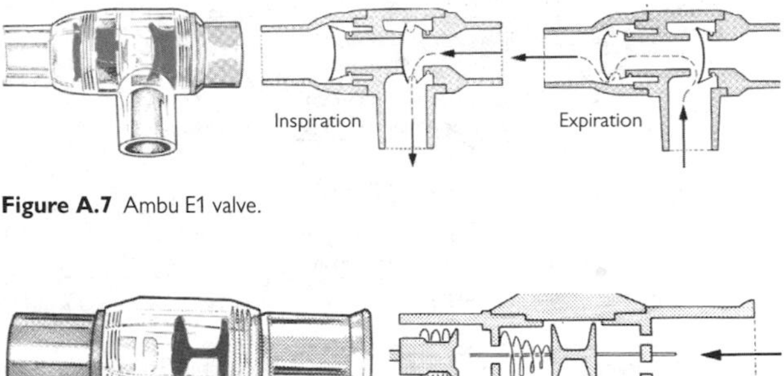

Figure A.7 Ambu E1 valve.

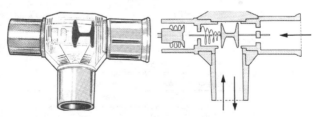

Figure A.8 Ruben valve.

Draw-over equipment checklist

Figure A.9 shows a checklist for draw-over anaesthetic equipment.

Checklist for Draw-over Anaesthetic Equipment 2019

Association of Anaesthetists Safety Guideline

Do checks at the start of every operating session
Do not use this equipment unless you have been trained

Check self-inflating bag available
Assemble equipment in accordance with instruction/diagram[1]

Check self-inflating bag available		Team brief notes
Power supply	• Power supply confirmed if available	Power limitations are:
Oxygen supply	Confirm supplementary oxygen source[1] (concentrator, cylinder, pipeline)	Oxygen limitations are:
Breathing system	• System checked, patent, with no foreign objects • Vaporisers filled with correct agent • Perform breathing system tests: • Correct function (2 bag) test • Pressure leak test • Confirm no volatile leak	Volatile anaesthetic stocks are:
Ventilator (if available)	• Working and configured correctly • Plugged in and/or battery status confirmed	Back-up ventilation is:
Suction	• Confirm ability to generate suction • Confirm back-up if possible (surgical)	Back-up suction is:
Scavenging	• Passive scavenging tube patent along length OR • Absorber connected and working	

DOCUMENT CHECK IN PATIENT'S ANAESTHETIC RECORD

Don't Forget	• Team brief limitations of equipment/supplies/environment • Alternate plans for oxygen/power/anaesthesia • Self inflating bag available • Difficult airway equipment and plan • Resuscitation equipment/emergency drugs

This guideline is not a standard of medical care. The ultimate judgement with regard to a particular clinical procedure or treatment plan must be made by the clinician in the light of the clinical data presented, the diagnostic and treatment options available, and the environmental limitations posed.

Association of Anaesthetists

Figure A.9 Checklist for draw-over anaesthetic equipment 2019. Safety guideline.

CHECKS BEFORE EACH CASE

Monitors	• Working and configured correctly • National minimum monitoring standards met (e.g. Association of Anaesthetists) • Alarm limits set
Airway equipment	• Checked as correct and available for the case, and working
Breathing system	• Whole system checked, patent, with no foreign objects • Vaporisers filled with correct agent
Ventilator (if available)	• Working and configured correctly • Plugged in and/or battery status confirmed
Suction	• Confirm clean • Confirm ability to generate suction
Scavenging	• Scavenging tubing connected and patent along length OR • Absorber connected and working

CHECKS BEFORE EACH CASE

- Equipment correctly configured for weight of child
- Correct size airway equipment available
- Specific limitations exist for draw-over in paediatrics - refer to full publication[1]

BREATHING SYSTEM TESTS

Breathing system tests should be performed after the breathing system, vaporisers and ventilator have been checked individually.

i. Correct function (two bag) test: with test lung or bag attached, squeeze the self-inflating bag or bellows and ensure action of test lung.
ii. Breathing system pressure test: Occlude the connector that joins the breathing valve to the patient. Squeeze the bag or bellows. No air should escape.
iii. Ensure no vaporiser leak detectable (sniff for volatile!).
iv. Ensure vaporiser filler cap correctly seated and firmly closed.

1. This is a concise version of the full *Checklist for Draw-over Anaesthesia 2019* (published by the Association of Anaesthetists). Scan the code below to access the full publication.

2. Video illustration of the use of the checklist to follow.

3. Scan the code below to access the e-learning for healthcare (e-LfH) module for draw-over anaesthesia.

Figure A.9 *(Contd.)*

Breathing systems

Anaesthetic breathing systems can be classified into **open** (e.g. air), **semi-open** (e.g. Hudson mask), **semi-closed** (Mapleson classification; Fig. A.10), and **closed** (circle; Fig. A.11). The FGFs required to prevent rebreathing in a Mapleson system are given in Table A.1 and the FGFs required in a circle system are given in Table A.2.

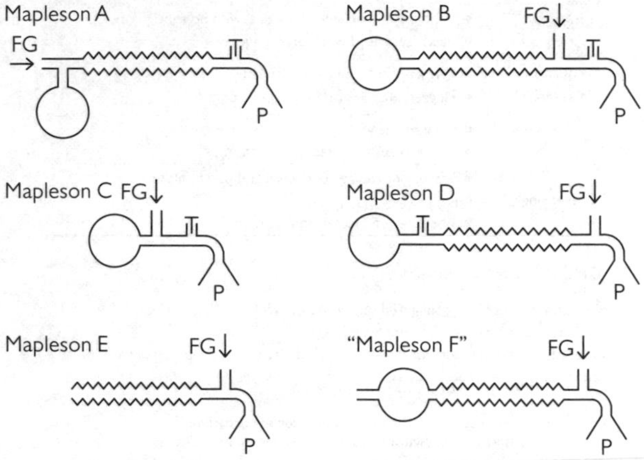

Figure A.10 Mapleson classification of breathing systems. FG, fresh gas; P, patient.

Reproduced from C. Gibson and F. Roberts. Anaesthesia Data. In: *Oxford Handbook of Anaesthesia*. K. Allman et al. (Eds.). Oxford, UK: Oxford University Press. Copyright © 2015, OUP. Reproduced with permission of the Licensor through PLSclear. DOI: 10.1093/med/9780198719410.001.0001.

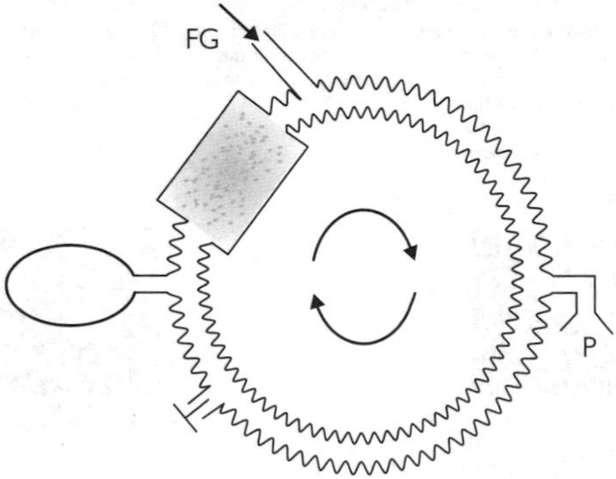

Figure A.11 The circle system.

Reproduced from C. Gibson and F. Roberts. Anaesthesia Data. In: *Oxford Handbook of Anaesthesia*. K. Allman et al. (Eds.). Oxford, UK: Oxford University Press. Copyright © 2015, OUP. Reproduced with permission of the Licensor through PLSclear. DOI: 10.1093/med/9780198719410.001.0001.

Table A.1 Fresh gas flows required in Mapleson breathing systems.

Breathing system	Spontaneous ventilation	Intermittent positive pressure ventilation
A (Lack or Magill)	Equal to V_A 70 ml/kg/min	2.5 × MV 250 ml/kg/min
D (Bain) E (Ayre's T-piece) F (Jackson Rees modification)	2 × MV 200 ml/kg/min*	70 ml/kg/min for $PaCO_2$ of 5.3 kPa (40 mmHg) or 100 ml/kg/min for $PaCO_2$ of 4.3 kPa (32 mmHg) Minimum of 3 l/min

*In young children, the greater MV/kg may require a fresh gas flow of up to 300 ml/kg/min.

MV, minute ventilation; V_A, alveolar minute ventilation.

Table A.2 Fresh gas flows required in a circle system.

Stage of case	Spontaneous ventilation or intermittent positive pressure ventilation
Initial uptake Rapid change in depth Washout (emergence)	Equal to MV 100 ml/kg/min
Maintenance	Fresh gas flow can be reduced, but the percentage of O_2 and volatile agent must be increased to produce same concentrations in the final inspired gas (due to patient uptake).* A total flow of at least 1 l/min is generally used

*O_2 and agent monitoring are essential at low flows.

MV, minute ventilation.

Medical gases

Table A.3 Pressure conversion chart.

100 kPa is equal to:
1 bar
750 mmHg (torr)
1020 cmH_2O
0.987 atm
14.5 p.s.i.

atm, Atmosphere; p.s.i, pounds per square inch.

Table A.4 Medical gases storage and properties

Medical gas	State in cylinder	Cylinder capacity (L)				Cylinder pressure when full (x100 Pa)	Critical temperature (°C)
		Type C	Type D	Type E	Type F		
Oxygen (O_2)	Gas	170	340	680	1360	137	–118.4
Nitrous oxide (N_2O)	Liquid	450	900	1800	3600	44*	36.4
O_2:N_2O 50:50 (Entonox®)	Gas		500		2000	137	–6†
Medical air	Gas			640	1280	137	
Carbon dioxide (CO_2)	Liquid	450		1800		50*	30
O_2:CO_2 95:5	Gas				1360	137	
Medical helium (He)	Gas		300		1200	137	–268
O_2:He 21:79	Gas				1200	137	
Water capacity of cylinder (L)		1.2	2.32	4.68	9.43		

* Where the contents are liquid, the pressure is not a reliable method of judging the contents.

†Entonox® separates into O_2 and N_2 O at —6°C—'pseudocritical' temperature.

Pressures quoted for full cylinders are at 15°C.

The colour and contents of cylinders varies country to country. Cylinders may not contain the stated contents, exercise caution!

Normal values

This section provides tables of pulmonary function tests (Table A.5), arterial/mixed venous blood gases (Table A.6), normal haematological blood results (Table A.7), and biochemical blood results (Table A.8).

Table A.5 Pulmonary function tests.

Age (year)	FEV_1 (l)		FVC (L)		FEV_1/FVC (%)		PEFR (l/min)	
	M	F	M	F	M	F	M	F
20	4.15	3.09	4.95	3.83	82.5	81.0	625	433
30	4.00	2.94	4.84	3.68	80.6	79.9	612	422
40	3.69	2.64	4.62	3.38	76.9	77.7	586	401
50	3.38	2.34	4.40	3.08	73.1	75.5	560	380
60	3.06	2.04	4.18	2.78	69.4	73.2	533	359
70	2.75	1.74	3.96	2.48	65.7	71.0	507	338

M, ♂ assuming height of 175 cm; F, ♀ assuming height of 160 cm.

Table A.6 Arterial/mixed venous blood gases.

	Mixed venous	Arterial
pH	7.32–7.42	7.36–7.44
PO_2	4.9–5.6 kPa (37–42 mmHg)	12.0–14.7 kPa (90–110 mmHg)
PCO_2	5.3–6.9 kPa (40–52 mmHg)	4.5–6.1 kPa (34–46 mmHg)
SaO_2	>75%	>97%
HCO_3^-	24–30 mmol/l	
Lactate	<2 mmol/l	
Base excess	± 2 mmol/l	
Anion gap	8–12 mmol/l (calculated from $(Na^+ + K^-) - (HCO_3^- + Cl^-)$)	

Table A.7 Normal blood results (haematology)

Measurement	Reference range
White cell count	4.0–11.0 × 10^9/L
Red cell count	♂ 4.5–6.5 × 10^{12}/L, ♀ 3.9–5.6 × 10^{12}/L
Haemoglobin	♂ 135–180g/L, ♀ 115–160g/L
Packed red cell volume (haematocrit)	♂ 0.4–0.54L/L, ♀ 0.37–0.47L/L
Mean cell volume	76–96fL
Mean cell haemoglobin	27–32pg
Neutrophils	2.0–7.5 × 10^9/L (40–75% of WCC)
Lymphocytes	1.3–3.5 × 10^9/L (20–45% of WCC)
Eosinophils	0.04–0.44 × 10^9/L (1–6% of WCC)
Basophils	0.0–0.10 × 10^9/L (0.1% of WCC)
Monocytes	0.2–0.8 × 10^9/L (2–10% of WCC)
Platelet count	150–400 × 10^9/L
Prothrombin time (factors I, II, VII, X)	10–14s
Activated partial thromboplastin time (VIII, IX, XI, XII)	35–45s
INR: Normal Anticoagulation targets: AF Treatment DVT/PE Prosthetic valve	 1 2.5 (± 0.5) 2.5 (± 0.5) 3.5 (± 0.5)

Table A.8 Normal blood results (biochemistry)

	Specimen	Reference interval
Adrenocorticotrophic hormone	P	<80ng/L
Alanine aminotransferase (ALT)	P	5–35IU/L
Albumin	P	35–50g/L
Aldosterone	P	100–500pmol/L
Alkaline phosphatase	P	30–300IU/L (adults)
Amylase	P	0–180 Somogyi units/dL
Antidiuretic hormone (ADH)	P	0.9–4.6pmol/L
Aspartate transaminase (AST)	P	5–35IU/L
Bicarbonate	P	24–30mmol/L
Bilirubin	P	3–17 micromoles/L
Calcitonin	P	<0.1 micrograms/L
Calcium (ionized)	P	1.0–1.25mmol/L
Calcium (total)	P	2.12–2.65mmol/L
Chloride	P	95–105mmol/L
Cholesterol	P	3.9–7.8mmol/L
Very-low-density lipoprotein (VLDL) Low-density lipoprotein (LDL) High-density lipoprotein (HDL)	P P P	0.128–0.645mmol/L 1.55–4.4mmol/L 0.9–1.93mmol/L
Cholinesterase	P	♂ 5900–12220U/L ♀ 4650–10440U/L
Cortisol	P	a.m. 450–700nmol/L Midnight 80–280nmol/L
Creatine kinase (CK)	P	25–195IU/L
Creatinine (related to lean body mass)	P	♂ 70–110 micromoles/L ♀ 60–100 micromoles/L
CRP	P	0–12mg/L
Ferritin	P	12–200 micrograms/L
Folate	S	2.1 micrograms/L
Gamma-glutamyl transpeptidase	P	11–51IU/L
Glucose (fasting)	P	3.5–5.5mmol/L
Growth hormone	P	<20mu/L
HbA1c (= glycosylated Hb)	B	2.3–6.5%
Iron	S	♂ 14–31 micromoles/L ♀11–30 micromoles/L

Reproduced from C. Gibson and F. Roberts. Anaesthesia Data. In: *Oxford Handbook of Anaesthesia*. K. Allman, et al. (Eds.). Oxford, UK: Oxford University Press. Copyright © 2015, OUP. Reproduced with permission of the Licensor through PLSclear. DOI: 10.1093/med/9780198719410.001.0001.

(*Continued*)

Table A.8 (*Contd.*)

	Specimen	Reference interval
Magnesium	P	0.7–1mmol/L
Osmolality	P	278–305mOsmol/kg
Parathyroid hormone (PTH)	P	<0.8–8.5pmol/L
Phosphate (inorganic)	P	0.8–1.45mmol/L
Potassium	P	3.5–5.0mmol/L
Protein (total)	P	60–80g/L
Red cell folate	B	0.36–1.44 micromoles/L (160–640 micrograms/L)
Renin (erect/recumbent)	P	2.8–4.5/1.1–2.7pmol/mL/hr
Sodium	P	135–145mmol/L
Thyroid-binding globulin (TBG)	P	7–17mg/L
Thyroid-stimulating hormone (TSH) Normal range widens with age	P	0.5–5.7mu/L
Thyroxine (T_4)	P	70–140mmol/L
Thyroxine (free)	P	9–22pmol/L
Total iron binding capacity	S	54–75 micromoles/L
Triglyceride	P	0.55–1.90mmol/L
Tri-iodothyronine (T_3)	P	1.2–3.0nmol/L
Troponin T (taken at least 12hr after onset of chest pain)	P	0–0.01 micrograms/L normal 0.01–0.1 micrograms/L suspicious >0.1 micrograms/L diagnostic of MI
Urate	P	♂ 210–480 micromoles/L ♀ 150–390 micromoles/L
Urea	P	2.5–6.7mmol/L
Vitamin B12	S	0.13–0.68nmol/L (>150ng/L)
Renal		
	Reference interval	
Glomerular filtration rate	4>120mL/min	
Renal blood flow	1200mL/min	
Urine output	0.5–1.0mL/kg/hr	
Urine osmolality	350–1000mOsmol/kg	

B, whole blood (edetic acid EDTA bottle); P, plasma (e.g. heparin bottle); S, serum (clotted; no anticoagulant).

Note: there is minor variation in the normal ranges quoted by different laboratories.

Anaesthesia cart: suggested equipment

Preparation of drugs + intravenous (IV) access

- Syringes 2 ml, 5 ml, 10 ml, 20 ml.
- Needles, different sizes.
- IV cannulae 24G though 16G.
- Three-way taps (useful, not essential).
- Adhesive tape for securing cannulae and labelling syringes.
- Gauze and disinfectant, e.g. iodine, for cleaning skin.
- Pen for labelling.
- Intraosseous access device (can use 19G hypodermic needle).

Miscellaneous

- Suction tubes CH10 through CH18.
- Nasogastric tubes CH10 through CH18.
- Urine bags and bladder syringe (50 ml).

Airway

- Self-inflating bags, adult and paediatric.
- Facemasks, neonatal to adult.
- Endotracheal tubes 3.0 mm though 8.0 mm (half sizes or full sizes with cuffs).
- Laryngeal masks, sizes 2 through 5.
- Oropharyngeal ('Guedel') airways, neonatal to adult.
- Nasopharyngeal airways, paediatric to adult.
- Laryngoscope handles, blades size 0 to 4 curved, size 0 to 1 straight.
- Magill forceps, large and small.
- Oxygen masks, adult and paediatric.
- Heat moisture exchanger (HME) filters.

Regional anaesthesia

- Regional anaesthesia needles.
- Spinal needles.
- Syringes 5 ml and 20 ml.
- Sterile drapes.
- Sterile gauze.

Emergency equipment

- Bougies, different sizes.
- Laryngeal masks, sizes 2 through 5.
- Cricotomy set or blade + forceps.
- Tracheotomy tubes, size 4–8.
- Laryngeal masks, sizes 2 through 5 (if not in Airway section).

World Health Organization (WHO) surgical safety checklist

The example checklist (Figure A.12) should be adapted to suit local circumstances.

World Health Organization

SURGICAL SAFETY CHECKLIST (FIRST EDITION)

Before induction of anaesthesia ▸▸▸▸▸▸▸▸▸ Before skin incision ▸▸▸▸▸▸▸▸▸▸▸▸▸ Before patient leaves operating room

SIGN IN

- ☐ **PATIENT HAS CONFIRMED**
  - IDENTITY
  - SITE
  - PROCEDURE
  - CONSENT
- ☐ **SITE MARKED/NOT APPLICABLE**
- ☐ **ANAESTHESIA SAFETY CHECK COMPLETED**
- ☐ **PULSE OXIMETER ON PATIENT AND FUNCTIONING**

DOES PATIENT HAVE A:

KNOWN ALLERGY?
- ☐ NO
- ☐ YES

DIFFICULT AIRWAY/ASPIRATION RISK?
- ☐ NO
- ☐ YES, AND EQUIPMENT/ASSISTANCE AVAILABLE

RISK OF >500ML BLOOD LOSS (7ML/KG IN CHILDREN)?
- ☐ NO
- ☐ YES, AND ADEQUATE INTRAVENOUS ACCESS AND FLUIDS PLANNED

TIME OUT

- ☐ **CONFIRM ALL TEAM MEMBERS HAVE INTRODUCED THEMSELVES BY NAME AND ROLE**
- ☐ **SURGEON, ANAESTHESIA PROFESSIONAL AND NURSE VERBALLY CONFIRM**
  - PATIENT
  - SITE
  - PROCEDURE

ANTICIPATED CRITICAL EVENTS

- ☐ **SURGEON REVIEWS:** WHAT ARE THE CRITICAL OR UNEXPECTED STEPS, OPERATIVE DURATION, ANTICIPATED BLOOD LOSS?
- ☐ **ANAESTHESIA TEAM REVIEWS**: ARE THERE ANY PATIENT-SPECIFIC CONCERNS?
- ☐ **NURSING TEAM REVIEWS:** HAS STERILITY (INCLUDING INDICATOR RESULTS) BEEN CONFIRMED? ARE THERE EQUIPMENT ISSUES OR ANY CONCERNS?

HAS ANTIBIOTIC PROPHYLAXIS BEEN GIVEN WITHIN THE LAST 60 MINUTES?
- ☐ YES
- ☐ NOT APPLICABLE

IS ESSENTIAL IMAGING DISPLAYED?
- ☐ YES
- ☐ NOT APPLICABLE

SIGN OUT

NURSE VERBALLY CONFIRMS WITH THE TEAM:

- ☐ **THE NAME OF THE PROCEDURE RECORDED**
- ☐ **THAT INSTRUMENT, SPONGE AND NEEDLE COUNTS ARE CORRECT** (OR NOT APPLICABLE)
- ☐ **HOW THE SPECIMEN IS LABELLED** (INCLUDING PATIENT NAME)
- ☐ **WHETHER THERE ARE ANY EQUIPMENT PROBLEMS TO BE ADDRESSED**
- ☐ **SURGEON, ANAESTHESIA PROFESSIONAL AND NURSE REVIEW THE KEY CONCERNS FOR RECOVERY AND MANAGEMENT OF THIS PATIENT**

THIS CHECKLIST IS NOT INTENDED TO BE COMPREHENSIVE. ADDITIONS AND MODIFICATIONS TO FIT LOCAL PRACTICE ARE ENCOURAGED.

Figure A.12 World Health Organization (WHO) surgical safety checklist.

Reproduced with permission of the World Health Organization. Surgical Safety Checklist. whqlibdoc.who.int/publications/2009/9789241598590_eng_Checklist.pdf.

Adult advanced life support

Figure A.13 shows an algorithm for advanced life support.

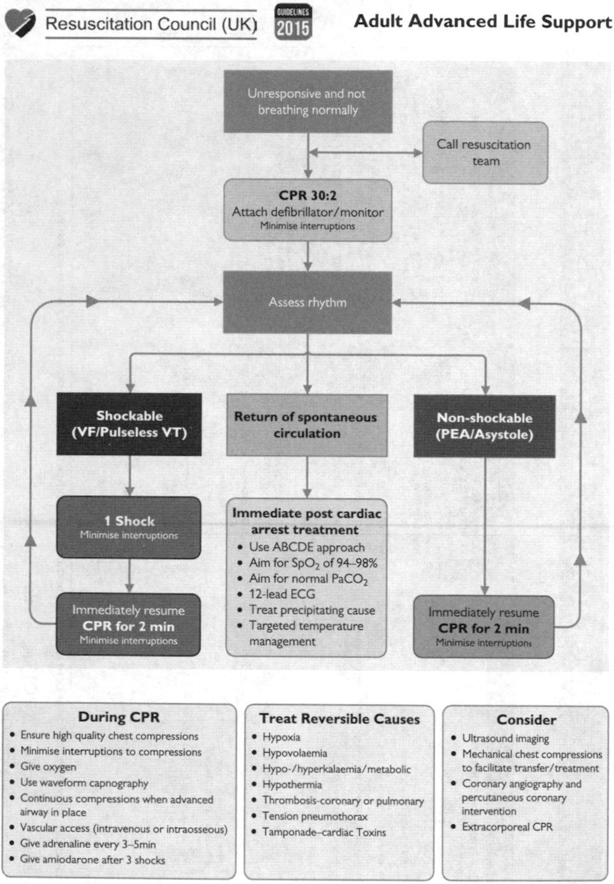
Resuscitation Council (UK)
GUIDELINES 2015
Adult Advanced Life Support
Unresponsive and not breathing normally
Call resuscitation team
CPR 30:2
Attach defibrillator/monitor
Minimise interruptions
Assess rhythm
Shockable (VF/Pulseless VT)
Return of spontaneous circulation
Non-shockable (PEA/Asystole)
1 Shock
Minimise interruptions
Immediately resume
CPR for 2 min
Minimise interruptions
Immediate post cardiac arrest treatment
• Use ABCDE approach
• Aim for SpO_2 of 94–98%
• Aim for normal $PaCO_2$
• 12-lead ECG
• Treat precipitating cause
• Targeted temperature management
Immediately resume
CPR for 2 min
Minimise interruptions
During CPR
• Ensure high quality chest compressions
• Minimise interruptions to compressions
• Give oxygen
• Use waveform capnography
• Continuous compressions when advanced airway in place
• Vascular access (intravenous or intraosseous)
• Give adrenaline every 3–5min
• Give amiodarone after 3 shocks
Treat Reversible Causes
• Hypoxia
• Hypovolaemia
• Hypo-/hyperkalaemia/metabolic
• Hypothermia
• Thrombosis-coronary or pulmonary
• Tension pneumothorax
• Tamponade–cardiac Toxins
Consider
• Ultrasound imaging
• Mechanical chest compressions to facilitate transfer/treatment
• Coronary angiography and percutaneous coronary intervention
• Extracorporeal CPR

Figure A.13 Adult advanced life support.

Reproduced with the kind permission of the Resuscitation Council (UK).

Paediatric advanced life support

Figure A.14 shows an algorithm for paediatric advanced life support.

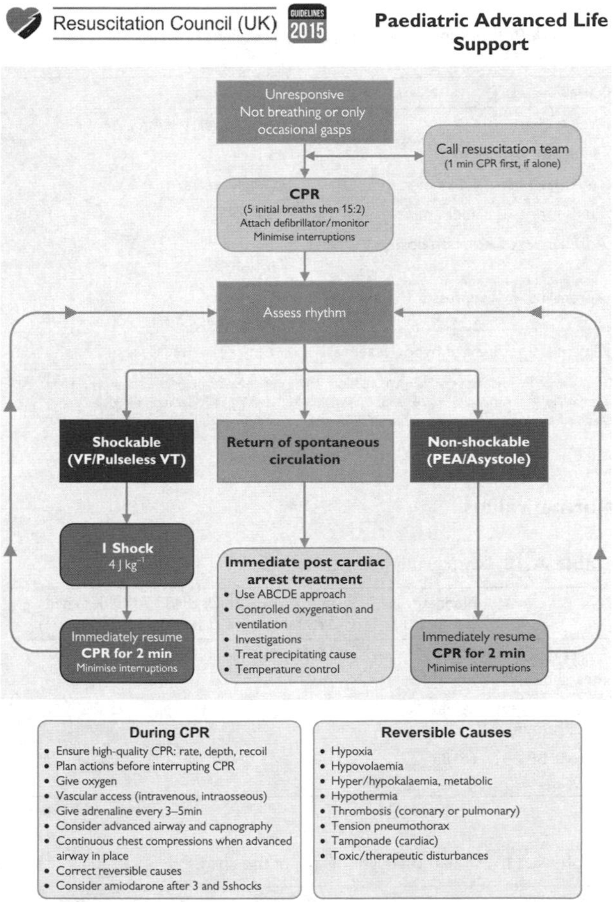
Resuscitation Council (UK)
GUIDELINES 2015
Paediatric Advanced Life Support
Unresponsive
Not breathing or only occasional gasps
Call resuscitation team
(1 min CPR first, if alone)
CPR
(5 initial breaths then 15:2)
Attach defibrillator/monitor
Minimise interruptions
Assess rhythm
Shockable
(VF/Pulseless VT)
Return of spontaneous circulation
Non-shockable
(PEA/Asystole)
1 Shock
4 J kg-1
Immediate post cardiac arrest treatment
• Use ABCDE approach
• Controlled oxygenation and ventilation
• Investigations
• Treat precipitating cause
• Temperature control
Immediately resume
CPR for 2 min
Minimise interruptions
Immediately resume
CPR for 2 min
Minimise interruptions
During CPR
• Ensure high-quality CPR: rate, depth, recoil
• Plan actions before interrupting CPR
• Give oxygen
• Vascular access (intravenous, intraosseous)
• Give adrenaline every 3–5min
• Consider advanced airway and capnography
• Continuous chest compressions when advanced airway in place
• Correct reversible causes
• Consider amiodarone after 3 and 5shocks
Reversible Causes
• Hypoxia
• Hypovolaemia
• Hyper/hypokalaemia, metabolic
• Hypothermia
• Thrombosis (coronary or pulmonary)
• Tension pneumothorax
• Tamponade (cardiac)
• Toxic/therapeutic disturbances

Figure A.14 Paediatric advanced life support.

Reproduced with the kind permission of the Resuscitation Council (UK).

Paediatric quick reference and formulary

Emergency calculations

Table A.9 Emergency calculations for children >1 year old: 'WETFLAG'.

Variable	Calculation
Weight (kg)	(Age in years + 4) × 2
Energy for defibrillation (J)	4 J/kg
Tube size (internal diameter, mm)	(Age in years/4) + 4.5
Fluids for resuscitation (ml/kg)	20 ml/kg
Adrenaline resuscitation dose	10 µg/kg 0.1 ml/kg of 1/10,000
Adrenaline as vasopressor bolus dose	1 µg/kg 0.1 ml/kg of 1/100,000
Glucose, treatment of hypoglycaemia	2 ml/kg of 10% glucose

Normal values

Table A.10 Normal physiological values.

	Neonate (<1 month)	Infant (<2 years)	Small child (2–5 years)	Older child (5–12 years)
Heart rate (beats/min)	110–160	100–140	80–120	60–100
Respiratory rate (breaths/min)	30–40	25–35	25–30	15–20
Systolic BP (mmHg)	65–85	80–100	95–110	100–115

Table A.11 Estimated weight by age of the child.

Age of child	Estimated weight (kg)
Term baby	3.0–3.5
<1 year	(Age in months × 0.5) + 4
1–5 years	(Age in years × 2) +8
6–12 years	(Age in years × 3) +7

Airway sizes

Table A.12 Laryngeal mask airway (LMA) size according to child's weight.

LMA size	Weight of child (kg)
1	<7.5
1½	7.5–12.5
2	12.5–20
2½	20–30
3	30–50
4	>50
5	70–100

Table A.13 Endotracheal tube size by age (weight).

Age	Tube size (uncuffed) (mm)	Tube size (cuffed) (mm)	Approx. length of tube at the lips (cm)
Neonate (3 kg)	3.0–3.5	2.5–3.0	9–10
6 months (6 kg)	3.5–4.0	3.0–3.5	9–12
1 year (10 kg)	4.0–4.5	3.5–4.0	12–13
Over 1 year	(Age/4.0) + 4.5	(Age/4) + 3.5	(Age/2) + 12

Paediatric formulary

Table A.14 Emergency drugs.

Drug	Dose	Route
Adrenaline: cardiac arrest	Cardiac arrest: 10 μg/kg (0.1 ml/kg of 1:10,000)	IV
Adrenaline: anaphylaxis	IM under 6 years 150 μg (0.15 ml of 1:1,000)	IM
	IM 6–12 years: 300 μg (0.3 ml of 1:1000)	IM
	IV: 1 μg/kg (0.1 ml/kg of 1:100,000)	IV
Adrenaline: as inotrope*	1 μg/kg (0.1 ml/kg of 1:100,000) bolus	IV
Atropine	20 μg/kg	IV
Suxamethonium	1–2 mg/kg	IV

*For inotropic infusion, see 'Cardiovascular Support' in Chapter 12 (p. 272).

IV, intravenous; IM, intramuscular.

Table A.15 Premedication.

Drug	Dose	Timing	Route
Atropine	10 μg/kg	Induction	IV
	20 μg/kg	30 min pre-op	IM
	40 μg/kg	60 min pre-op	PO
Chloral hydrate	25–50 mg/kg	60 min pre-op	PO
Clonidine	4 μg/kg	30–60 min pre-op	PO
	2–4 μg/kg	30–60 min pre-op	IM
Ketamine	5–10 mg/kg	10–20 min pre-op	PO
	3–5 mg/kg	5 min pre-op	IM
Midazolam	0.5 mg/kg (max. 20 mg)	30 min pre-op	PO
	0.05–0.1 mg/kg	5 min pre-op	IV
	0.2 mg/kg (max. 20 mg)	20–30 min pre-op	Buccal
Lorazepam (>12 years)	0.05 mg/kg (max. 2 mg)	20 min pre-op	PO
Temazepam (>12 years)	0.3 mg/kg	30–60 min pre-op	PO

IV, intravenous; IM, intramuscular; PO, per oram.

Table A.16 Induction.

Drug	Dose	Route
Etomidate	0.3 mg/kg	IV
Ketamine	1–2 mg/kg over 1 year; 0.5–1 mg/kg under 1 year	IV
	5–10 mg/kg	IM
Propofol	2–3 mg/kg	IV
Thiopental	2–4 mg/kg (neonate), 5–6 mg/kg (child)	IV

IV, intravenous; IM, intramuscular.

Table A.17 Muscle relaxants (intubating dose).

Drug	Dose	Route
Atracurium	0.3–0.6 mg/kg	IV
Cisatracurium	0.1–0.2 mg/kg	IV
Mivacurium	0.1–0.2 mg/kg	IV
Pancuronium	0.1 mg/kg	IV
Rocuronium	0.6–1.2 mg/kg	IV
Suxamethonium	1–2 mg/kg	IV
Vecuronium	0.1 mg/kg	IV

IV, intravenous.

Table A.18 Antiemetics.

Drug	Dose	Frequency	Route
Cyclizine	1 mg/kg	8 hourly	IV
Dexamethasone	0.1 mg/kg	6 hourly	IV
Droperidolss	0.03–0.07 mg/kg: max. 1.25 mg	6 hourly	IV
Metoclopramide	0.15 mg/kg	8 hourly	IV/PO
Ondansetron	0.15 mg/kg	8 hourly	IV/PO
Prochlorperazine (>10 kg)	0.25 mg/kg	8 hourly	PO
	0.1–0.2 mg/kg	8 hourly	IM

IV, intravenous; IM, intramuscular; PO, per oram.

Table A.19 Intraoperative analgesia.

Drug	Dose		Route
Alfentanil	5–20 μg/kg slow bolus, then 10 μg/kg supplemental doses		IV
Diclofenac (>1 year)	1 mg/kg (max 50 mg)		PR
Fentanyl	1–5 μg/kg (up to 50 μg/kg if ventilating postoperatively)		IV
Morphine sulfate	50–100 μg/kg boluses		IV
Paracetamol	Neonates	10 mg/kg	IV
		20 mg/kg (loading dose)	PR
	Others	15 mg/kg	IV
		30 mg/kg (loading dose)	PR
Pethidine (>12 years)	0.5–1 mg/kg (max. 100 mg)		IV
Remifentanil	0.5–1 μg/kg slow bolus		IV
	0.1–0.5 μg/kg/min infusion		
Tramadol (>1 year)*	1 mg/kgσ		IV

*Warning: unpredictable analgesic effect. There is potential for rapid metabolism, leading to a more potent effect and respiratory depression.

IV, intravenous; PR, per rectum.

Table A.20 Reversal drugs.

Drug	Dose	Route
Atropine	0.2 mg/kg	IV
Glycopyrronium	0.01 mg/kg	IV
Neostigmine	0.05–0.07 mg/kg	IV
Sugammadex	2 mg/kg (if T2 present train of four)	IV

IV, intravenous.

Table A.21 Antagonists.

Drug	Dose	Route
Naloxone	0.01 mg/kg incrementally	IV
Flumazenil	0.01–0.02 mg/kg (max dose 0.1 mg)	IV

IV, intravenous.

Table A.22 Postoperative analgesia.

Drug	Dose	Frequency	Route
Codeine phosphate (>12 years)*	1 mg/kg 6 hourly (max. 240 mg/day)	6 hourly	PO/PR
σ	*Avoid in children under 12 years*		
Diclofenac (>1 year)	1 mg/kg	8 hourly	PO/PR
Ibuprofen (>3 months)	5–10 mg/kg (max. 30 mg/kg/day)	8 hourly	PO
Morphine sulfate: infant 1–3 months	50–100 μg/kg	4 hourly	PO
Morphine sulfate: > 3 months	100–200 μg/kg	4 hourly	PO
Paracetamol: neonates	10–15 mg/kg (max. 60 mg/kg/day)	6 hourly	PO
	10 mg/kg (max. 30 mg/kg/day)	6 hourly	IV
Paracetamol: others	15 mg/kg (max. 75 mg/kg/day or 4g/day)	6 hourly	PO/PR
	15 mg/kg (max. 60 mg/kg/day)	6 hourly	IV
Tramadol (>1 year)* σ	1 mg/kg If >50 kg: 50–100 mg (max. 400 mg/day)	6 hourly	PO/IV

*Warning: unpredictable analgesic effect. There is potential for rapid metabolism, leading to a more potent effect and respiratory depression.

IV, intravenous; PO, per oram; PR, per rectum.

Essential anaesthetic drugs

The following is adapted from the 19th WHO Model List of Essential Medicines April 2015.

Anaesthetic

- Halothane.
- Isoflurane.
- Nitrous oxide.
- Oxygen.
- Ketamine.
- Propofol (thiopental may be used as an alternative).
- Bupivacaine.
- Lidocaine.
- Lidocaine + adrenaline.
- Atropine.
- Midazolam (diazepam is an alternative).
- Morphine.

Inotropes

- Adrenaline.
- Ephedrine (optional), phenylephrine (optional).

Medicines for pain and palliative care

- Ibuprofen.
- Paracetamol.
- Codeine.
- Morphine.

Muscle relaxants and cholinesterase inhibitors

- Atracurium.
- Neostigmine.
- Suxamethonium.
- Vecuronium.

Medical treatment

- Hydralazine.
- Furosemide.
- Metoprolol.
- Salbutamol.
- Glyceryl trinitrate (GTN).
- Glucose 50%.
- Hydrocortisone.
- Calcium chloride 10%.
- Potassium chloride 20%.
- Tranexamic acid.

Consider if resources allow

- Naloxone.
- Cyclizine or ondansetron.
- Tramadol.

Drug formulary

Table A.23 Drug formulary

Drug	Description and perioperative indications	Cautions and contraindications	Side effects	Dose (paediatric)	Dose (adult)
Abciximab	Synthetic monoclonal antibody. Glycoprotein IIb/IIIa inhibitor (powerful antiplatelet action). Used to prevent ischaemic complications before or during PCI	Intracranial or intraspinal surgery within 2 months, stroke within 2yr, trauma, or neoplasm. Major surgery. Ongoing haemorrhage. Hypertensive retinopathy. Can only be given once	Haemorrhage. Bradycardia, hypotension, nausea and vomiting. Chest and back pain. May provoke hypersensitivity reactions. Increased bleeding in hepatic/renal impairment		250 micrograms/kg bolus over 1 min, then infuse at 0.125 micrograms/kg/min (max 10 micrograms/min). Start 10–60min before coronary intervention, and continue for at least 12hr; unstable angina, start 24hr prior to PCI
Acetazolamide	Carbonic anhydrase inhibitor used for acute reduction of intraocular pressure. Weak diuretic	Extravasation causes necrosis. Hypokalaemia/hyponatraemia. Hyperchloraemic acidosis. Avoid in severe hepatic impairment	Thrombocytopenia, nausea, vomiting, flushing, paraesthesiae, rash	1 month–12yr: PO/IV 5mg/kg 2–4 times daily (max 750mg). 12–18yr 250mg 2–4 times daily	IV/PO: 0.25–1g daily in divided doses

Adenosine	Endogenous nucleoside with antiarrhythmic activity. Slows conduction through AV node. Treatment of acute paroxysmal SVT (including WPW) or differentiation of SVT from VT. Duration 10s	2nd– or 3rd–degree heart block. Long QT. Asthma/COPD. Reduce dose in heart transplant or dipyridamole treatment	Flushing, dyspnoea, headache, AV block, angina—transient	1 month–1yr: 0.1mg/kg fast IV bolus, increasing by 0.05–0.1 mg/kg every 1–2 min to max 0.5mg/kg (max 12mg). >12yr: as adult	6mg fast IV bolus, followed by 12mg at 1–2min, then further 12mg at 1–2min, as necessary. Reduce to quarter of dose if giving with dipyridamole
Adrenaline	Endogenous catecholamine with α and β action: 1. Treatment of anaphylaxis 2. Bronchodilator 3. Positive inotrope 4. Given by nebulizer for croup 5. Prolongation of LA action. 1:1000 contains 1mg/mL, 1:10 000 contains 100 micrograms/mL, 1:200 000 contains 5 micrograms/mL 6. Cardiac arrest	Arrhythmias, especially with halothane. Caution in elderly. Via central catheter whenever possible	Hypertension, tachycardia, anxiety, hyperglycaemia, arrhythmias. Reduces uterine blood flow	1. Refer to paediatric anaphylaxis emergency (see ➔ p. 937) 2. ETT 0.1mL/kg of 1:1000 (100 micrograms/kg) 3. Infusion 0.05–1 micrograms/kg/min 4. Neb 0.5mL/kg (up to 5mL) 1:1000 5. Maximum dose for infiltration 2 micrograms/kg 6.10 micrograms/kg refer to cardiac arrest (see ➔ p. 926)	1–3. IV/IM/ET 1mL aliquots of 1:10 000 up to 5–10mL (0.5–1mg). Infusion 2–20 micrograms/min (0.04–0.4 micrograms/kg/min) 4. Nebulization 5mL 1:1000 (max 5mg) 5. Maximum dose for infiltration 2 micrograms/kg 6. 1mg(10mL of 1:10 000), every 3–5 min

IV, intravenous. IM, intramuscular. SC, subcutaneous. PO, *per os* (oral). SL, sublingual. ET, endotracheal. od, once daily. bd, twice daily. tds, three times daily. qds, four times daily. NR, not recommended. Doses are IV and dilutions in 0.9% NaCl unless otherwise stated.

(*Continued*)

Table A.23 *(Contd.)*

Drug	Description and perioperative indications	Cautions and contraindications	Side effects	Dose (paediatric)	Dose (adult)
Alcohol	See ethanol				
Alfentanil	Short–acting, potent, opioid analgesic. Duration 10min Sedation in ICU		Respiratory depression, bradycardia, hypotension. Prolonged half–life in neonates Use IBW	Injection: 5–20 micrograms/kg, then 10 micrograms/kg boluses Infusion: 10–100 micrograms/kg over 10min, then 0.5–1 micrograms/kg/min	250–750 micrograms (5–10 micrograms/ kg). Attenuation of CVS response to intubation: 10–20 micrograms/kg Sedation: infusion 2mg/hr
Alimemazine (trimeprazine)	Sedative antihistamine (paediatric pre med)			PO: 2mg/kg 1–2hr preop Ametop® (over 2yr) max 100mg daily	
Am etop®	See tetracaine				
Aminophylline	Methylxanthine bronchodilator used in prevention and treatment of asthma. Converted to theophylline, a phosphodiesterase inhibitor. Serum levels 10–20mg/L (55–110 micromoles/L)	Caution in patients already receiving oral or IV theophyllines. Where serum level known, aminophylline 0.6mg/kg should increase level by 1mg/L	Palpitations, tachycardia, tachypnoea, seizures, nausea, arrhythmias	IV 5mg/kg over 20min, then 0.5–1 mg/kg/hr infusion according to levels	5mg/kg over 20min, then 0.5mg/kg/hr infusion according to levels

Amiodarone	Mainly class III antiarrhythmic useful in treatment of supraventricular and ventricular arrhythmias	Via central catheter. Sinoatrial heart block, thyroid dysfunction, pregnancy, porphyria, iodine sensitivity. Dilute in dextrose 5% not saline	Commonly causes thyroid dysfunction and reversible corneal deposits	>1yr IV: 5mg/kg over 20–120min. Infusion: 5 micrograms/kg/min, max 1.2g/24hr. 5mg/kg slow IV bolus for defib–resistant VF/VT	5mg/kg over 20–120min, followed by infusion if required, maximum 1.2g in 24hr. 300mg slow IV bolus for defib–resistant VF/VT
Amoxicillin	Broad–spectrum penicillin antibiotic 1. UTI/CAP/infections 2. *Listeria* meningitis or endococcal endocarditis	History of allergy	Nausea, diarrhoea, rash	1. IV/IM: 20–30mg/kgtds (double in severe infections) 2. 50mg/kg max 2g every 4hr	1. PO/IM/IV: 500mg tds, increased to 1g qds in severe infections 2. 2g every 4hr
Atenolol	Cardioselective β–blocker. Long–acting	Asthma, heart failure, AV block, verapamil treatment	Bradycardia, hypotension, and decreased contractility	0.05mg/kg every 5min—max four doses	5–10mg over 10min
Atracurium	Benzylisoquinolinium non–depolarizing muscle relaxant. Undergoes temperature– and pH–dependent Hofmann elimination (to laudanosine), plus non–specific enzymatic ester hydrolysis. Useful in severe renal or hepatic disease. Duration 20–35min	NMB potentiated by aminoglycosides, loop diuretics, magnesium, lithium, ↓ temp, ↓ K^+, ↓ pH, prior use of suxamethonium, volatile agents. Store at 2–8°C	Mild histamine release and rash common with higher doses. Flush with saline before and after	Intubation: 0.3–0.6mg/kg Maintenance: 0.1–0.2mg/ kg Infusion: 0.3–0.6mg/kg/hr, monitor NMB	Intubation: 0.3–0.6mg/kg Maintenance: 0.1–0.2mg/ kg Infusion: 0.3–0.6mg/kg/hr, monitor neuromuscular blockade Use IBW

IV, intravenous. IM, intramuscular. SC, subcutaneous. PO, *per os* (oral). SL, sublingual. ET, endotracheal. od, once daily. bd, twice daily. tds, three times daily. qds, four times daily. NR, not recommended. Doses are IV and dilutions in 0.9% NaCl unless otherwise stated.

(Continued)

Table A.23 (*Contd.*)

Drug	Description and perioperative indications	Cautions and contraindications	Side effects	Dose (paediatric)	Dose (adult)
Atropine	Muscarinic acetylcholine antagonist. Vagal blockade at AV and sinus node increases heart rate (transient decrease at low doses due to weak agonist effect). Tertiary amine, therefore crosses blood–brain barrier	Obstructive uropathy and CVS disease. Glaucoma, myasthenia gravis	Decreases secretions and lower oesophageal sphincter tone, relaxes bronchial smooth muscle. Confusion in elderly	IV: 10–20 micrograms/kg. Control of muscarinic effects of neostigmine: 20 micrograms/kg. IM/ SC: 10–30 micrograms/kg. PO: 40 micrograms/kg	300–600 micrograms. Prevention of muscarinic effects of neostigmine: 600–1200 micrograms
Benzylpenicillin	Broad–spectrum antibiotic	History of allergy	Nausea, diarrhoea, rash	25mg/kg qds. 50mg/kg qds for severe infections (max 2.4g 4–hourly)	600mg–1.2g qds. Higher doses may also be used (max 2.4g 4–hourly)
Bicarbonate (sodium)	Alkaline salt used for correction of acidosis and to enhance onset of action of LAs. 8.4%, 1000mmol/L. Dose (mmol) in acidosis: weight (kg) x base deficit x 0.3	Precipitation with calcium–containing solutions, increased CO_2 production, necrosis on extravasation. Via central catheter if possible	Alkalosis, hypokalaemia, hypernatraemia, hypocalcaemia	Dependent on degree of acidosis. 1mL/kgof 8.4% solution (1mmol/kg)	Dependent on degree of acidosis. Resuscitation: 50mL 8.4%, then recheck blood gases. Bicarbonation of LA 1mL 8.4% to 20mL bupivacaine. 1 mL of 8.4% to 10mL lidocaine/prilocaine
Bupivacaine	Amide–type LA used for infiltration, epidural, and spinal anaesthesia. Slower onset than lidocaine. Duration 3–6hr (slightly prolonged by adrenaline), pKa 8.1	Greater cardiotoxicity than other local agents. Do not use for IVRA. Adrenal ine–containi ng solutions contain preservative and do not prolong action	Toxicity: tongue/circumoral numbness, restlessness, tinnitus, seizures, cardiac arrest	Infiltration/epidural: maximum dose dependent upon injection site—2mg/kg/4hr recommended	0.25–0.75% solution. Infiltration/epidural: maximum dose dependent upon injection site—2mg/kg/ 4hr (2mg/kg with adrenaline). 0.75% solution contraindicated in pregnancy

Buprenorphine	Opioid with both agonist and antagonist actions. Duration 6hr	May precipitate withdrawal in opioid–dependent patients. Only partially reversed by naloxone	Nausea, respiratory depression, constipation	6 months–12yr: IV 3–6 micrograms/kg tds (max 9 micrograms/kg) 12–18yr: IV 300–600 micrograms tds	Slow IV/IM: 300–600 micrograms qds. SL: 200–400 micrograms qds
Caffeine citrate	Mild stimulant effective in the treatment of post–dural puncture headache. IV preparation available as caffeine sodium benzoate	Monitor levels in neonates	Insomnia, weakly diuretic, excitation, tachycardia	SCBU: loading dose 20mg/kg, then 5mg/kg od	IV/PO: 300–500mg bd. One cup of coffee contains 50–100mg. Soft drinks contain up to 35–50mg
Calcium chloride	Electrolyte replacement, positive inotrope, hyperkalaemia, hypermagnesaemia. Calcium chloride 10% contains Ca^{2+} 680 micromoles/mL	Necrosis on extravasation. Incompatible with bicarbonate	Arrhythmias, hypertension, hypercalcaemia	0.1 mL/kg 10% solution, slow IV	2–10 mL 10% solution (10mg/kg, 0.07mmol/kg)
Calcium gluconate	As calcium chloride. Calcium gluconate 10% contains Ca^{2+} 225 /mL	Less phlebitis than calcium chloride	As calcium chloride	0.3–0.5 mL/kg10% solution (max 20mL)	6–15mL of 10% solution (30mg/kg, 0.07mmol/kg)

IV, intravenous. IM, intramuscular. SC, subcutaneous. PO, *per os* (oral). SL, sublingual. ET, endotracheal. od, once daily. bd, twice daily. tds, three times daily. qds, four times daily. NR, not recommended. Doses are IV and dilutions in 0.9% NaCl unless otherwise stated.

(*Continued*)

Table A.23 (*Contd.*)

Drug	Description and perioperative indications	Cautions and contraindications	Side effects	Dose (paediatric)	Dose (adult)
Carboprost	Synthetic PGF2α analogue used to treat severe post–partum haemorrhage due to uterine atony (after ergometrine and oxytocin failed)	Asthma, diabetes,epilepsy, jaundice,anaemia, glaucoma. Large doses may cause uterine rupture	Fever, bronchospasm, Nausea, vomiting, flushing. May cause CVS collapse		NEVER GIVE IV. 250 micrograms deep IM or directly into the myometrium. Repeat, if needed, after at least 15min. Max dose 2mg/24hr
Cefotaxime	3rd–generation cephalosporin broad–spectrum antibiotic	10% cross–sensitivity with penicillin allergy		Neonate: 25mg/kg bd. Child: 50mg/kg bd/tds. 50mg/kg qds in severe infections (max 12g daily)	1g bd (up to 12g daily in divided doses in severe infections)
Cefuroxime	2nd–generation cephalosporin broad–spectrum antibiotic	10% cross–sensitivity with penicillin allergy		20–30mg/kg tds (max 1 –5g tds)	750mg–1.5g tds
Celecoxib	NSAID with selective inhibition of cyclo–oxygenase 2 (COX–2) enzyme. Reduced gastric, asthma, and platelet side effects	Hypersensitivity to sulfonamides and aspirin, severe renal impairment, peptic ulceration, IHD, inflammatory bowel disease		NR	PO: 100–200mg bd
Cetirizine	Non–sedative antihistamine. Relief of allergy, urticaria	Prostatic hypertrophy, urinary retention, glaucoma, porphyria	Dry mouth	PO: 1–2yr 0.25 mg/kg bd. 2–6yr: 2.5mg bd. >6yr: 5mg bd	PO: 10mg od. Half dose if eGFR <50mL/min/m^2

Chloral hydrate	Formerly a popular hypnotic in children	Avoid prolonged use. Caution in elderly, gastritis, and porphyria	Gastric irritation, ataxia	PO: 30–50mg/kg as single dose for sedation (up to 1g)	
Chlorphenamine	Sedative antihistamine. Relief of allergy, urticaria, anaphylaxis (see ➔ p. 920 for doses)	Prostatic hypertrophy, urinary retention, glaucoma, porphyria	Drowsiness, dry mouth	PO 0.1mg/kg up to 4mg qds	Slow IV/IM: 10mg qds. PO: 4mg qds
Chlorpromazine	Phenothiazine, antipsychotic. Mild a blocking action. Potent antiemetic and used for chronic hiccups	Hypotension	Extrapyramidal and anticholinergic symptoms, sedation, hypotension	1–6yr: IM/PO 0.5mg/ kg tds (max 40mg/d). 6–12yr: IM/PO 0.5mg/ kg tds (max 75mg/d). >12yr: adult dose	PO: 10–25 mg tds/75mg ON. Deep IM: 25–50mg 6– to 8–hourly
Cisatracurium	Single isomer of atracurium with greater potency, longer duration of action, and less histamine release. Duration 55min	Neuromuscular block potentiated by aminoglycosides, loop diuretics, magnesium, lithium, ↓ temp, ↓ K^+, ↓ pH, prior use of suxamethonium, volatile agents. Store at 2–8°C	Enhanced effect in myasthenia gravis, effects antagonized by anticholinesterases, e.g. neostigmine. Monitor response with peripheral nerve stimulator	Intubation: (>1 month) 150 micrograms/kg. Maintenance (>2yr) 30 micrograms/kg every 20min. Infusion: (>2yr) 0.06–0.18mg/kg/hr	Intubation: 150 micrograms/kg. Maintenance: 30 micrograms/kg every 20–30min. Infusion: 0.06–0.18mg/ kg/hr
Citrate (sodium)	Non–particulate antacid oral premedication. Aspiration prophylaxis				PO: 30mL 0.3M solution

IV, intravenous. IM, intramuscular. SC, subcutaneous. PO, *per os* (oral). SL, sublingual. ET, endotracheal. od, once daily. bd, twice daily. tds, three times daily. qds, four times daily. NR, not recommended. Doses are IV and dilutions in 0.9% NaCl unless otherwise stated.

(*Continued*)

Table A.23 (*Contd.*)

Drug	Description and perioperative indications	Cautions and contraindications	Side effects	Dose (paediatric)	Dose (adult)
Clonidine	Centrally acting α_2–agonist. Reduces requirement for opioids and volatile anaesthetics. Enhances epidural analgesia	Rebound hypertension on acute withdrawal of chronic therapy	Hypotension, sedation	Over 6 months: 1–3 micrograms/kg slowly. PO premed: 4 micrograms/kg. Caudal: 1 microgram/kg	150–300 micrograms over 5min. Epidural: 75–150 micrograms in 10mL saline
Co–amoxiclav	Mixture of amoxicillin and clavulanic acid. 1.2g contains 1g amoxicillin	See amoxicillin	Cholestatic jaundice, see amoxicillin	30mg/kg (max 1.2g) tds	1.2g tds
Cocaine	Ester–type LA and potent vasoconstrictor. Topical anaesthesia of mucous membranes (nasal passages). Duration 20–30min	Topical use only. Caution with other sympathomimetic agents, halothane, anticholinesterase deficiency. Porphyria, MAOIs	Hypertension, arrhythmias, euphoria	1–3mg/kg topical	4–10% solution. Maximum topical dose 3mg/kg
Co–codamol 8/500	Combination oral analgesic containing codeine 8mg and paracetamol 500mg	See paracetamol		NR	PO: 1–2 tablets qds (maximum eight tablets per day)
Co–codamol	Combination oral analgesic containing codeine and paracetamol (available as 8/500 or 30/500)	See paracetamol and codeine		NR	PO: 1–2 tablets qds (maximum eight tablets per day)

Co–codaprin	Combination oral analgesic containing codeine 8mg and aspirin 400mg	See ibuprofen and codeine		NR	PO: 1–2 tablets qds (maximum eight tablets per day)
Codeine phosphate	Opioid used for mild to moderate pain. Wide variation in capacity to metabolize	<12yr, <18yr with tonsillectomy/ adenoid ectomy for OSA	Nausea, vomiting, dysphoria, drowsiness, constipation	>12yrPO/IM/PR: 1mg/ kg 6–hourly (max 240mg/d for 3 days total)	PO/IM: 30–60mg 4–hourly (maximum 240mg/d)
Co–dydramol	Combination oral analgesic containing dihydrocodeine 10mg and paracetamol 500mg	See paracetamol		NR	PO: 1–2 tablets qds (maximum eight tablets per day)
Cyclizine	Antihistamine, anti muscarinic, anti–emetic agent	Caution in severe heart failure	Drowsiness, dry mouth, blurred vision, tachycardia	IV/IM/PO: 1mg/kgupto 50 mg tds	IV/IM/PO: 50mgtds
Dabigatran	Direct inhibitor of factor Xa. Uses: 1. Prophylaxis of VTE after major orthopaedic surgery 2. Prophylaxis of stroke in AF	Risk of major bleeding, severe liver disease. Reduce dose in elderly or concomitant use of verapamil or amiodarone. No routine monitoring required	Nausea, haemorrhage	NR	1. PO: 110mg 1–4hr post–operatively, then 220mg daily for 9d 2. PO:150mgbd

IV, intravenous. IM, intramuscular. SC, subcutaneous. PO, *per os* (oral). SL, sublingual. ET, endotracheal. od, once daily. bd, twice daily. tds, three times daily. qds, four times daily. NR, not recommended. Doses are IV and dilutions in 0.9% NaCl unless otherwise stated.

(*Continued*)

Table A.23 *(Contd.)*

Drug	Description and perioperative indications	Cautions and contraindications	Side effects	Dose (paediatric)	Dose (adult)
Dalteparin	LMWH used in prevention and treatment of VTE. No routine monitoring required. Complete risk assessment, and follow local policy	Risk of bleeding, renal impairment	HIT rarely	SC prophylaxis: 100U/kg od. >12yr: adult dose	SC prophylaxis: 2500–5000U od. High risk—see local policy
Dantrolene	Direct-acting skeletal muscle relaxant used in treatment of malignant hyperthermia and neuroleptic malignant syndrome. 20mg/ vial—reconstitute in 60mL warm water, and give via blood set	Avoid combination with calcium channel blockers (verapamil), as may cause hyperkalaemia and CVS collapse. Crosses placenta	Skeletal muscle weakness (22%), phlebitis (10%)	1mg/kg, repeated every 5min to a maximum of 10mg/kg	1mg/kg, repeated every 5min to a maximum of 10mg/kg. Usually 2.5mg/kg
Desmopressin	Synthetic analogue of vasopressin (ADH) with longer duration of action and reduced pressor effect. Used for neurogenic diabetes insipidus and haemophilia (enhances factor VIII activity)	Caution in hypertension and CVS disease	Hypertension, angina, abdominal pain, flushing, hyponatraemia	Diabetes insipidus: IV/ IM/SC 0.5–2 micrograms/d (not per kg). Haemophilia: 0.3 micrograms/kg (in 50mL saline over 30min IV)	Diabetes insipidus: IV/ IM/SC 0.5–2 micrograms/d (not per kg). Haemophilia: 0.3 micrograms/kg (in 50mL saline over 30min IV)

Dexamethasone	Prednisolone derivative corticosteroid. Less sodium retention than hydrocortisone. Cerebral oedema, oedema prevention, antiemetic	Interacts with anticholinesterase agents to increase weakness in myasthenia gravis. Dexamethasone 0.75mg, prednisolone 5 mg	See prednisolone	IV/IM/SC: 200–400 micrograms/kg bd. Cerebral oedema: see *BNFc*. Croup: 150 micrograms/kg, ± repeat at 12h. Antiemetic: 150 micrograms/kg (max 8mg)	IV/IM/SC: 4–8mg. Cerebral oedema: 8–16mg initially, then 5mg qds. Antiemesis 2–8 mg
Diamorphine	Potent opioid analgesic	Spinal/epidural use associated with risk of respiratory depression, pruritus, nausea	Histamine release, hypotension, bronchospasm, nausea, vomiting, pruritus, dysphoria	IV/SC: 20–100 micrograms/kg, then 15 micrograms/kg/hr. Epidural: 2.5mg in 60mL 0.125% bupivacaine at 0.1–0.4mL/kg/hr. Intranasal: 100 micrograms/ kg in 0.2mL saline	IV/IM/SC: 2.5–5mg 4–hourly. Epidural: 2.5mg diluted in 10mL LA/saline, then 0.1–0.5mg/hr. Spinal: 0.25–0.5mg
Diazepam	Long–acting benzodiazepine. Sedation or termination of status epilepticus. Alcohol withdrawal	Thrombophlebitis: emulsion (Diazemuls®) less irritant to veins. Reduce in elderly	Sedation, circulatory depression	0.2–0.3 mg/kg. Rectal: 0.5mg/kg as Stesolid® or may use IV preparation	IV/IM/PO: 2–1 Omg, repeat if required (max tds)
Diclofenac sodium	Potent NSAID analgesic for mild to moderate pain	Hypersensitivity to aspirin, asthma, severe renal impairment, peptic ulceration, proctitis	GI upset or bleeding, bronchospasm, tinnitus, fluid retention, platelet inhibition, thrombotic events	>1yr: PO/PR: 1mg/kg tds. Maximum 150mg/d. PR: NR <6 months	PO/PR: 25–50mg tds (or 100mg 18–hourly). Maximum 150mg/d

IV, intravenous. IM, intramuscular. SC, subcutaneous. PO, *per os* (oral). SL, sublingual. ET, endotracheal. od, once daily. bd, twice daily. tds, three times daily. qds, four times daily. NR, not recommended. Doses are IV and dilutions in 0.9% NaCl unless otherwise stated.

(Continued)

Table A.23 *(Contd.)*

Drug	Description and perioperative indications	Cautions and contraindications	Side effects	Dose (paediatric)	Dose (adult)
Digoxin	Cardiac glycoside. Weak inotrope and control of ventricular response in supraventricular arrhythmia. Therapeutic levels 0.8–2 micrograms/L (1.2–2.6nmol/L)	Reduce dose in elderly. Enhanced effect/toxicity in hypokalaemia. Avoid cardioversion in toxicity	Anorexia, nausea, fatigue, arrhythmias, blurred/yellow vision	Rapid IV/PO loading: 20–35 micrograms/kg stat	Rapid IV loading: 250–500 micrograms over30min. Maximum 1mg/24hr. PO loading: 1–1.5mg in divided doses over 24hr. PO maintenance: 125–250 micrograms/d
Di hydrocodeine tartrate	Opioid used for mild to moderate pain		Nausea, vomiting, dysphoria, drowsiness	PO/IM/PR:+0.5–1 mg/kg 4–hourly (max dose 60mg 4–hourly)	PO/IM: 30–60mg 4–hourly
Dobutamine	β_1–adrenergic agonist, positive inotrope and chronotrope Cardiac failure	Arrhythmias and hypertension. Phlebitis, but can be administered peripherally	Tachycardia. Decreased peripheral and pulmonary vascular resistance	Infusion: 2–20 micrograms/kg/min	Infusion: 2.5–10 micrograms/kg/min
Domperidone	Antiemetic acting on chemo receptor trigger zone and peripheral D_2 receptors	Renal impairment, QT interval prolongation. Not recommended for PONV prophylaxis	Raised prolactin. Rarely acute dystonic reactions	PO: 200–400 micrograms/kg 6– to 8–hourly	PO: 10–20 mg 4– to 6–hourly. PR: 30–60mg 4– to 6–hourly
Dopamine	Naturally occurring catecholamine with α, β_1, and dopaminergic activity. Inotropic agent	Via central catheter. Phaeochromocytoma (due to noradrenaline release)	Tachycardia, dysrhythmias	Infusion: 2–20 micrograms/kg/min	Infusion: 2–5 micrograms/kg/min

Dopexamine	Catecholamine with β2 and dopaminergic activity. Inotropic agent	Via central catheter. Phaeochromocytoma, hypokalaemia	Tachycardia	Infusion: 0.5–6 micrograms/kg/min	Infusion: 0.5–6 micrograms/kg/min
Doxapram	Respiratory stimulant acting through carotid chemoreceptors and medulla. Duration 12min	Epilepsy, airway obstruction, acute asthma, severe CVS disease	Risk of arrhythmia. Hypertension	1mg/kg slowly. Infusion: 0.5–1mg/kg/hr for 1hr. NR<12yr	1–1.5mg/kg over >30s. Infusion: 2–4mg/min
Droperidol	Butyrophenone related to haloperidol. Neuroleptic anaesthesia and potent antiemetic. Duration 4hr	α–adrenergic blocker. Parkinson's disease	Vasodilatation, hypotension. Dystonic reactions	Antiemetic: 25–50 micrograms/kg (max dose 1.25 mg qds)	Antiemetic: 0.5–2.5mg
Edrophonium	Anticholinesterase used in diagnostic assessment of myasthenia gravis; 15 times less potent than neostigmine	Short–acting (10min)	Bradycardia, AV block	20 micrograms/ kg test dose, then 80 micrograms/kg. >12yr: adult dose	1mg slow IV every 2–4min. Maximum 10mg. Reversal: 0.5mg/kg with anticholinergic
EMLA®	Eutectic mixture of 2.5% lidocaine and 2.5% prilocaine. Topical anaesthesia	Absorption of anaesthetic depends on surface area and duration of application. Avoid use on abrasions or mucous membranes	Methaemoglobinaemia in high doses	NR premature neonates. Apply 1–2g under occlusive dressing 1–5hr before procedure (max two doses/24hr)	Apply under occlusive dressing 1–5hr before procedure (max 60g)

IV, intravenous. IM, intramuscular. SC, subcutaneous. PO, *per os* (oral). SL, sublingual. ET, endotracheal. od, once daily. bd, twice daily. tds, three times daily. qds, four times daily. NR, not recommended. Doses are IV and dilutions in 0.9% NaCl unless otherwise stated.

(*Continued*)

Table A.23 (*Contd.*)

Drug	Description and perioperative indications	Cautions and contraindications	Side effects	Dose (paediatric)	Dose (adult)
Enoxaparin	LMWH used in prevention of VTE	Once–daily dosing and monitoring not usually required		SC prophylaxis: 500 micrograms/kg bd (max 40mg daily)	SC prophylaxis: 20mg (2000U) od (40mg if high–risk)
Enoximone	Type III phosphodiesterase inhibitor used in cardiac failure with increased filling pressures. Inodilator	Stenotic valvular disease, cardiomyopathy	Arrhythmias, hypotension, nausea	Initial loading dose 500 micrograms/kg, then infusion: 5–20 micrograms/kg/min for 24hr	Infusion: 90 micrograms/kg/min for 10–30min, then 5–20 micrograms/kg/min (max 24mg/kg/d)
Ephedrine	Direct and indirect sympathomimetic (α– and β–adrenergic action). Vasopressor, safe in pregnancy. Duration 10–60min	Caution in elderly, hypertension, and CVS disease. Tachyphylaxis. Avoid with MAOI	Tachycardia, hypertension		3–6mg repeated (dilute 30mg in 10mL saline, 1mL increments). IM: 30mg
Ergometrine	Ergot alkaloid used to control uterine hypotony or bleeding. Syntometrine® = ergometrine 500 micrograms/mL and oxytocin 5U/mL	Severe cardiac disease and hypertension	Vasoconstriction, hypertension, vomiting		IM: 1mL as Syntometrine®. Careful SLOW IV: 250–500 micrograms, with antiemetic cover recommended
Erythromycin	Macrolide antibiotic with spectrum similar to penicillin	Arrhythmias with cisapride, terfenadine, astemizole	Nausea, diarrhoea	12.5mg/kg qds over 20–60min. >8yr: adult dose	250–500mg (6–hourly in divided doses). Max four doses

Esmolol	Short–acting cardioselective β–blocker. Metabolized by red cell esterases. Treatment of SVT or intraoperative hypertension. Duration 10min	Asthma, heart failure, AV block, verapamil treatment	Hypotension, bradycardia. May prolong action of suxamethonium	SVT: 0.5mg/kg over 1 min, then 50–200 micrograms/kg/min	SVT: 0.5mg/kg over 1min, then 50–200 microgram s/kg/min. Hypertension: 25–100mg, then 50–300 micrograms/kg/min
Ethanol	Useful sedative/hypnotic. Has been tried as an IV induction agent in doses of up to 44g	Administered as dehydrated absolute alcohol BP. Refer to TOXBASE	Diuretic effect		2g (2mL) diluted to 5–10% solution in saline or glucose, repeated as necessary
Etomidate	IV induction agent. Cardiostable in therapeutic doses. Available in lipid emulsion	Pain on injection. Adrenocortical suppression	Nausea and vomiting. Myoclonic movements	0.3mg/kg	0.15–0.3mg/kg
Fentanyl	Synthetic phenylpiperidine derivative opioid analgesic. High lipid solubility and cardiostability. Duration 30–60min	Reduce dose in elderly. Delayed respiratory depression and pruritus if epidural/spinal	Circulatory and ventilatory depression. High doses may produce muscle rigidity	1–5 micrograms/kg, up to 50 micrograms/ kg if ventilating post–operatively. Infusion: 2–4 micrograms/kg/hr	1–5 micrograms/kg (up to 50 micrograms/kg). Epidural: 50–100 micrograms (diluted in 10mL saline/LA). Spinal: 5–20 micrograms
Flecainide	Class 1c antiarrhythmic agent used for VT, WPW, and 'chemical cardioversion' of paroxysmal AF	Rise in pacemaker threshold. AV block, heart failure, previous MI	Nausea and vomiting. Pro–arrhythmic effects, AV block	2mg/kg (max dose 150mg) over 15min, with ECG monitoring	'Chemical cardioversion': 2mg/kg up to 150mg (over 15min with ECG monitoring). PO: 200–300mg

IV, intravenous. IM, intramuscular. SC, subcutaneous. PO, *per os* (oral). SL, sublingual. ET, endotracheal. od, once daily. bd, twice daily. tds, three times daily. qds, four times daily. NR, not recommended. Doses are IV and dilutions in 0.9% NaCl unless otherwise stated.

(*Continued*)

Table A.23 (*Contd.*)

Drug	Description and perioperative indications	Cautions and contraindications	Side effects	Dose (paediatric)	Dose (adult)
Flucloxacillin	Penicillinase–resistant antibiotic active against staphylococci	Hypotension on rapid IV administration	Thrombophlebitis, cholestatic jaundice	12.5–50mg/kg qds (max dose 2g qds)	500mg–2g qds slow IV. Surgical prophylaxis: 1–2g slow IV
Flumazenil	Benzodiazepine receptor antagonist. Duration 45–90min	Benzodiazepine dependence (acute withdrawal), resedation if long–acting benzodiazepine	Arrhythmia, seizures	10 micrograms/kg (max 200 micrograms), repeat if required (max 50 micrograms/ kg). Infusion: 2–10 m i crog ram s / kg/hr	200 micrograms, then 100 micrograms at 60s intervals (up to max 1mg). Infusion: 100–400 micrograms/hr
Fondaparinux	Synthetic pentasaccharide which inhibits activated factor X. DVT prophylaxis after major lower limb orthopaedic surgery	Active bleeding, severe renal impairment, bacterial endocarditis. Caution with spinal and epidural (see ➲ p. 1141)	Haemorrhage, thrombocytopenia, oedema, deranged LFTs	NR	Prophylaxis SC: 2.5mg od started 6hr post–operatively for up to 5d. Do not give IM or IV. Monitor platelet count
Fosphenytoin	Prodrug of phenytoin. Can be administered more rapidly. Dosages in phenytoin equivalents (PE): fosphenytoin 1.5mg, phenytoin 1mg	See phenytoin—monitor ECG/BP. Infusion rate: 50–100 mg (PE)/ min (status 100–150mg (PE)/min)	See phenytoin	>5yr: 10–20 mg (PE)/ kg, then 4–5mg (PE)/kg daily in 1–4 divided doses. Infusion rate: 1–2mg (PE)/ kg/min	Infusion: 10–15 mg (PE)/ kg, then 4–5mg (PE)/ kg daily. Status: 20mg (PE)/kg. Can also be administered IM. Infusion rate 50–100mg (PE)/min
Furosemide (frusemide)	Loop diuretic used in treatment of hypertension, CCF, renal failure, fluid overload		Hypotension, tinnitus, ototoxicity, hypokalaemia, hyperglycaemia	0.5–1.5mg/kg bd	10–40mg slowly

Gabapentin	Structural analogue GABA. Indications post–herpetic neuralgia, neuropathic pain, focal seizures	Avoid abrupt withdrawal, elderly, renal impairment	Nausea, vomiting, abdominal pain, malaise	Seizures: day 1 10mg/kg (max 300mg) od, then bd, then tds max 70mg/kg	Pain: day 1 300mg od, day 2 300mg bd, then 300mg tds to max 3.6g/d
Gentamicin	Aminoglycoside antibiotic active against Gram–negative bacteria. Peak level 6–1 Omg/ L. Trough level <1–2mg/L	Impairs neuromuscular transmission—avoid in myasthenia	Ototoxicity, nephrotoxicity	2mg/kg tds or 5mg/ kg/d as a single dose (administered over 5min)	3–5mg/kg divided doses or 5–7mg/kg/d as a single dose (administered over 5 min)
Glucagon	Polypeptide hormone used in treatment of hypoglycaemia and overdose of |3–blocker. Hyperglycaemic action lasts 10–30min. 1U = 1mg	Glucose must be administered as soon as possible. Phaeochromocytoma	Hypertension, hypotension, nausea, vomiting	<25kg: 0.5U (0.5mg). >25kg: 1U(1mg)	SC/IM/IV: 1U(1mg). |3–blocker overdose unresponsive to atropine: 2–1 Omg (max 10mg) in glucose 5%
Glucose	Treatment of hypoglycaemia in unconscious patient	50% solution irritant, therefore flush after administration into large vein. <20% peripherally		0.5mL/kg of 50% solution; use more dilute solutions: bolus 5mL/kg 10%, repeat PRN	25–50g (50–100mL 50% solution). Can use more dilute solutions
Glyceryl trinitrate	Organic nitrate vasodilator. Controlled hypotension, angina, CCF	Remove patches before defibrillation to avoid electrical arcing	Tachycardia, hypotension, headache, nausea, flushing, methaemoglobinaemia	10–30 micrograms/kg/ hr, starting dose up to 300 micrograms/kg/hr. Max 600 micrograms/kg/hr	Infusion: 0.5–10mg/ hr. SL tabs: 0.3–1mg PR.N. SL spray: 400 micrograms PRN. Patch: 5–10mg/24hr

IV, intravenous. IM, intramuscular. SC, subcutaneous. PO, *per os* (oral). SL, sublingual. ET, endotracheal. od, once daily. bd, twice daily. tds, three times daily. qds, four times daily. NR, not recommended. Doses are IV and dilutions in 0.9% NaCl unless otherwise stated.

(*Continued*)

Table A.23 (*Contd.*)

Drug	Description and perioperative indications	Cautions and contraindications	Side effects	Dose (paediatric)	Dose (adult)
Glycopyrronium bromide (glyco pyrrolate)	Quaternary ammonium anticholinergic agent. Bradycardia, blockade of muscarinic effects of anticholinesterases, antisialogogue	Caution in glaucoma, CVS disease. Unlike atropine, does not cross blood–brain barrier	Paradoxical bradycardia in small doses. Reduces lower oesophageal sphincter tone	4–10 micrograms/kg	200–400 micrograms. Control of muscarinic effects of neostigmine: 200 micrograms for each 1mg neostigmine
Granisetron	5–HT_3 receptor antagonist. Antiemetic. Long–acting	Pregnancy, breastfeeding, QT interval prolongation	Reduces colonic motility. Headache	NR<12yr	1 mg diluted to 5mL with saline. Give over 30s. Max 9mg/d
Haloperidol	Butyrophenone derivative antipsychotic. Useful antiemetic	Neuroleptic malignant syndrome. Half dose in elderly	Extrapyramidal reactions	NR	IM/IV: 2–10mg 4–to 8–hourly (max 18mg/d). Antiemetic: 0.5–2mg IV. PO: 0.5–3mg
Heparin (unfractionated)	Endogenous mucopolysaccharide used for anticoagulation. Half–life 1–3hr. 100U, 1mg	Monitor APTT. Reversed with protamine	Haemorrhage, thrombocytopenia, hyperkalaemia	Low dose: 50–75U/ kg IV, then 10–15U/kg/ hr. Full dose: 200U/kg IV, then 15–30U/kg/hr, Anticoagulation for bypass 300–400U/kg IV	Low dose SC: 5000U bd. Full dose IV: 5000U, then 18U/kg/hr infusion. Anti coagulation for bypass: 300–400U/kg
Human prothrombin complex (Beriplex®, Octaplex®)	Dried prothrombin complex, prepared from human plasma. Rapid reversal of warfarin anticoagulation.		Risk of thrombotic events	Discuss with haematologist	Discuss with haematologist

Hyaluronidase	Enzyme used to enhance permeation of injected fluids and LAs. Treatment of extravasation. Hypodermoclysis: 1500U/L	Not for IV administration	Occasional severe allergy	LA: 15U/mL solution	Ophthalmology: 10–15U/mL local. Extravasation: 1500U in 1mL saline infiltrated to affected area
Hydralazine	Direct–acting arteriolar vasodilator used to control arterial pressure. Duration 2—4hr	Higher doses required in rapid acetylators. SLE	Increased HR, cardiac output, stroke volume	0.1–0.5 mg/kg 4– to 6–hourly	5mg every 5min to a max of 20mg
Hydrocortisone (cortisol)	Endogenous steroid with antiinflammatory and potent mineralocorticoid action (steroid of choice in replacement therapy—active form of cortisone). Treatment of allergy	Hydrocortisone 20mg, prednisolone 5mg	Hyperglycaemia, hypertension, psychiatric reactions, muscle weakness, fluid retention	4mg/kg, then 2–4mg/kg qds	IV/IM: 50–200mg qds. Adrenal suppression and surgery: 25mg at induction, then 25mg qds. PO: 10–30mg/d
Hydro morphone hydrochloride	Opioid used for moderate to severe pain in cancer	As morphine	Nausea, vomiting, dysphoria, drowsiness	<12yr: NR. >12yr: adult dose	PO: 1.3mg4–hourly, increased as necessary. PO slow release: 4mg bd
Hyoscine butyl bromide	Antimuscarinic agent used as an antispasmodic (racemic hyoscine)	See atropine	See atropine	2–6yr: IV/IM: 5mg. 6–12yr: IV/IM: 5–10mg. >12yr: adult dose	IV/IM: 20mg slowly, repeated if necessary

IV, intravenous. IM, intramuscular. SC, subcutaneous. PO, *per os* (oral). SL, sublingual. ET, endotracheal. od, once daily. bd, twice daily. tds, three times daily. qds, four times daily. NR, not recommended. Doses are IV and dilutions in 0.9% NaCl unless otherwise stated.

(*Continued*)

Table A.23 *(Contd.)*

Drug	Description and perioperative indications	Cautions and contraindications	Side effects	Dose (paediatric)	Dose (adult)
Hyoscine hydrobromide	Antimuscarinic sedative, anti emetic agent used as premedication (L–isomer of hyoscine)	See atropine. Avoid in elderly—delirium	See atropine. Sedation	IM/SC: 15 micrograms/kg (max 600 micrograms)	IV/IM/SC: 200–600 micrograms. PO: 300 micrograms tds
Ibuprofen	NSAID analgesic for mild to moderate pain. Best side effect profile of NSAIDs	Hypersensitivity to aspirin, asthma, severe renal impairment, peptic ulceration	GI upset or bleeding, bronchospasm, tinnitus, fluid retention, platelet inhibition	NR. <3months/<5kg. PO: 10mg/kg tds or 5mg/kg qds (max 30mg/kg tds)	PO: 400mg qds
Imipenem	Carbapenem broad–spectrum antibiotic. Administered with cilastatin to reduce renal metabolism	Caution in renal failure and pregnancy	Nausea, vomiting, diarrhoea, convulsions, thrombophlebitis	>3 months: 15mg/kgover 30min qds (25mg/kg in severe infections)	Slow IV (1hr): 250–500mg qds. Surgical prophylaxis: 1g at induction, repeated after 3hr
Indometacin	NSAID analgesic for moderate pain. High incidence of side effects. Also used for neonatal ductus arteriosus closure	Hypersensitivity to aspirin, asthma, severe renal impairment, peptic ulceration	GI upset or bleeding, bronchospasm, tinnitus, fluid retention, platelet inhibition	Ductus closure: 200 micrograms/kg, three doses	PO/PR: 25–50mg tds. PR: 100mg bd
Insulin (soluble)	Human soluble pancreatic hormone facilitating intracellular transport of glucose and anabolism. Diabetes mellitus, ketoacidosis, and hyperkalaemia	Monitor blood glucose and serum potassium. Store at 2–8°C	Hypoglycaemia, hypokalaemia	Ketoacidosis: 0.1–0.2U/kg (max 20U), then 0.1U/kg/hr (max 5–10U/hr)	Ketoacidosis: 10–20U, then 5–10U/hr. Sliding scale (see ➔ p. 148). Hyperkalaemia (see ➔ p.176)

Intralipid®	20% emulsion used in the treatment of severe LA toxicity	See ➔ p. 1148 for LA toxicity guidelines		1.5mL/kg bolus, followed by 15mL/kg/hr	1.5mL/kg bolus, followed by 15mL/kg/hr
Isoprenaline	Synthetic catecholamine with potent β_1–adrenergic agonist activity. Emergency treatment of heart block and bradycardia unresponsive to atropine. β–blocker overdose	IHD, hyperthyroidism, diabetes mellitus. MHRA: NR, unless special requirements	Tachycardia, arrhythmias, sweating, tremor	Bolus: 5 micrograms/kg. Infusion: 0.02–1 micrograms/kg/min	Infusion: 0.5–10 micrograms/min (0.2mg in 500mL 5% glucose at 2–20mL/min or 1mg in 50mL at 1.5–30mL/hr)
Ketamine	Phencyclidine derivative producing dissociative anaesthesia. Induction/maintenance of anaesthesia in high–risk and hypovolaemic patients	Emergence delirium reduced by benzodiazepines. Caution in hypertension. Control excess salivation with anti muscarinic agent	Bronchodilation. Increased ICP, BP, uterine tone, salivation. Respiratory depression if given rapidly	Induction: 0.5–2mg/ kg IV, 5–10mg/kg IM. Infusion: 10–45 micrograms/kg/min. Caudal: 0.5mg/kg (preservative–free only)	Induction: 1–2mg/ kg IV, 5–10mg/kg IM. Infusion: 1–3mg/kg/hr (analgesia only 0.25mg/ kg/hr)
Ketorolac	NSAID analgesic for mild to moderate pain. Not licensed for perioperative use	Hypersensitivity to aspirin, asthma, severe renal impairment, peptic ulceration	GI upset or bleeding, bronchospasm, tinnitus, fluid retention, platelet inhibition	>6 months: slow IV/IM: 0.5mg/kg up to 30mg tds (max 60mg/d)	Slow IV/IM: 10mg, then 10–30mg every 4–6hr (max daily dose 90mg, but 60mg in elderly)
Labetalol	Combined α– (mild) and β–adrenergic receptor antagonist. BP control without reflex tachycardia. Duration 2–4hr	Asthma, heart failure, AV block, verapamil treatment	Hypotension, bradycardia, bronchospasm. liver damage	0.2 mg/kg boluses up to 0.5mg/kg (max 20mg <12yr). Infusion: 0.5–3mg/kg/hr	5mg increments up to 100mg. Infusion: 20–160mg/hr (in glucose)

IV, intravenous. IM, intramuscular. SC, subcutaneous. PO, *per os* (oral). SL, sublingual. ET, endotracheal. od, once daily. bd, twice daily. tds, three times daily. qds, four times daily. NR, not recommended. Doses are IV and dilutions in 0.9% NaCl unless otherwise stated.

(*Continued*)

Table A.23 (*Contd.*)

Drug	Description and perioperative indications	Cautions and contraindications	Side effects	Dose (paediatric)	Dose (adult)
Lansoprazole	PPI. Reduction of gastric acid secretion	Liver disease, pregnancy	Headache, diarrhoea	PO: 0.5–1 mg/kg (max 15–30 mg) od	PO: 15–30mgod
Levobupivacaine	Levorotatory (S) enantiomer of bupivacaine with reduced cardiotoxicity	See bupivacaine	See bupivacaine and use IBW	See bupivacaine. 2mg/kg	See bupivacaine. Max dose: 2mg/kg
Lidocaine	Amide–type LA: 1. Treatment of ventricular arrhythmias. 2. Reduction of pressor response to intubation. 3. LA—rapid onset, duration 30–90min (prolonged by adrenaline), pKa 7.7	Adrenaline–containing solutions contain preservative. Max dose dependent upon injection site—3mg/kg/4hr (6mg/kg with adrenaline)	Toxicity: tongue/circumoral numbness, restlessness, tinnitus, seizures, cardiac arrest. Prolongs action of neuromuscular blockers. Use IBW	1. Antia rrhythmic: 0.5–1 mg/kg, then 10–50 micrograms/kg/min. 2. Attenuation of pressor response: 1.5mg/kg. 3. LA: 0.5–2% solution	1. Antiarrhythmic: 1mg/kg, then 1–4mg/min. 2. Attenuation of pressor response: 1.5mg/kg. 3. LA: 0.5–2% solution
Loratadine	Non–sedative antihistamine. Relief of allergy, urticaria	Prostatic hypertrophy, urinary retention, glaucoma, porphyria	Dry mouth	<2yr: NR. PO: <30kg: 5mg od. >30kg: 10mg od	PO: 10mg/d

Lorazepam	Benzodiazepine: 1. Sedation or premedication 2. Status epilepticus. Duration 6–1 0hr	Decreased requirement for anaesthetic agents. Half in elderly	Respiratory depression , in combination with opioids. Amnesia	Status 0.1 mg/kg; max 4mg	1. PO: 1–4mg 1–2hr pre operatively. IV/ IM: 1.5–2.5mg 2. Status: 4mg IV, repeat after 10min if required
Lormetazepam	Benzodiazepine hypnotic sedative premed	Decreased requirement anaesthetic agents	Respiratory depression for in combination with opioid. Amnesia	NR	0.5–1.5mg1–2hr preoperatively (elderly 0.5mg)
Magnesium sulfate	Essential mineral used to treat: 1. Hypomagnesaemia 2. Arrhythmias 3. Eclamptic seizures 4. Severe asthma. Magnesium sulfate 50%, 500mg/mL, 2 mmo l Mg^{2+}/mL. Normal plasma level Mg^{2+}0.75–1.05mmol/L. Therapeutic level 2–4mmol/L	Potentiates muscle relaxants. Monitoring of serum level essential during treatment. Myasthenia and muscular dystrophy. Heart block. Magnesium sulfate 1g = Mg^{2+} 4mmol	CNS depression, hypotension, muscle weakness	1. Hypomagnesaemia: 0.2–0.4mmol/kg (max 20mmol/d)—check levels 2. Arrhythmias: 25–50mg/kg over 10min (max dose 2g) once if necessary	1. Hypomagnesaemia: 0.5–1 mmol/kg (max 160mmol/5d), check levels. 2. Arrhythmias/asthma: 2g (8mmol) over 10min, repeat once if necessary. 3. Eclampsia: 4g (16mmol) over 10min, then lg/hrfor 24hr (see ➔ p. 760)
Mannitol	Osmotic diuretic used for renal protection and reduction of ICP. 20% solution, 20g/100mL	Extracellular volume expansion, caution in severe renal and CVS disease	Diuresis, ARF, hypertonicity	0.25–1.5g/kg	0.25–2g/kg (typically 0.5g/kg of 20% solution)

IV, intravenous. IM, intramuscular. SC, subcutaneous. PO, *per os* (oral). SL, sublingual. ET, endotracheal. od, once daily. bd, twice daily. tds, three times daily. qds, four times daily. NR, not recommended. Doses are IV and dilutions in 0.9% NaCl unless otherwise stated.

(*Continued*)

Table A.23 (*Contd.*)

Drug	Description and perioperative indications	Cautions and contraindications	Side effects	Dose (paediatric)	Dose (adult)
Metaraminol	Potent direct/indirect acting α–adrenergic sympathomimetic. Treatment of hypotension. Duration 20–60min	MAOIs, pregnancy. Caution in elderly and hypertensives. Extravasation can cause necrosis	Hypertension, reflex bradycardia, arrhythmias, decreased renal and placental perfusion	10 micrograms/kg, then 0.1–1 micrograms/kg/min, >12yr	0.5–2mg. Dilute 10mg in 20mL saline, and give 0.5–1 mL increments (increase dilution in elderly)
Methohexital	Short–acting barbiturate induction agent useful for ECT. Duration 5–10min. 1% solution, 10mg/mL	Porphyria. Premedication reduces excitation at induction	Excitatory phenomenon, hypotension, respiratory depression, hiccups	1–2mg/kg	1–1.5 mg/kg. Infusion: 50–150 micrograms/kg/min
Methylthioninium chloride (methylene blue)	1. Treatment of methaemoglobinaemia 2. Ureteric identification during surgery (renally excreted) 3. Identification of parathyroid glands during surgery 4. Identification of sentinel node during cancer surgery	G6PD deficiency. Blue coloration causes acute changes in pulse oximetry readings	Tachycardia, nausea, stains skin, allergy reported	1mg/kg slow IV(max 7mg/kg)	1 mg/kg slow IV (max 7mg/kg)
Metoclopramide	Dopaminergic antiemetic which increases gastric emptying and lower oesophageal sphincter tone	Hypertension in phaeochromocytoma. Inhibits plasma cholinesterase. Increases IOP	Extrapyramidal/dystonic reactions (treat with benztropine or procyclidine)	PO/IM/IV: 0.15mg/kg, up to 5mg tds (>60kg, up to 10mg tds)	PO/IM/IV: 10mg tds

Metoprolol	Cardioselective β–blocker	Asthma, heart failure, AV block, verapamil treatment	Causes bradycardia, hypotension, and decreased cardiac contractility	0.1mg/kg up to 5mg over 10min	1–5mg over 10min, repeat if required (max 15 mg)
Metronidazole	Antibiotic with activity against anaerobic bacteria	Disulfiram (Antabuse®)–like effect with alcohol consumption		7.5mg/kg tds (max dose 500mg tds)	500mg tds
Midazolam	Short–acting benzodiazepine. Sedative, anxiolytic, amnesic, anticonvulsant. Duration 20–60min. Oral administration of IV preparation effective, though larger dose required	Reduce dose in elderly (very sensitive)	Hypotension, respiratory depression, apnoea	IV: 0.1–0.2mg/ kg. PO: 0.5mg/kg (use IV preparation in orange squash). Intranasal: 0.2–0.3mg/ kg (use 5mg/ mL IV preparation). Infusion: 0.5–20 micrograms/kg/min	Sedation: 0.5–5mg, titrate to effect. PO: 0.5mg/kg (use IV preparation in orange squash). IM: 2.5–1 Omg (0.1 mg/kg)
Milrinone	Selective phosphodiesterase inhibitor used in cardiac failure with increased filling pressures. Inodilator used after cardiac surgery	Stenotic valvular disease, cardiomyopathy	Arrhythmias, hypotension, nausea	50 micrograms/kg over 30–60min, then 0.375–0.75 micrograms/ kg/min. Max 1.13mg/kg/d	50 micrograms/kg over 10min, then 0.375–0.75 micrograms/kg/min. Max 1.13mg/kg/d

IV, intravenous. IM, intramuscular. SC, subcutaneous. PO, *per os* (oral). SL, sublingual. ET, endotracheal. od, once daily. bd, twice daily. tds, three times daily. qds, four times daily. NR, not recommended. Doses are IV and dilutions in 0.9% NaCl unless otherwise stated.

(*Continued*)

Table A.23 (*Contd.*)

Drug	Description and perioperative indications	Cautions and contraindications	Side effects	Dose (paediatric)	Dose (adult)
Mivacurium	Short–acting non–depolarizing muscle relaxant. Metabolized by plasma cholinesterase. Duration 6–16min (often variable). Enhanced duration if low plasma cholinesterase. Antagonized by neostigmine— but avoid giving too early to avoid inhibiting drug metabolism	See cisatracurium. Avoid in asthma	See cisatracurium. Some histamine release	Intubation: 0.15–0.2mg/ kg. Maintenance: 0.1 mg/ kg. Infusion: 8–10 micrograms/kg/min	Intubation: 0.07–0.25mg/ kg (doses of 0.07, 0.15,0.2, and 0.25mg/ kg produce block for 13,16,20, and 23min, respectively). Maintenance: 0.1 mg/ kg. Infusion: 0.4–0.6mg/ kg/ hr
Morphine	Opioid analgesic. Half–life 2–4hr	Prolonged risk of respiratory depression, pruritus, nausea when used via spinal/epidural	Histamine release, hypotension, bronchospasm, nausea, vomiting, pruritus, dysphoria	PO: 0.05–0.3mg/kg 4–hourly. IV boluses: 50–100 micrograms/ kg. For PCA, NCA, infusion, see ➔ p. 808	IV: 2.5–10mg. IM/ SC: 5–10mg 4–hourly. PO: 10–30mg 4–hourly. PCA: 1mg 5min lockout. Infusion: 1–3.5 mg/ hr. Epidural: 2–5mg preservative–free. Spinal: 0.1–1 mg preservative–free

Naloxone	Pure opioid antagonist. Can be used in low doses to reverse pruritus associated with epidural opioids and as depot IM injection in newborn of mothers given opioids	Beware renarcotization if reversing long–acting opioid. Caution in opioid–dependent patients—may precipitate acute withdrawal. Duration of action 30min		5–10 micrograms/kg. Infusion: 5–20 micrograms/kg/hr. IM depot in newborn: 200 micrograms. Pruritus: 0.5 micrograms/kg	200–400 micrograms, titrated to desired effect. Treatment of opioid/epidural pruritus: 100 micrograms bolus plus 300 micrograms added to IV fluids
Naproxen	NSAID analgesic for mild to moderate pain. Juvenile idiopathic arthritis	See ibuprofen	See ibuprofen. Low thrombotic risk profile	5–10 micrograms/kg. Infusion: 5–20 micrograms/kg/hr. IM depot in newborn: 200 micrograms. Pruritus: 0.5 micrograms/kg	PO: 500mg bd. Max 1.25g/d
Neostigmine	Anticholinesterase used for: 1. Reversal of non–depolarizing muscle relaxant 2. Treatment of myasthenia gravis Duration 60min IV (2–4hr PO)	Administer with anti muscarinic agent	Bradycardia, nausea, excessive salivation (muscarinic effects)	50 micrograms/kg with atropine 20 micrograms/kg or glycopyrronium 10 micrograms/kg	1. 50–70 micrograms/kg (max 5mg) with atropine 10–20 micrograms/kg or glycopyrronium 10–15 micrograms/kg 2. PO:15–30mg at suitable intervals
Neostigmine and glycopyrronium	Combination of neostigmine metilsulfate (2.5mg) and glycopyrronium (500 micrograms) per 1mL	See neostigmine	See neostigmine	0.02mL/kg (dilute 1mL with 4mL saline, give 0.1mL/kg). Max 2mL	1–2mL over 30s

IV, intravenous. IM, intramuscular. SC, subcutaneous. PO, *per os* (oral). SL, sublingual. ET, endotracheal. od, once daily. bd, twice daily. tds, three times daily. qds, four times daily. NR, not recommended. Doses are IV and dilutions in 0.9% NaCl unless otherwise stated.

(*Continued*)

Table A.23 *(Contd.)*

Drug	Description and perioperative indications	Cautions and contraindications	Side effects	Dose (paediatric)	Dose (adult)
Nimodipine	Calcium channel blocker used to prevent vascular spasm after subarachnoid haemorrhage (treat for 21 days)	Via central catheter. Cerebral oedema, raised ICP, grapefruit juice. Incompatible with PVC	Hypotension, flushing, headache	Infusion: 0.1–0.5 micrograms/kg/min (increased max 2mg/hr)	PO: 60mg 4–hourly (max 360mg/d). Infusion: 1mg/hr, increasing after 2hr to 2mg/hr
Nitroprusside (sodium—SNP)	N_2O generating potent peripheral vasodilator. Controlled hypotension	Protect solution from light. Metabolism yields cyanide which is then converted to thiocyanate	Methaemoglobinaemia, hypotension, tachycardia. Cyanide causes tachycardia, sweating, acidosis	Infusion: 0.3–1.5 micrograms/kg/min, increase if required (max 4–8 micrograms/kg/min)	Infusion: 0.3–1.5 micrograms/kg/min (up to 8 micrograms/ kg/ min). Max total dose: 1.5mg/kg (acutely)
Noradrenaline	Potent catecholamine α–adrenergic agonist. Vasoconstriction	Via central catheter only. Potentiated by MAOI and tricyclic antidepressants	Reflex bradycardia, arrhythmia, hypertension	Infusion: 0.02–0.5 micrograms/kg/min	Infusion: 0.04–0.4 micrograms/kg/min
Octreotide	Somatostatin analogue used in treatment of carcinoid, acromegaly, and variceal bleeding (unlicensed use)	Pituitary tumour expansion, reduced need for antidiabetic treatments	GI disturbance, gallstones, hyper– and hypoglycaemia	SC: 1–5 micrograms/kg 6– to 8–hourly	SC: 50 micrograms od/ bd, increased up to 200 micrograms tds. IV: 50 micrograms diluted in saline (ECG monitoring)

Omeprazole	PPI. Reduction in gastric acid secretion	Liver disease max 20 mg od	Headache, diarrhoea, prolonged QT	PO: 0.7–1.4mg/kg up to 40mg od. IV: 0.5mg/kg od	PO/slow IV: 20–40mg od. Premedication PO: 40mg. Bleeding peptic ulcer: 80mg bolus, then 8mg/hr for 3d
Ondansetron	Serotonin (5–HT_3) receptor antagonist antiemetic	QT interval prolongation	Hypotension, headache, flushing	>1/12: slow IV: 100 micrograms/kg (max 4mg) qds	Slow IV/IM/PO: 4mgtds
Oxybuprocaine	LA. Topical anaesthesia to cornea				0.4% solution. 0.5mL eye drops
Oxycodone	Opioid used for moderate pain, often in palliative care. IV preparation available: dose 1–10mg 4–hourly	Porphyria, acute abdomen	Nausea, vomiting, dysphoria, drowsiness	PO: Oxynorm® >1 month: initially 200 micrograms/kg (max 5mg) 4– to 6–hourly. >12yr: adult doses	PO: Oxy no rm® 5 mg 4– to 6–hourly, increased as required. Oxycontin® 10mg bd, increased as required
Oxytocin	Nonapeptide hormone which stimulates uterine contraction. Induction of labour and prevention of post–partum haemorrhage	Avoid rapid administration. Fetal distress	Vasodilatation, hypotension, flushing, tachycardia		Post–partum slow IV: 5U, followed, if required, by infusion 10U/hr(40U in 40mL 0.9% saline)

IV, intravenous. IM, intramuscular. SC, subcutaneous. PO, *per os* (oral). SL, sublingual. ET, endotracheal. od, once daily. bd, twice daily. tds, three times daily. qds, four times daily. NR, not recommended. Doses are IV and dilutions in 0.9% NaCl unless otherwise stated.

(*Continued*)

Table A.23 (*Contd.*)

Drug	Description and perioperative indications	Cautions and contraindications	Side effects	Dose (paediatric)	Dose (adult)
Pancuronium	Long–acting aminosteroid non–depolarizing muscle relaxant. Little histamine release. Duration 45–65min	See cisatracurium	See cisatracurium. Increased HR and BP due to vagolysis and sympathetic stimulation	Intubation: 0.1 mg/kg. Maintenance: 0.02mg/kg, as required	Intubation: 0.1 mg/kg. Maintenance: 0.02mg/kg, as required
Pantoprazole	PPI used to inhibit gastric acid secretion	Liver disease, pregnancy. Renal disease	Headache, pruritus, bronchospasm	NR	PO/slow IV: 40mg od (max 80mg)
Paracetamol	Mild to moderate analgesic and antipyretic	Neonates: PO: 10–15mg/kg 6–hourly (5mg/kg if jaundiced). Max 60 mg/kg/d. <10kg: IV: 7.5mg/kg 6–hourly. Max 30mg/ kg/d	Liver damage in overdose	Slow IV: 15mg/kg qds (max 60mg/kg/d) (10–50kg max 60mg/ kg, >50kg max 4g/d). PO/PR: 20mg/kg qds (max 75mg/ kg/d up to 4g/d). PR loading dose. 30–40mg/kg (>44 wk post–conception)	Slow IV: >50kg 1g qds, <50kg 15mg/kg qds. PO: 0.5–1g qds
Paraldehyde	Status epilepticus	Dilute neat solution with equal volume of olive oil before PR administration		Deep IM: 0.2mL/kg. PR: 0.3mL/kg	Deep IM: 5–10mL. PR: 10–20mL
Parecoxib	See celecoxib. Prodrug of valdecoxib. COX–2 inhibitor. Licensed for acute pain	See celecoxib. Reconstitute with 0.9% saline	GI upset, thrombotic events		IV/IM: 40mg, then 20–40mg 6– to 12–hourly (max 80mg/d)

Pethidine	Synthetic opioid: 1. Analgesia 2. Post–operative shivering	Seizures possible in high dosage—max daily dose 1g/d (20mg/kg/d). MAOI	Respiratory depression, hypotension, dysphoria	>12yr: IV/IM/SC: 0.5–1 mg/kg (max 100mg). Infusion: 5mg/kg in 50mL 5% glucose at 1–3 mL/hr (100–300 micrograms/kg/hr)	IM/SC: 25–100mg 3–hourly. IV: 25–50mg. PCA: 10mg/5min lockout. Shivering: 10–25mg
Phentolamine	α_1– and α_2–adrenergic antagonist. Peripheral vasodilatation and controlled hypotension. Treatment of extravasation. Duration 10min	Treat excessive hypotension with noradrenaline or methoxamine (not adrenaline/ephe– drine due to β effects)	Hypotension, tachycardia, flushing	0.1 mg/kg, then 5–50 micrograms/kg/min	2–5mg (10mg in 10mL saline, 1mL aliquots)
Phenylephrine	Selective direct–acting α–adrenergic agonist. Peripheral vasoconstriction and treatment of hypotension. Duration 20min	Caution in elderly and CVS disease. Hyperthyroidism	Reflex bradycardia, arrhythmias	2–10 micrograms/kg, then 0.1–0.5 micrograms/kg/min	20–100 micrograms increments (10mg in 500mL saline, 1mL aliquots). IM: 2–5mg. Infusion: 30–60 micrograms/min (5mg in 50mL saline at 0–30mL/hr)
Phenytoin	Anticonvulsant and treatment of digoxin toxicity. Serum levels 10–20mg/L (40–80 micromoles/L)	Avoid in AV heart block, pregnancy, and porphyria. Monitor ECG/BP on IV administration	Hypotension, AV conduction defects, ataxia. Enzyme induction	IV loading dose: 20mg/kg over 1 hr	20mg/kg (max 2g) over 1hr (dilute to 10mg/mL in saline), then 100mg tds. Arrhythmia: 3.5–5mg/kg (rate <50mg/min)

IV, intravenous. IM, intramuscular. SC, subcutaneous. PO, *per os* (oral). SL, sublingual. ET, endotracheal. od, once daily. bd, twice daily. tds, three times daily. qds, four times daily. NR, not recommended. Doses are IV and dilutions in 0.9% NaCl unless otherwise stated.

(*Continued*)

Table A.23 (*Contd.*)

Drug	Description and perioperative indications	Cautions and contraindications	Side effects	Dose (paediatric)	Dose (adult)
Pipecuronium	Piperazinium derivative long–acting non–depolarizing muscle relaxant. Duration 45–120min	See cisatracurium	See cisatracurium		Intubation: 0.08mg/kg. Maintenance: 0.01–0.04mg/kg
Piroxicam	NSAID analgesic for inflammatory or degenerative joint pain. High incidence of side effects	Hypersensitivity to aspirin, asthma, severe renal impairment, peptic ulceration. Avoid in porphyria	GI upset or bleeding, bronchospasm, tinnitus, fluid retention, platelet inhibition, skin reactions	NR	PO/PR: 10–20mg od
Potassium chloride	Electrolyte replacement (see ➲ p. 1053 and p. 174)	Dilute solution before administration	Rapid infusion can cause cardiac arrest. High concentration causes phlebitis	0.5mmol/kg over 1 hr. Maintenance: 1–2mmol/kg/d	10–20mmol/hr (max concentration 40mmol/L peripherally). With ECG monitoring: up to 20–40mmol/hr via central line (max 200mmol/d)
Pregabalin	Binds to voltage–dependent calcium channels and decreases release neurotrans mitters. Adjunct for focal seizures.	Avoid abrupt withdrawal, severe CCF, renal impairment	Dry mouth, constipation, oedema, dizziness		Pain >18yr: 150mg 2–3 divided doses with slow increase. Epilepsy >18yr: 25mg bd increasing

Prednisolone	Orally active corticosteroid. Less mineralocorticoid action than hydrocortisone	Adrenal suppression, severe systemic infections	Dyspepsia and ulceration, osteoporosis, myopathy, psychosis, impaired healing, diabetes mellitus	PO: 1–2mg/kg od. Croup: 4mg/kg, then 1 mg/kg tds	PO: initially 20–60mg od, reduced to 2.5–15mg od for maintenance
Prilocaine	Amide–type LA. Less toxic than lidocaine. Used for infiltration and IVRA. Rapid onset. Duration 30–90min (prolonged by adrenaline), pKa 7.9	Adrenaline–containing solutions contain preservative. Significant methaemoglobinaemia if dose >600mg. Use IBW	Toxicity: tongue/ circumoral numbness, restlessness, tinnitus, seizures, cardiac arrest	NR <6 months	LA: 0.5–2% solution. Max dose dependent upon injection site—6mg/ kg/4hr (9mg/kg with adrenaline)
Prochlorperazine	Phenothiazine antiemetic	Hypotension on rapid IV administration. Neuroleptic malignant syndrome	Tardive dyskinesia and extrapyramidal symptoms	>10kg: PO: 0.25mg/kg tds. IM: 0.1–0.2mg/kg tds	IM: 12.5mg tds. PO: 20mg, then 5–10mg tds
Procyclidine	Antimuscarinic used in acute treatment of drug–induced dystonic reactions (except tardive dyskinesia)	Glaucoma, GI obstruction. Lower dose in elderly	Urinary retention, dry mouth, blurred vision	<2yr: 0.5–2mg. 2–1 Oyr: 2–5 mg. >10yr: adult dose	IV/IM: 5–10mg, repeat after 20min if needed
Promethazine	Phenothiazine, antihistamine, anticholinergic, antiemetic sedative. Paediatric sedation		Extrapyramidal reactions	>2yr: sedation/premed. PO: 1–2mg/kg	PO/IM: 10–25 mg tds

IV, intravenous. IM, intramuscular. SC, subcutaneous. PO, *per os* (oral). SL, sublingual. ET, endotracheal. od, once daily. bd, twice daily. tds, three times daily. qds, four times daily. NR, not recommended. Doses are IV and dilutions in 0.9% NaCl unless otherwise stated.

(*Continued*)

Table A.23 (*Contd.*)

Drug	Description and perioperative indications	Cautions and contraindications	Side effects	Dose (paediatric)	Dose (adult)
Propofol	Di–isopropylphenol IV induction agent. Rapid recovery and little nausea. Agent of choice for day surgery, sedation, or laryngeal mask insertion—can be used for ECT	Reduce dose in elderly or haemodynamically unstable. Caution in severe allergy to eggs, peanuts, soya, soybean oil. Caution in epilepsy	Apnoea, hypotension, pain on injection. Myoclonic spasms, rarely convulsions	Induction: 2–4mg/kg. Infusion: 4–15mg/kg/hr. NR induction <1 month. NR maintenance <3yr	Induction: 2–3mg/kg. Infusion: 6–10mg/kg/hr. TCI: initially 4–8 micrograms/mL, then 3–6 micrograms/mL (reduce in elderly)
Propranolol	Non–selective β–adrenergic antagonist. Controlled hypotension, symptomatic treatment of thyrotoxicosis	Asthma, heart failure, AV block, verapamil treatment	Bradycardia, hypotension, AV block, bronchospasm	0.1mg/kg over 5min	1mg increments, up to 5–10mg
Protamine	Basic protein produced from salmon sperm. Heparin antagonist	Weakly anticoagulant and marked histamine release. Risk of allergy	Severe hypotension, pulmonary hypertension bronchospasm, flushing	Slow IV: 1 mg per 1 mg , heparin (100U) to be reversed	Slow IV: 1 mg per 1 mg heparin (100U) to be reversed
Proxymetacaine (proparacaine)	LA. Topical anaesthesia to cornea	Less stinging than with other eye drops		Avoid preterms. One drop/eye, then one drop/eye every 10min, max 5–7 doses	0.5% solution. 0.5mL eye drops
Pyridostigmine	Long–acting anticholinesterase used in treatment of myasthenia gravis	See neostigmine	See neostigmine	PO: 1–1.5mg/kg at intervals (4– to 12–hourly)	PO: 30–120mg at intervals through day (maximum 1.2g/d)

Ranitidine	Histamine (H_2) receptor antagonist. Reduction in gastric acid secretion	Porphyria	Tachycardia	IV: 1 mg/kg slowly tds (max 50mg). PO: 2–4mg/kg bd	IV: 50mg (diluted in 20mL saline, given over 2min) qds. IM: 50mg qds. PO: 150mg bd or 300mg od
Remifentanil	Ultrashort–acting opioid used to supplement GA. Metabolized by non–specific esterases (not plasma cholinesterase). Duration 5–10min. Can be used as PCA in labour: 25–75 micrograms bolus, 3min lockout (0.5–1.5mL of 50 micrograms/mL). May be mixed with propofol: 125 micrograms/50mL SV, 250–500 micrograms/50 mL IPPV		Muscle rigidity, respiratory depression, hypotension, bradycardia. Use IBW	Slow bolus: up to 1 microgram/kg. Infusion (IPPV): 0.1–0.5 micrograms/kg/min. Start at 0.1 micrograms/kg/min, and adjust dose as necessary	Slow bolus: up to 1 microgram/kg. Infusion (IPPV): 0.1–0.5 micrograms/kg/min. Infusion (SV): 0.025–0.1 micrograms/kg/min. Start at 0.1 micrograms/kg/min, and adjust dose as necessary
Rivaroxaban	Direct inhibitor of factor Xa. Uses: 1. Prophylaxis of VTE after major orthopaedic surgery 2. Prophylaxis of stroke in AF 3. Treatment of VTE and prevention of recurrent VTE	Risk of major bleeding, renal impairment, severe liver disease. No routine monitoring required	Nausea, haemorrhage	NR	1. PO: 10mg od for 14d 2. PO: 20mg od 3. PO: 15mg bd for 21d, then 20mg od

IV, intravenous. IM, intramuscular. SC, subcutaneous. PO, *per os* (oral). SL, sublingual. ET, endotracheal. od, once daily. bd, twice daily. tds, three times daily. qds, four times daily. NR, not recommended. Doses are IV and dilutions in 0.9% NaCl unless otherwise stated.

(*Continued*)

Table A.23 *(Contd.)*

Drug	Description and perioperative indications	Cautions and contraindications	Side effects	Dose (paediatric)	Dose (adult)
Rocuronium	Rapidly acting aminosteroid See cisatracurium non–depolarizing muscle relaxant. RSI (avoiding suxamethonium). Duration 10–40min (variable). Intubating conditions within 1min	See cisatracurium	Mild tachycardia. See cisatracurium	Intubation: 0.6–1 mg/kg. Maintenance: 0.1–0.15mg/kg. Infusion: 0.3–0.6mg/kg/hr	Intubation: 0.6–1 mg/kg. Maintenance: 0.1–0.15mg/kg. Infusion: 0.3–0.6mg/kg/hr
Ropivacaine	Amide–type LA agent. Possibly less motor block than other agents. Duration similar to bupivacaine, but lower toxicity. pKa 8.1		Toxicity: tongue/circumoral numbness, restlessness, tinnitus, seizures, cardiac arrest	0.2–1% solution. Maximum dose dependent upon injection site—3–4mg/kg/4hr	0.2–1% solution. Infiltration/epidural: max dose dependent upon injection site, 3–4mg/kg/4hr
Salbutamol	β_2 receptor agonist. Treatment of bronchospasm, Larger doses now suggested in paediatrics or IV	Monitor potassium concentration with higher doses	Tremor, vasodilatation, tachycardia, hypokalaemia	Slow IV: 1 month–2 yr 5 micrograms/kg, >2yr 15 micrograms/kg (max 250 micrograms). Infusion: 1–5 micrograms/kg/min. Nebulizer: <5yr 2.5mg, >5yr 2.5–5mg	250 micrograms slow IV, then 5 micrograms/min (up to 20 micrograms/min). Nebulizer: 2.5–5mg PRN
Sufentanil	More potent thiamyl analogue See fentanyl of fentanyl (five times potency). Analgesia. Duration 20–45min	See fentanyl	See fentanyl	Analgesia: 10–30 micrograms (0.2–0.6 micrograms/kg). Anaesthesia 0.6–8 micrograms/kg	Analgesia: 10–30 micrograms (0.2–0.6 micrograms/kg). Anaesthesia 0.6–8 micrograms/kg

Sugammadex	Specific cyclodextrin reversal agent for rocuronium and vecuronium	Wait 24hr after use before using rocuronium/ vecuronium in patient; fusidic acid or flucioxacillin may displace relaxant from sugammadex within 6hr	Binds with contraceptive pill	T2 present 2mg/kg. Full reversal NR at present	T2 present 2mg/kg. To reverse full dose of rocuronium or vecuronium immediately 16mg/kg
Suxamethonium	Depolarizing muscle relaxant. Rapid short–acting muscle paralysis. Phase II block develops with repeated doses (>8mg/kg). Store at 2–8°C	Prolonged block in plasma cholinesterase deficiency, hypokalaemia, hypocalcaemia. MH, neuromuscular disorders. Increased serum K^+ (normally 0.5mmol/L, greater in burns, trauma, upper motor neuron injury)	Increased intraocular pressure. Bradycardia with 2nd dose	IV: 1–2mg/kg. IM: 3–4mg/kg	1–1.5 mg/kg. Infusion: 0.5–10mg/min
Tapentadol	Moderate to severe pain managed only by opioids	Reduce in hepatic impairment	Diarrhoea, dyspepsia, weight loss	Consult tertiary consultant	>18yr PO: 50mg 4– to 6–hourly, max 700mg

IV, intravenous. IM, intramuscular. SC, subcutaneous. PO, *per os* (oral). SL, sublingual. ET, endotracheal. od, once daily. bd, twice daily. tds, three times daily. qds, four times daily. NR, not recommended. Doses are IV and dilutions in 0.9% NaCl unless otherwise stated.

(*Continued*)

Table A.23 (*Contd.*)

Drug	Description and perioperative indications	Cautions and contraindications	Side effects	Dose (paediatric)	Dose (adult)
Teicoplanin	Glycopeptide antibiotic with activity against aerobic and anaerobic Gram–positive bacteria	Renal impairment	Allergic reactions, blood disorders, ototoxicity, nephrotoxicity	>1 month: 10mg/kg for three doses 12–hourly, then 6mg/kg od	IV/IM: 400mg for three doses 12–hourly, then 400mg od
Temazepam	Benzodiazepine. Sedation or premedication. Duration 1–2hr	Decreased requirement for anaesthetic agents	Respiratory depression in combination with opioids. Amnesia	PO: 0.3mg/kg preoperatively. NR <12yr	PO: 10–40mg1hr preoperativevly (elderly 10–20mg)
Tenoxicam	NSAID analgesic for mild to moderate pain	Hypersensitivity to aspirin, asthma, severe renal impairment, peptic ulceration	GI upset or bleeding, bronchospasm, tinnitus, fluid retention, platelet inhibition	NR	PO: 20mg od. IV/ IM: 20mg od
Tetracaine (amethocaine)	Ester–type LA. Topical analgesia prior to venepuncture. Ametop® gel contains 4% amethocaine. (Also available as eye drops, but has temporary disruptive effect on corneal epithelium). Duration 4hr	Apply only to intact. skin under occlusive dressing. Remove after 45min. Rapid absorption through mucosa		As adult. <1 month NR	Each tube expels 1.5g (sufficient for area 6 x 5cm)

Thiopental	Short–acting thiobarbiturate. Induction of anaesthesia, anticonvulsant, cerebral protection. Recovery due to redistribution	Accumulation with repeated doses. Caution in hypovolaemia and elderly. Porphyria	Hypotension. Necrosis if intra–arterial	Induction: neonate 2–4mg/kg, child 5–6mg/kg. Status: 2–4mg/kg, then 8mg/kg/hr	Induction/cerebral protection: 3–5mg/kg. Anticonvulsant: 0.5–2mg/ kg PRN
Tramadol	Analgesic thought to have less respiratory depression, constipation, euphoria, and abuse potential than other opioids. Has opioid and non–opioid mechanisms of action	Only 30% antagonized by naloxone. Caution in epilepsy. Previously not recommended for intraoperative use. MAOI	Nausea, dizziness, dry mouth. Increased side effects in conjunction with other opioids	>12yr: adult dose	PO: 50–100mg 4–hourly. Slow IV/IM: 50–100mg 4–hourly (100mg initially, then 50mg increments to max 250mg). Max 600mg/d
Tranexamic acid	Inhibits plasminogen activation, reducing fibrin dissolution by plasmin. Reduced haemorrhage in major trauma, prostatectomy, and dental extraction	Avoid in thromboembolic disease, renal impairment, and pregnancy	Dizziness, nausea	Slow IV: 10–15mg/kg tds. PO: 10–25 mg/kg tds	Slow IV: 0.5–1g tds. PO: 15–25 mg/kg tds

IV, intravenous. IM, intramuscular. SC, subcutaneous. PO, *per os* (oral). SL, sublingual. ET, endotracheal. od, once daily. bd, twice daily. tds, three times daily. qds, four times daily. NR, not recommended. Doses are IV and dilutions in 0.9% NaCl unless otherwise stated.

(*Continued*)

Table A.23 (*Contd.*)

Drug	Description and perioperative indications	Cautions and contraindications	Side effects	Dose (paediatric)	Dose (adult)
Triamcinolone acetonide	Relatively insoluble corticosteroid for depot injection. Epidural unlicensed use. Triamcinolone 4mg, prednisolone 5mg	Dose depends upon site of injection. Strict asepsis essential. Dilute 40mg/mL solution prior to use	See prednisolone	Intra–articular or intrasynovial: 2 mg/kg, max 40 mg	Intra–articular or intrasynovial: 5–40 mg. Epidural: 40–60mg diluted with LA
Trimeprazine	See alimemazine				
Vancomycin	Glycopeptide antibiotic with activity against aerobic and anaerobic Gram–positive bacteria. Peak level <30mg/L. Trough level 10–15mg/L	Avoid rapid infusion (hypotension, wheezing, urticaria, 'red man' syndrome). Reduce dose in renal impairment/elderly	Ototoxicity, nephrotoxicity, phlebitis, neutropenia	>1 month: 15mg/kgover 2hr tds (max 2g daily)	1–1.5g over 100min bd (check blood levels after 3rd dose). Reduce 500mg bd elderly
Vasopressin	Synthetic ADH used in treatment of diabetes insipidus, resistant vasodilatory shock, variceal bleeding	Extreme caution in coronary vascular disease	Pallor, coronary vasoconstriction, water intoxication	Diabetes insipidus SC/IM: <12yr0.1–0.4 micrograms/d. >12yr1–4 micrograms/d. See *BNFc* for specific indications	Diabetes insipidus SC/IM: 5–20U 4–hourly. Septic shock infusion: 1–4U/hr. Variceal bleed: 20U over 15min

Vecuronium	Aminosteroid non–depolarizing muscle relaxant. Cardiostable and no histamine release. Duration 30–45min	See cisatracurium	See cisatracurium	Intubation: 80–100 micrograms/kg. Maintenance: 20–30 micrograms/kg. Infusion: 0.8–1.4 micrograms/kg/min	Intubation: 80–100 micrograms/kg. Maintenance: 20–30 micrograms/kg. Infusion: 0.8–1.4 micrograms/kg/min
Warfarin	Coumarin derivative oral anticoagulant. Target INR: 2.5—treatment DVT/ PE, AF, mitral valve disease; 3.5—recurrent DVT/PE while on warfarin, mechanical heart valves (lower INR. acceptable with low–risk valves)	Previous haemorrhagic stroke, severe renal or liver disease, pregnancy, peptic ulcer disease. Reduce dose in elderly	Haemorrhage	PO: 0.2mg/kg up to 10mg od for 2d, then 0.05–0.2mg/kg od	PO: 10mg od for 2d, then 3–9mgod, dependent on INR
Zolpidem	Short–acting imidazopyridine hypnotic with little hangover effect	OSA, myasthenia gravis	Nausea, dizziness	NR	PO: 10mg nocte (elderly 5 mg)
Zopiclone	Short–acting cyclopyrrolone hypnotic with little hangover effect	OSA, myasthenia gravis	Nausea, bitter taste in mouth	NR	PO: 7.5mg nocte (elderly 3.75mg)

IV, intravenous. IM, intramuscular. SC, subcutaneous. PO, *per os* (oral). SL, sublingual. ET, endotracheal. od, once daily. bd, twice daily. tds, three times daily. qds, four times daily. NR, not recommended. Doses are IV and dilutions in 0.9% NaCl unless otherwise stated.

Infusion regimes

Table A.24 Infusion regimes

Drug	Indication	Diluent	Dose	Suggested regime (60kg adult)	Infusion range	Initial rate (adult)	Comments
Adrenaline	Treatment of hypotension	0.9% NaCl, 5% glucose	2–20 micrograms/min (0.04–0.4 micrograms/kg/min)	5mg/50mL (100 micrograms/mL)	1.2–12+ mL/hr	5mL/hr	Via central catheter. Suggest 1mg/50mL for initial intra-operative use (or 1 mg/500mL if no central access)
Alfentanil	Analgesia	0.9% NaCl, 5% glucose	0.5–1 micrograms/kg/min	Undiluted (500 micrograms/mL)	0–8mL/hr	4mL/hr	1 –2mg can be added to 50mL propofol for infusion
Aminophylline	Bronchodilation	0.9% NaCl, 5% glucose	0.5 mg/kg/hr	250mg/50mL (5mg/ mL)	0–6mL/hr	6mL/h	After 5mg/kg slow bolus
Amiodarone	Treatment of arrhythmias	5% glucose only	Loading infusion 5mg/kg over 20–120min, then 900mg over 24hr	300mg/50mL (6mg/ mL)	25–50mL/hr, then 6mL/hr	25mL/hr	Via central line (peripherally '*in extremis*'). Max 1.2g in 24hr. Adjust to therapeutic levels

Atracurium	Muscle relaxant	0.9% NaCl, 5% glucose	0.3–0.6mg/kg/hr	Undiluted (10mg/mL)	1.5–4mL/hr	3mL/hr	Assess rate with nerve stimulator
Cisatracurium	Muscle relaxant	0.9% NaCl, 5% glucose	0.06–0.18mg/kg/hr	Undiluted (2mg/mL)	2–5 mL/hr	5mL/hr	Assess rate with nerve stimulator
Digoxin	Rapid control of ventricular rate	0.9% NaCl, 5% glucose	250–500 micrograms over 30–60min; 0.75–1 mg over 2hr	250–500 micrograms/50mL	0–100m L/hr	50mL/hr	ECG monitoring suggested
Dobutamine	Cardiac failure/ inotrope	0.9% NaCl, 5% glucose	2.5–10 micrograms/kg/ min	250mg/50mL (5mg/ mL)	2–7mL/hr	2mL/hr	
Dopamine	Inotrope	0.9% NaCl, 5% glucose	2–10 micrograms/ kg/min	200mg/50mL (4mg/ mL)	2–9 mL/hr	2mL/hr	Via central line
Dopexamine	Inotrope	0.9% NaCl, 5% glucose	0.5–6 micrograms/ kg/min	50mg/50mL (1mg/ mL)	2–22mL/hr	2mL/hr	May be given via large peripheral vein
Doxapram	Respiratory stimulant	0.9% NaCl, 5% glucose	2–4mg/min	200mg/50mL (4mg/ mL)	30–60mL/hr	30mL/hr	Max dose 4mg/kg. NR child
Alternative regimes for any infusion	3mg/kg/50mL, then 1mL/hr = 1 microgram/kg/min; 3mg/50mL, then 1mL/hr = 1 microgram/min. Rate (mL/hr) = 60 x rate (micrograms/kg/min) x weight (kg)/concentration (micrograms/mL)						

(Continued)

Table A.24 (*Contd.*)

Drug	Indication	Diluent	Dose	Suggested regime (60kg adult)	Infusion range	Initial rate (adult)	Comments
Enoximone	1 nodilator	0.9% NaCl only	90 micrograms/kg/min for 10–30min, then 5–20 micrograms/kg/min	100mg/50mL (2mg/mL)	9–36mL/hr	162mL/hrfor 10–30min	Max 24mg/kg/d
Esmolol	β–blocker	0.9% NaCl, 5% glucose	50–200 micrograms/kg/min	2.5g/50mL (50mg/mL)	3–15mL/hr	3mL/hr	ECG monitoring
Glyceryl trinitrate	Controlled hypotension	0.9% NaCl, 5% glucose	0.5–12mg/hr	50mg/50mL (1mg/mL)	0.5–12mL/hr	5mL/hr	
Heparin	Anti coagulation	0.9% NaCl, 5% glucose	24 000–48 000U per24hr	50 000U/50mL (1000U/mL)	1–2mL/hr	2mL/hr	Check APTT after 12hr. See local guidelines
Insulin (soluble)	Diabetes mellitus	0.9% NaCl	Sliding scale	50U/50mL (1U/mL)	Sliding scale	Sliding scale	
Isoprenaline	Treatment of heart block or bradycardia	0.9% NaCl, 5% glucose	1.5–10 micrograms/min	1mg/50mL(20 micrograms/mL)	0.5–30mL/hr	7mL/hr	Special order request required
Ketamine	GA	0.9% NaCl, 5% glucose	1–3mg/kg/hr	500mg/50mL (10mg/mL)	6–18m L/hr	10mL/hr	Induction 0.5–2mg/kg

Ketamine	Analgesia	0.9% NaCl, 5% glucose	0.2mg/kg/hr	200mg/50mL (4mg/ mL)	0–6mL/hr	3mL/hr	With midazolam 2–5 mg/hr
Ketamine	'Trauma' mixture	0.9% NaCl	0.5mL/kg/hr	50mL mixture (4mg/ mL ketamine)	15–45mL/hr	30mL/hr	200mg ketamine + 10mg midazolam + 10mg vecuronium in 50mL
Lidocaine (lignocaine)	Ventricular arrhythmias	0.9% NaCl	4mg/min for 30min, 2mg/min for 2hr, then 1mg/ min for 24hr	500mg/50mL (10mg/mL, 1%)	6–24mL/hr	24mL/hr	After 50–100mg, slow IV bolus. ECG monitoring
Milrinone	Inodilator	0.9% NaCl, 5% glucose	50 micrograms/ kg over 10min, then 0.375–0.75 microgram s/kg/min	10mg/50mL (0.2mg/ mL)	7–14m L/hr	90mL/hrfor 10min	Max 1.13mg/kg/d
Mivacurium	Muscle relaxant	0.9% NaCl, 5% glucose		0.4–0.6 mg/kg/h r	Undiluted (2mg/mL)	12–18mL/hr	18mL/hr Assess rate with nerve stimulator
Morphine	Analgesia	0.9% NaCl	0–3.5mg/hr	50mg/50mL (1mg/ mL)	0–3.5mL/hr	2mL/hr	Monito r respiratin and sedation hourly. Administer O_2
Alternative regimes for any infusion	3mg/kg/50mL, then 1mL/hr = 1 microgram/kg/min; 3mg/50mL, then 1mL/hr = 1 microgram/min. Rate (mL/hr) = 60 x rate (micrograms/kg/min) x weight (kg)/concentration (micrograms/mL)						

(*Continued*)

Table A.24 (*Contd.*)

Drug	Indication	Diluent	Dose	Suggested regime (60kg adult)	Infusion range	Initial rate (adult)	Comments
Naloxone	Opioid antagonist	0.9% NaCl, 5% glucose	>1 microgram/kg/hr	2mg/500mL (4 micrograms/mL)		100mL/hr	Rate adjusted according to response
Nimodipine	Prevention of vasospasm after SAH	0.9% NaCl, 5% glucose	1mg/hr, increasing to 2mg/hr after 2hr	Undiluted (0.2mg/mL)	5–10mL/hr	5mL/hr	Via central line. Incompatible with polyvinyl chloride
Nitroprusside (sodium)	Controlled hypotension	5% glucose	0.3–1.5 micrograms/kg/min	25mg/50mL (500 micrograms/mL)	2–10mL/hr	5mL/hr	Max dose 1.5mg/kg. Protect from light
Noradrenaline	Treatment of hypotension	5% glucose	2–20 micrograms/min (0.04–0.4 micrograms/kg/min)	4mg/40mL(100 micrograms/mL)	1.2–12+ mL/hr	5mL/hr	Via central line
Octreotide	Somatostatin analogue	0.9% NaCl	25–50 micrograms/hr	500 micrograms/50mL (10 micrograms/mL)	2–5 mL/hr	5mL/hr	Use in variceal bleeding unlicensed
Oxytocin	Prevention of uterine atony	0.9% NaCl, 5% glucose	0.02–0.125U/min (10U/hr)	30U in 500mL (0.06U/mL)	30–125mL/hr	125mL/hr	Individual unit protocols vary
Phenylephrine	Treatment of hypotension	0.9% NaCl, 5% glucose	30–60 micrograms/min	5mg in 50mL (100 micrograms/mL)	18–36mL/hr	30mL/hr	Gaining popularity for regional Caesarean

Phenytoin	Anticonvulsant prophylaxis	0.9% NaCl	20 mg/kg	900mg/90mL (administer via 0.22–0.5 micron filter)	Up to 50mg/min	180mL/hr	ECG and BP monitoring. Complete within 1hr of preparation
Propofol	Anaesthesia		6–10mg/kg/hr	Undiluted (10mg/mL)	36–60mL/hr		TCI: initially 4–8 micrograms/mL, then 3–6 micrograms/mL
Propofol	Sedation		0–3mg/kg/hr	Undiluted (10mg/mL)	0–20mL/hr		TCI: 0–2.5 micrograms/mL
Remifentanil	Analgesia during GA	0.9% NaCl, 5% glucose	0.1–1.0 micrograms/kg/min	2mg/40mL (50 micrograms/ mL)	5–40mL/hr IPPV. 2–7mL/hr SV	8mL/hrIPPV. 2mL/hrSV	Suggest starting at 0.1 micrograms/kg/min (8mL/hr), then adjust up to 0.25 micrograms/kg/min (20mL/hr) as required
Rocuronium	Muscle relaxant	0.9% NaCl, 5% glucose	0.3–0.6mg/kg/hr	Undiluted (10mg/mL)	1.5–4mL/hr	3mL/hr	Assess rate with nerve stimulator
Alternative regimes for any infusion	3mg/kg/50mL, then 1mL/hr = 1 microgram/kg/min; 3mg/50mL, then 1mL/hr = 1 microgram/min. Rate (mL/hr) = 60 x rate (micrograms/kg/min) x weight (kg)/concentration (micrograms/mL)						

(Continued)

Table A.24 (*Contd.*)

Drug	Indication	Diluent	Dose	Suggested regime (60kg adult)	Infusion range	Initial rate (adult)	Comments
Salbutamol	Bronchospasm	5% glucose	5–20 micrograms/min	1mg/50mL(20 micrograms/ mL)	15–60mL/hr	30mL/hr	After 250 micrograms, slow IV bolus
Sodium bicarbonate	Acidosis		(Weight (kg) x base deficit x 0.3) mmol	Undiluted (8.4% solution)			8.4%, 1000mmol/L. Via central line, if possible
Vancomycin	Antibiotic	0.9% NaCl, 5% glucose	1–1.5g 12–hourly	1g/500mL	500mL/100min	500mL/100min	Elderly 500mg 12–hourly
Vecuronium	Muscle relaxant	0.9% NaCl, 5% glucose	0.05–0.08mg/kg/hr	Undiluted (2mg/mL)	1.5–3mL/hr	2.5mL/hr	Assess rate with nerve stimulator
Alternative regimes for any infusion	3mg/kg/50mL, then 1mL/hr = 1 microgram/kg/min; 3mg/50mL, then 1mL/hr = 1 microgram/min. Rate (mL/hr) = 60 x rate (micrograms/kg/min) x weight (kg)/concentration (micrograms/mL)						

Minimum alveolar concentration values

Table A.25 Properties of inhalational agents

	MAC in O_2/air[1] (%)			MAC in 67% N_2O (%)			BP (°C)	SVP (kPa)	Oil:gas part. coeff.	Blood:gas part. coeff	MW	Biotrans. (%)
	1yr	40yr	80yr	1yr	40yr	80yr						
Halothane	0.95	0.75	0.58	0.47	0.27	0.1	50.2	32.5	224	2.3	197.4	25
Enflurane	2.08	1.63	1.27	1.03	0.58	0.22	56.5	22.9	96	1.91	184.5	3
Isoflurane	1.49	1.17	0.91	0.74	0.42	0.17	48.5	31.9	91	1.4	184.5	0.2
Sevoflurane	2.29	1.8	1.4	1.13	0.65	0.25	58.5	21.3	53	0.59	200	2.5
Desflurane	8.3	6.6	5.1	4.2	2.4	0.93	23.5	88.5	18.7	0.42	168	Minimal
Nitrous oxide	133	104	81	NA	NA	NA	-88	5080	1.4	0.47	44	0
Xenon	92	72	57	NA	NA	NA	-107.1	5800	20	0.14	131.3	0

Potency (MAC) correlates with oil:gas partition coefficient (hence lipid solubility).

Speed of onset correlates with blood:gas partition coefficient (lower, faster).

SVP, saturated vapour pressure at 20°C; part, coeff., partition coefficient at 37°C; MW, molecular weight; BP, boiling point; biotrans., biotransformation.

[1] Nickalls RWD, Mapleson WW (2003). Age-related iso-MAC charts for isoflurane, sevoflurane and desflurane in man. *Br J Anaesth* 91,170—4.

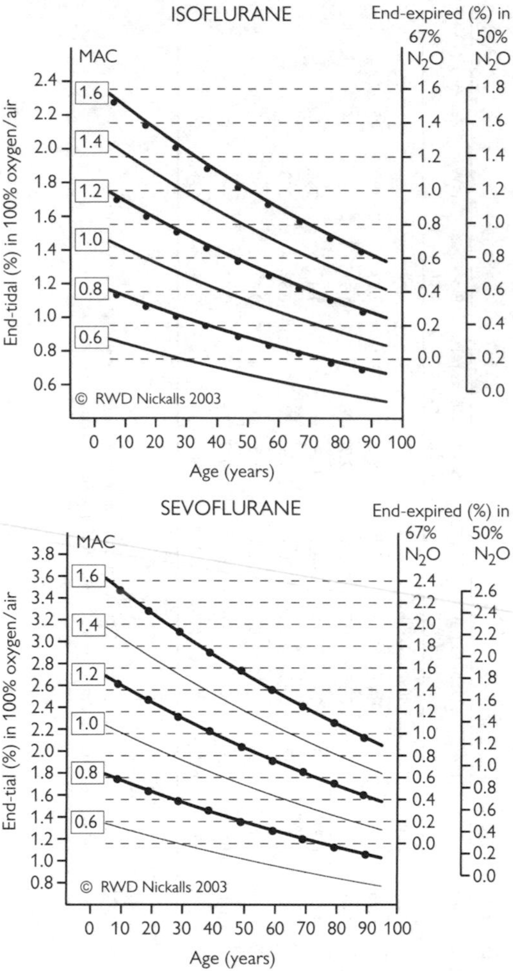

Figure A.15 Age-related iso-MAC charts for isoflurane, sevoflurane, and desflurane.

Reprinted from *British Journal of Anaesthesia*, 2, 5, R. W. D. Nickalls and W. W. Mapleson. Age-related iso-MAC charts for isoflurane, sevoflurane and desflurane in man. pp. 170–174. https://doi.org/10.1093/bja/aeg132.

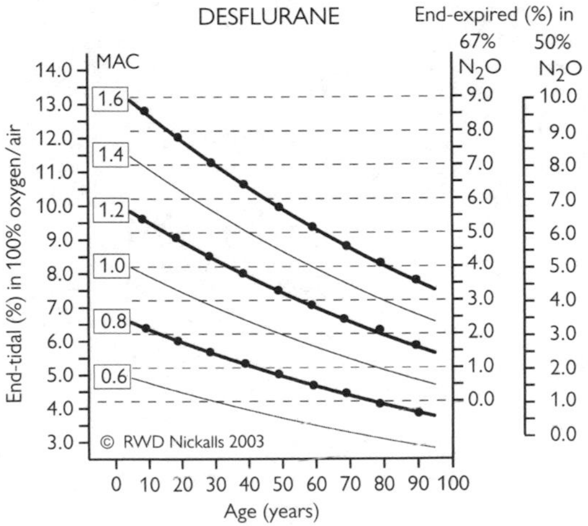

Figure A.15 *(Contd.)*

Index

Tables, figures and boxes are indicated by *t*, *f* and *b* following the page number

U

V

W

Y

Z